Managing Older People in Primary Care
A practical guide

Edited by

Professor Margot Gosney
Professor of Elderly Care Medicine
University of Reading and Royal Berkshire NHS Foundation Trust

and

Dr Tess Harris
Senior Lecturer in Primary Care
St George's University of London
and General Practitioner
Sonning Common Health Centre, Reading

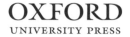
OXFORD
UNIVERSITY PRESS

OXFORD
UNIVERSITY PRESS

Great Clarendon Street, Oxford ox2 6DP

Oxford University Press is a department of the University of Oxford.
It furthers the University's objective of excellence in research, scholarship,
and education by publishing worldwide in

Oxford New York

Auckland Cape Town Dar es Salaam Hong Kong Karachi
Kuala Lumpur Madrid Melbourne Mexico City Nairobi
New Delhi Shanghai Taipei Toronto

With offices in

Argentina Austria Brazil Chile Czech Republic France Greece
Guatemala Hungary Italy Japan Poland Portugal Singapore
South Korea Switzerland Thailand Turkey Ukraine Vietnam

Oxford is a registered trade mark of Oxford University Press
in the UK and in certain other countries

Published in the United States
by Oxford University Press Inc., New York

© Oxford University Press, 2009

The moral rights of the author have been asserted
Database right Oxford University Press (maker)

First published 2009

British Library Cataloguing in Publication Data
Data available

Library of Congress Cataloging in Publication Data
Data available

Typeset in Minion by Cepha Imaging Private Ltd.,
Banglore, India
Printed in Great Britain
on acid-free paper by the MPG Books Group, Bodmin and King's Lynn

ISBN 978-0-19-954-6589

10 9 8 7 6 5 4 3 2 1

Foreword

Professor David Haslam, CBE, FRCP, FFPH, PRCGP

I'm getting older every day. However young you might be, you are getting older too, as is the whole UK population. For whatever reason—whether lifestyle, or public health, or the remarkable advances of modern medicine—the British population is changing quite dramatically. For the first time ever, we now have more pensioners than children, and the impact for everyone working in health care will be profound.

I have a patient who is a quite remarkable man. He was a professional locally in my small town, and retired six months after I joined my practice in 1976. Despite having a number of long-term conditions, and taking a handful of pills every day, he still plays golf several times a week, and has a brain that seems as sharp now as it ever did. It struck me a while ago that his retirement is likely to be longer than my career, and if anything exemplifies the changing demographics of our country, it is him.

The ageing population is sometimes seen as a problem—a 'pensions crisis', or a 'demographic time bomb', phrases that cannot be good for anyone's morale. But as someone who hopes to look forward to a long and active old age, I'm delighted we are faced with such 'problems'.

And as the population ages, the role of the generalist doctor becomes evermore important. In the past, patients all too frequently died of acute conditions. Now, frequently thanks to the skill of our specialist colleagues, they survive and live with their long-term conditions. 'Dying of' has been replaced by 'living with'. And as more and more people survive with more and more conditions, the role of the specialist becomes less clear-cut. The role of the generalist becomes central. If a patient has ischaemic heart disease, diabetes, osteoarthritis, hyperlipidaemia, and (hardly surprisingly) depression, which specialist can offer the care that he or she needs? The future lies with generalists.

Indeed, I well remember being contacted by a man whom I will call Mr Atkins; a patient who exemplified perfectly how health care has become increasingly complex.

Mr Atkins is a patient of mine who is 77 years old, and who has lived in my area for only three or four years. He has prostate cancer—but he also has hypertension, diabetes, and an arthritic right hip. For these, he takes 17 tablets a day—not unusual for someone with hypertension and diabetes. He recently wrote to me before a consultation enclosing copies of a couple of papers from the New England Journal of Medicine and The Lancet about prostate cancer, and in his letter he said that he thought I'd like to read these before our next consultation.

Just this single case vignette beautifully demonstrates the importance of an ageing population, an increasingly mobile population, comorbidity, polypharmacy, the information explosion, the pressure of time on professionals, and the increasing complexity of our consultations.

And so, when he came in to see me, I thanked him for the papers. 'I've had a look at them,' I said, 'but you have to understand that I'm not an expert in prostate cancer. You really need to discuss these with your urologist.'

He smiled and looked at me. 'I know you aren't an expert in prostate cancer,' he said. 'That's not why I come to see you. You are an expert in me.'

It was a comment that put a tingle down my spine, as incisive a description of the role of the general practitioner (GP) as I have ever heard. But it does present us with a huge challenge. The remarkable levels of trust that patients have in their family doctors is quite astonishing, but absolutely behoves us to be as good as we can, to go that extra mile.

That is why I welcome this book so warmly. Most chapters are co-authored by a GP and a specialist, highlighting perfectly the teamwork that we will need to care for the increasingly complex problems that our elderly patients will present to us.

Few aspects of health care can be more gratifying. GPs can make a huge difference to our patients' lives, and we owe it to our patients to get it right. After all, with luck, one day we too will be on the receiving end. As the old saying goes, 'Do as you would be done by.' Nothing less—that's the challenge.

dementia works very well in epidemiological studies, but education, previous intellectual capacity, visual and hearing deficits, depression and acute illness may all influence individual scores. False-positive scores are particularly likely when such a threshold is applied to large populations with a relatively low incidence of dementia, such as well older people living independently in the community.[8] In this group, it may be better to interpret the MMSE using three ranges, with a score of ≤20 making dementia very likely (likelihood ratio (LR) 14.5), a score of ≥26 effectively ruling out dementia (LR: 0.1) and scores of 21–25 relatively inconclusive (LR: 2.2).[9] It is also important that screening tests such as the MMSE are not used in isolation to define decision-making capacity: being unable to draw intersecting pentagons or not knowing the name of the Prime Minister, for example, are not of themselves relevant to capacity.

Impairment of visuospatial function and of verbal fluency develop relatively early in AD. Other simple tests that are helpful in assessing cognition include the clock-drawing test and asking the patient to generate word lists. The former tests visuospatial function in addition to planning. In a common approach, the patient is presented a pre-drawn circle and asked to 'draw a clock'. Clock-drawing is correct if the patient has included most of the 12 numbers in a clockwise orientation; minor spacing errors are acceptable.[10] A number of formal scoring systems are available, but complicated grading systems defeat the test's fundamental simplicity; abnormalities are usually obvious and can be followed with serial testing. Also, unlike the MMSE, clock-drawing is relatively insensitive to the patient's level of education.

The most common word list test is to ask the patient to generate the names of as many animals as possible in a minute. Most normal people can generate 15 names or more, although allowance must again be made for prior education and linguistic skills.[11] Apart from the total score, repetition of common domestic animals is often an ominous feature.

Delirium or dementia?

Delirium is characterized by a change of cognition that develops over a period of hours or days.[12] Symptoms tend to fluctuate over the course of a day and are worst at night. Disturbed consciousness and impaired ability to attend to the environment are cardinal features. Patients are often disoriented with rambling, incoherent speech.

Almost any acute illness or medication can trigger delirium. However, delirium is almost invariably multifactorial in older people, and it is often as inappropriate to isolate a single precipitant as 'the cause' as it would be to place the entire blame for breaking the camel's back on the final straw. Prior cognitive impairment, older age, severity of illness and psychoactive drug use have consistently emerged as the most important risk factors for delirium.

A history from a carer of the onset and course of the cognitive disturbance is invaluable in distinguishing between dementia and delirium (Table 3.1). However, even when such a history is unavailable, delirious patients can often be easily recognized from the bedside from their characteristic distractibility and difficulty in focusing or sustaining concentration during conversation.[13] If there is doubt, the default diagnosis should be delirium, since a delay in diagnosis of delirium is more likely to have serious consequences.

Physical examination

As with the history, physical examination of older people often presents a number of challenges. There may be practical physical difficulties in examining those who are extremely immobile or are wearing multiple layers of clothing, and assistance from a nurse or carer is often essential. Patients may be reluctant to allow examination due to cognitive impairment, modesty or embarrassment about their state of hygiene. Space may be limited when patients are seen at home.

Table 3.1 Distinguishing delirium and dementia

	Delirium	Dementia
Onset	Acute	Gradual
Attentiveness	Impaired	Normal
Consciousness	Reduced	Normal
Hallucinations/delusions	Common	Late feature
Short-term fluctuations	Yes	No
Outcome	Recovery/death	Chronic, progressive

Some degree of compromise is often needed, and a limited examination of the patient in a chair or focusing on the areas suggested by the history is better than no examination. Nevertheless, it is important to check for pressure sores in immobile patients; dentures should be removed to allow inspection of the mouth; a full bladder should always be sought in those with urinary incontinence or delirium; and digital rectal examination is essential in those with urinary retention, constipation or diarrhoea.

Even in the most difficult and hurried circumstances, an enormous amount of information can be gleaned by inspection of the patient's posture, gait, hygienic status and general demeanour. Because of its importance, gait assessment will be dealt with in more detail. Asking the patient to clap his hands loudly over his head is a useful catch-all test of hearing, comprehension, mood, neurological and musculoskeletal function in the upper limb that can be used even in the bed-bound patient.

Pitfalls in physical examination of the older patient

The principles of conducting a physical examination are the same in old as in young patients, although positive findings, some of dubious significance, are more common. This section highlights some of the potential difficulties that may arise.

Blood pressure should always be measured with the appropriate cuff size. A significant minority of older people with hypertension have an auscultatory gap (disappearance then reappearance of Korotkoff sounds);[14] failure to inflate the cuff beyond initial disappearance of the sounds leads to significant underestimation of systolic blood pressure.

The skin in older people is often thin and transparent with 'senile' purpura and small bruises, and lesions such as seborrhoeic keratoses, cherry angiomas and skin tags are common and harmless. However, basal and squamous-cell carcinomas are also common incidental findings, and unexplained bruises may indicate unreported falls or even abuse. Facial pallor in the older patient is as often due to staying indoors as to anaemia.

Wasting of the abdominal musculature is common in inactive patients, and it may be possible to palpate a normal aorta or stool in the colon. Basal crackles may be heard in the chest of immobile patients, presumably due to closure of small airways; coughing or deep inspiration should lead to considerable clearing.[15] Gravitational oedema is also common in immobile patients, especially if long hours are spent sitting (or sleeping) in a chair.

Ejection systolic murmurs are common in the very old. Such murmurs are often due to aortic sclerosis, are of no haemodynamic significance and are not transmitted to the carotid arteries.[16] However, careful assessment of such patients is required, because significant aortic valve stenosis may occur with a soft murmur and, because of reduced vascular compliance, without narrowing of the pulse pressure. Although a fourth heart sound is common among apparently normal older people, this may reflect the high frequency of subclinical cardiac disease.

Many classical neurological signs have relatively poor predictive power in older people. As a general rule, symmetrical findings that are not accompanied by functional loss, symptoms or other neurological signs are less likely to be significant. Older people often have small pupils and sluggish pupillary light reflexes. An inexplicably absent corneal reflex is found unilaterally in 8% of healthy older people.[17] A decline in muscle mass is a common age-related finding, especially in those who are relatively inactive; generalized symmetrical wasting of hand muscles is a common non-specific finding. Although deep tendon reflexes are generally preserved with age, ankle jerks are absent bilaterally in 6–50% of neurologically normal older people in different series;[18,19] a plantar strike technique, where the examiner strikes his own hand as it lies on the ball of the foot, is often helpful when arthritis limits hip rotation.[20] Symmetrical reduction of touch and vibratory sensation below the knees is a common asymptomatic finding; diabetes mellitus should always be sought in such patients, although often no explanation is found.

Assessment of gait and balance

Examination of the patient's gait and balance is an essential part of the physical examination that provides important information about the patient's overall functional status and prognosis as well as about neurological, visual and musculoskeletal disease. It is an excellent screening test since it is uncommon to find major neurological or musculoskeletal problems in the legs of someone who can rise unaided from a chair and walk back and forth quickly without difficulty. Conversely, it is not uncommon to find patients who have difficulty walking despite examination in the bed having revealed no neurological or musculoskeletal problems.

The 'get up and go' test has been well studied in older people as a measure of functional status: the doctor measures the time taken to rise from a standard chair, walk 3 m, return and sit down.[21] Slowness of walking in older people is a good predictor of falls risk and of the risk of functional decline. In a nursing home population, stopping walking when starting to talk was a strong predictor of falls risk over the following 6 months.[22]

In examining gait, attention must be paid in particular to posture, speed, step length, symmetry of gait and arm swing. Ageing is in general associated with a reduction in speed, a stooped posture and shorter step length. The first step in walking is getting up from the bed or chair. A common contributor to problems in getting up is that the bed or chair is too low or the surface too soft. Rising is also impaired by weakness of the gluteal and quadriceps muscles, parkinsonism, arthritis of leg joints or balance problems. Examination of the gait also requires investigation of the aids used and their provenance. The proper length of a walking stick is from the distal palmar crease to the ground; in practice, many use sticks of the wrong length.[23] While Zimmer frames provide improved stability for some patients, it is not uncommon to see patients where they represent a hindrance to walking safely.

Balance requires that the brain receives good sensory information from proprioceptors in the legs, from the vestibular system and from the eyes. Walking requires also that joints, muscles, and peripheral motor system and the cerebral control of postural and locomotor responses are functioning well. Problems in any of these areas give rise to gait dysfunction.

The 'classical' gait patterns, summarized in Table 3.2, are commonly seen in older patients. However, gait disturbance in this population is often multifactorial and not easily broken down into the constituent pathologies. Poorly fitting footwear is a common and easily remediable cause of poor gait. Fear of falling, not always in those with a history of falls, may be associated with dramatic grabbing at nearby people and objects and with premature and dangerous attempts to sit down.[2] Finally, many patients with vascular or other dementias have a 'higher-order' or 'frontal' gait disorder characterized by some combination of difficulty initiating walking ('ignition failure' or, where gait starts with small steps that gradually increase in length, the 'slipping clutch'),

Table 3.2 Classical gait disorders

Condition	Gait description
Sensory ataxia	Unsteady, looks to ground, feet slap on the ground, positive Romberg's sign
Antalgic (painful) gait	Limp, minimizes weight-bearing on affected side. Trendelenberg gait with painful hip: trunk leans to affected side on weight-bearing
Motor weakness	Proximal myopathy gives waddling gait; foot drop leads to exaggerated foot-lifting and foot-slapping on the ground
Hemiplegic gait	Leg swings out and around from hip (circumduction), ankle plantar flexed, foot drags on ground
Parkinsonism	Reduced arm swing, stooped posture, narrow base, small shuffling steps, whole body turns together 'en bloc', involuntary acceleration forward (festination) and falls backwards (retropulsion)
Cerebellar ataxia	Wide-based, staggering, unsteady gait; less often positive Romberg's sign than sensory ataxia

a shuffling, wide-based gait (*'marche à petit pas'*) and difficulty lifting the feet from the floor ('magnetic feet').[24] In contrast to PD, arm swing is normal (hence 'lower-half parkinsonism'), posture is more upright and the base is wide. The condition may be described as 'gait apraxia' when motor function is greatly improved when the patient is supine. Potentially reversible causes such as subdural haematoma and normal pressure hydrocephalus are rarely found.

Conclusion

The history and physical examination are essential to the clinician in forming a differential diagnosis and management plan for his patient. However, it is also essential to consider the goals of care when dealing with the very frail older patient with multiple problems. Ultimately the goals of care should be those of the patient rather than of the clinician or the family, and this requires open discussion with the patient about their expectations and preferences. For many people, managing disease and maintaining function and quality of life is as important as curing disease and maximizing duration of life. This is not to encourage therapeutic nihilism: older people have as much if not more to gain from many medical advances. However, it is no triumph for medical science to investigate and treat every symptom, sign and laboratory abnormality without regard to the goals and preferences of that individual. Finding the correct balance is never easy and remains the ultimate challenge for all clinicians caring for older people.

References

1. Jarrett PG, Rockwood K, Carver D, Stolee P, Cosway S. Illness presentation in elderly patients. *Arch Intern Med* 1995;155:1060–4.
2. Isaacs B. *The Challenge of Geriatric Medicine*. Oxford: Oxford University Press; 1992.
3. Mahoney JE, Sager MA, Jalaluddin M. New walking dependence associated with hospitalization for acute medical illness: incidence and significance. *J Gerontol A Biol Sci Med Sci* 1998;53:M307–12.
4. Chen YF, Dewey ME, Avery AJ. Self-reported medication use for older people in England and Wales. *J Clin Pharm Ther* 2001;26:129–40.
5. Zhan C, Correa-de-Araujo R, Bierman AS, *et al.* Suboptimal prescribing in elderly outpatients: potentially harmful drug-drug and drug-disease combinations. *J Am Geriatr Soc* 2005;53:262–7.
6. Feldman HH, Jacova C. Mild cognitive impairment. *Am J Geriatr Psychiatr* 2005;13:645–55.

7. Tombaugh TN, McIntyre NJ. The mini-mental state examination: a comprehensive review. *J Am Geriatr Soc* 1992;40:922–35.

8. Tangalos EG, Smith GE, Ivnik RJ, *et al*. The Mini-Mental State Examination in general medical practice: clinical utility and acceptance. *Mayo Clin Proc* 1996;71:829–37.

9. Kay DW, Henderson AS, Scott R, Wilson J, Rickwood D, Grayson DA. Dementia and depression among the elderly living in the Hobart community: the effect of the diagnostic criteria on the prevalence rates. *Psychol Med* 1985;15:771–88.

10. Paganini-Hill A, Clark LJ, Henderson VW, Birge SJ. Clock drawing: analysis in a retirement community. *J Am Geriatr Soc* 2001;49:941–7.

11. Minett TS, Da Silva RV, Ortiz KZ, Bertolucci PH. Subjective memory complaints in an elderly sample: a cross-sectional study. *Int J Geriatr Psychiatry* 2008;23:49–54.

12. Nayeem K, O'Keeffe S. Delirium. *Clin Med* 2003;3:412–5.

13. O'Keeffe ST, Gosney MA. Assessing attentiveness in older hospital patients: global assessment versus tests of attention. *J Am Geriatr Soc* 1997;45:470–3.

14. Cavallini MC, Roman MJ, Blank SG, Pini R, Pickering TG, Devereux RB. Association of the auscultatory gap with vascular disease in hypertensive patients. *Ann Intern Med* 1996;124:877–83.

15. Forgacs P. *Lung Sounds*. London: Ballière Tindall; 1978.

16. Aronow WS, Kronzon I. Prevalence and severity of valvular aortic stenosis determined by Doppler echocardiography and its association with echocardiographic and electrocardiographic left ventricular hypertrophy and physical signs of aortic stenosis in elderly patients. *Am J Cardiol* 1991;67:776–7.

17. Rai GS, Elias-Jones A. The corneal reflex in elderly patients. *J Am Geriatr Soc* 1979;27:317–8.

18. Bowditch MG, Sanderson P, Livesey JP. The significance of an absent ankle reflex. *J Bone Joint Surg Br* 1996;78:276–9.

19. Impallomeni M, Kenny RA, Flynn MD, Kraenzlin M, Pallis CA. The elderly and their ankle jerks. *Lancet* 1984;1:670–2.

20. O'Keeffe ST, Smith T, Valacio R, Jack CI, Playfer JR, Lye M. A comparison of two techniques for ankle jerk assessment in elderly subjects. *Lancet* 1994;344:1619–20.

21. Podsiadlo D, Richardson S. The timed "Up & Go": a test of basic functional mobility for frail elderly persons. *J Am Geriatr Soc* 1991;39:142–8.

22. Lundin-Olsson L, Nyberg L, Gustafson Y. "Stops walking when talking" as a predictor of falls in elderly people. *Lancet* 1997;349:617.

23. George J, Binns VE, Clayden AD, Mulley GP. Aids and adaptations for the elderly at home: underprovided, underused, and undermaintained. *Br Med J (Clin Res Ed)* 1988;296:1365–6.

24. Nutt JG, Marsden CD, Thompson PD. Human walking and higher-level gait disorders, particularly in the elderly. *Neurology* 1993;43:268–79.

Chapter 4

Pharmacokinetics and pharmacodynamics

Vincent Riley, Tony Avery, and Stephen Jackson

Introduction

The world's population is ageing and by the year 2031 it is predicted that people aged >65 years will represent 30% of the world's total population.[1] With the ageing of the population there is a higher prevalence of chronic illnesses such as cardiovascular disease, cancers, diabetes, and dementia. The advancement in medical technology and a greater understanding of disease processes have led to improvement in disease outcomes and quality of life in elderly patients affected by chronic illnesses. Drug therapy is very important in managing chronic disease but this can be a double-edged sword.[2] The ageing process is characterized by structural and functional changes affecting all organ systems and is associated with reduced homeostatic capacity. The combined effects of ageing, chronic disease and pharmacotherapy in elderly patients have created a highly complex situation both for the patient and health care team.[3]

Pharmacokinetics

Pharmacokinetics describes the liberation, absorption, distribution, metabolism and excretion of drugs and their metabolites. The physiological changes that accompany ageing result in changes in pharmacokinetics (Table 4.1).

Absorption

Ageing itself does not appear to be associated with significantly reduced rate or extent of absorption.[4] When reduced rate of absorption is evident it probably represents the effects of pathology. Drugs may reduce the rate of gastric emptying, which is an important determinant of rate of absorption as the stomach does not contribute much to absorption. A number of drugs that are used as prokinetics may increase the rate of absorption (e.g. metoclopramide, erythromycin) and others may delay absorption (e.g. anticholinergic agents). These agents do not change the extent of absorption.

Distribution

Distribution occurs when the drug reaches the circulation. Ageing is associated with a relative increase in the proportion of body fat and decrease in proportion of water, and thus fat-soluble drugs have a large volume of distribution compared to that in younger people and the converse for water-soluble drugs.

Table 4.1 Age-related changes in pharmacokinetics

Pharmacokinetic process	Physiological changes	Clinical relevance	Examples
Liberation	No effect of ageing— process determined by formulation	None	–
Absorption	No clinically relevant change	None	–
Distribution	Decreased proportion of body water. Increased proportion of body fat	Higher concentration of water-soluble drugs. Increased volume of distribution for lipid-soluble drugs leading to prolonged elimination half-life.	Prolonged half-life of: ◆ benzodiazepines (metabolized) ($\uparrow$V, $\downarrow$CL) ◆ morphine (metabolized) ($\uparrow$V, $\downarrow$CL) ◆ active metabolite of morphine (renally cleared) ($\uparrow$CL) ◆ digoxin (renally cleared) ($\uparrow$CL) ◆ lithium (renally cleared) ($\uparrow$CL)
Metabolism	Reduced liver volume	Reduced clearance of lipid-soluble drugs. Multiplicative (with reduced volume of distribution) effect on prolonging half-life.	
Elimination	Reduced GFR. Decreased tubular secretion	Reduced renal clearance of water-soluble drugs	

V, volume of distribution; CL, clearance; GFR, glomerular filtration rate.

The importance of these physiological changes is the effect they have on elimination half-life ($t_{1/2}z$), which is is the time taken for the plasma concentration of the drug to decrease by half and is determined by volume of distribution (V) and clearance (CL):

$$t_{1/2}z \propto V/CL$$

Thus the increase in volume of distribution that is seen for lipid-soluble drugs (e.g. benzodiazepines, morphine) with increasing age results in prolongation of half-life. Another factor that affects volume of distribution is protein binding. Serum albumin falls only minimally with age but in the presence of chronic disease the amount of drug bound to albumin will fall due to the fall in serum albumin. This results in distribution of drug out of the plasma volume into the tissues, increasing volume of distribution and hence elimination half-life. It therefore also results in greater free concentration of the drug which, as it is the free drug that is active, increases the activity of the drug. For example, ibuprofen is 99.5% bound to serum albumin. A 0.5% reduction in binding would double the amount of free drug (from 0.5% to 1%). By contrast, a 0.5% reduction for a drug that is 50% bound would increase the free drug by only 1% (from 50% to 50.5%). Thus this effect is relevant only for heavily protein-bound drugs.

Clearance

Clearance of a drug is defined as the volume of plasma that appears to be cleared of drug per unit time. For example a creatinine clearance of 120 ml/min means that the clearance is equal to the amount of creatinine present in 120 ml every minute. Clearance is independent of concentration, so the creatinine clearance would not change if the serum creatinine were artificially increased.

The predominant clearance mechanism of lipid-soluble drugs is hepatic metabolism and for water-soluble drugs clearance is via renal excretion.

Hepatic metabolism

The metabolism of drugs occurs primarily in the liver, and liver volume can decrease by 20–40% from early adulthood to old age.[5,6] Thus the metabolism of benzodiazepines, morphine and lipid-soluble beta-blockers such as propranolol, metoprolol, and labetalol is reduced as a result of age-related reduction in liver volume. This reduction results in an equivalent prolongation of elimination half-life. The practical implications of this are that lower doses are needed in older patients to produce plasma concentrations similar to those of younger patients.

Renal clearance

Although the kidney plays a very small role in drug metabolism it is entirely responsible for excretion of water-soluble drugs and metabolites. Ageing is associated with a reduction in renal function, resulting in an average of ~10% per decade decrease in glomerular filtration rate (GFR).[7] The decrease in glomerular filtration rate affects the clearance of many commonly used drugs, e.g digoxin, lithium, respiridone, atenolol, angiotensin-converting enzyme inhibitor (ACEI) active metabolites, e.g ramiprilat, gabapentin, penicillin, cephalosporins, and quinolones.

GFR is now automatically estimated by laboratories using the Modification of Diet in Renal Disease (MDRD) formula, which uses serum creatinine, gender, age and ethnic group (see Chapter 14).[8] This has superseded the Cockcroft and Gault equation (which uses serum creatinine, weight, gender, and age) since patients' weight data are not available to laboratories.[9] These equations do not allow for the muscle bulk of the patient other than by allowing for the effect of age. They will therefore overestimate renal function in patients with low muscle bulk. This is particularly important in frail older people.

Bioavailability

Bioavailability is defined as the fraction of unchanged drug reaching the systemic circulation following administration. Graphically, the bioavailability of a drug is measured by the area under the curve of the blood concentration versus time curve given by a particular route expressed as a percentage of that of a comparator, e.g. after intravenous administration. Bioavailability may be reduced by incomplete absorption or first pass metabolism in the gut wall or liver. For example, digoxin taken orally has a reduced bioavailability due to poor absorption from the gut whereas glyceryl trinitrate has a reduced bioavailability due to first pass metabolism. For this reason it is given sublingually or sprayed into the mouth, thus avoiding first pass metabolism. Ageing itself has little effect on bioavailability.

Pharmacodynamics

Pharmacodynamics describe the effects of a drug on the body. When these effects are measured in relation to the dose used, sensitivity can be derived. Ageing may result in changes in sensitivity to drugs. Changes in sensitivity are independent of any changes in pharmacokinetics that might also be present. Thus, for example, ageing is associated with an increase in volume of distribution and decrease in clearance of lipid-soluble drugs such as benzodiazepines. Both of these effects lead to a prolongation of elimination half-life. In addition, however, ageing is also associated with an increased sensitivity to benzodiazepines. Both the pharmacokinetic and pharmacodynamic effects of ageing will lead to impairment of balance and an increased risk of falls. Thus, for the same serum concentration, older patients are more sensitive to the effects of these and other drugs (Table 4.2).

Table 4.2 Examples of age-related changes in sensitivity to drugs

Drug	Pharmacodynamic effect	Age-related change in sensitivity
Benzodiazepines	Sedation, postural way	↑
Hyoscine and other anticholinergics	Cognitive function	↑
Warfarin	Anticoagulant effect	↑
Furosemide	Diuresis; sodium excretion	↓
Morphine	Analgesic effect	↑
Propranolol	Chronotropic effect	↓
β-Antagonists	Chronotropic effect	↓
NSAIDs	Gastrointestinal toxicity	↑

↑, increase; ↓, decrease; NSAIDs, non-steroidal anti-inflammatory drugs.

Polypharmacy and appropriate prescribing

Polypharmacy refers to the coprescription of multiple medications to an individual patient. It is associated with negative outcomes.[10] The risk of adverse drug reactions is increased in proportion to the number of drugs. Polypharmacy is also associated with reduced compliance with agreed treatment regimens, nursing home placement, malnutrition, fractures, impaired mobility and falls. Although some classes of drugs can impair balance and genuinely increase the risk of falls (e.g. benzodiazepines) much of the associated burden relates to the underlying pathology seen in patients taking multiple medication rather than to the medications themselves. Thus frail older patients with multiple pathology (and taking multiple drugs) tend to experience problems such as malnutrition, falls and fractures and are more likely to need nursing home placement.

The traditional approach to polypharmacy was that multiple drug treatments in older patients were to be avoided. The concept of appropriate prescribing, however, not only encompasses the notion that drug treatments that are not indicated or contraindicated should be discontinued, but also that additional drugs may need to be prescribed where there is an indication. This is highly relevant in the management of asymptomatic conditions such as osteoporosis. The recently published Hypertension in the Very Elderly Trial (HYVET) trial showed substantial benefit from treatment of patients with sustained systolic blood pressures of ≥160 mmHg for those aged >80 years.[11] Another example is the benefit of stroke prophylaxis in atrial fibrillation. It is, of course, important that the patient is fully involved in the decision-making process wherever possible.

Medication review

Undertaking regular medication review is an important approach to enhancing appropriate prescribing. The National Service Framework for Older People[12] recommends that medication review is carried out six-monthly in those taking four or more drugs and annually in those taking fewer. This will not only identify unnecessary and potentially harmful medications, but will also identify indications for appropriate new prescriptions. Patients should always be given the opportunity to discuss any changes relating to discontinuation of existing medication and introduction of any new medication. Where there is a strong evidence base,[13–16] prescribers can be confident of their advice. Where the evidence base involves extrapolation from data based on younger patients, this should be explained to patients to help them come to a decision. For example, stroke prophylaxis in high risk patients with atrial fibrillation has not been unequivocally established in patients in their eighties, but the evidence base strongly suggests that both aspirin 300 mg and warfarin are effective.

Medication reviews can be performed by various healthcare professionals, such as GPs, specialist nurses, pharmacists and geriatricians. Medication review without access to clinical records or the patient will identify areas for further consideration; however, these must subsequently be acted upon by a prescriber. It is clearly most efficient if circumstances permit, for medication review to be undertaken by someone able to review the clinical records, patient and current prescriptions at the same time.

Several studies have investigated the effect of reviews by pharmacists on a variety of end points. In a systematic review of studies in primary care aimed at reducing medication-related adverse events that result in morbidity, hospital admissions and/or mortality, 38 studies met the inclusion criteria.[17] Of these, five were conducted in the UK including patients living at home as well as in care homes. A variety of end points were used including hospital admission rate, falls rates, cognition, depression, behaviour and adverse drug events. None showed benefit from interventions including pharmacist-led medication review on any end point. A meta-analysis of the pharmacist-led interventions (17 studies) found that they were effective in reducing hospital admissions with a statistically significant odds ratio of 0.64. When only randomized controlled trials were included the effect lost its statistical significance.

Improvements reported in patients' quality of life were more variable and no study has examined the overall health of the patients concerned. Whether reducing numbers of medications and saving money on such reductions is of overall benefit remains to be seen.

Conclusion

Prescribing medications to older people is challenging due to age-related pharmacokinetic and pharmacodynamic changes, multiple co-morbidities and increased risk of adverse drug reactions and interactions. This is further complicated by the frequent need to extrapolate efficacy and, sometimes, adverse effect data, from middle age to old age.

References

1. Azeem M, Aylin P. *The Ageing Population of the United Kingdom and Cardiovascular Disease*. London: Office of Health Economics; 2005.

2. Mallet L, Spinewine A, Huang A. The challenge of managing drug interactions in elderly people. *Lancet* 2007;370:185–91.

3. Mangoni AA, Jackson SHD. Age related changes in pharmacokinetics and pharmacodynamics: basic principles and practical applications. *Br J Clin Pharmacol* 2003;57:6–14.

4. Gainsborough N, Maskrey VL, Nelson ML, *et al*. The association of age with gastric emptying. *Age Ageing* 1993;22:37–40.

5. Swift CG, Homeida M, Halliwell M, Roberts CJC. Antipyrine disposition and liver size in the elderly. *Eur J Clin Pharmacol* 1978;14:149–52.

6. Wynne HA, Cope LH, Herd B, *et al*. The association of age and frailty with paracetamol conjugation in man. *Age Ageing* 1990;19:419–24.

7. Linderman RD, Tobin J, Shock NW. Longitudinal studies on the rate of decline of renal function with age. *J Am Geriatr Soc* 1985;33:278–85.

8. Levey AS, Bosch JP, Lewis JB, Graeme T, Rogers N, Roth D. A more accurate method to estimate glomerular filtration rate from serum creatinine: a new prediction equation. Modification of Diet in Renal Disease Study Group. *Arch Intern Med* 1999;130:461–70.

9. Cockcroft TW, Gault MW. Prediction of creatinine clearance from serum creatinine. *Nephron* 1976;16:31–4.

10. Milton JC, Jackson SHD. Inappropriate polypharmacy: reducing the burden of multiple medication. *Clin Med* 2007;7:514–17.

11. Beckett NS, Peters R, Fletcher AE, *et al.* Treatment of hypertension in patients 80 years of age or older. *N Engl J Med* 2008;358:1887–98.

12. Department of Health. *Medicines and Older People: Implementing Medicines-related Aspects of the NSF for Older People 2001.* London: DoH; 2001. Available at: www.hcsu.org.uk/index.php

13. Mangoni AA, Jackson SHD. The implications of a growing evidence base for drug use in elderly patients. Part 1. Statins for primary and secondary cardiovascular prevention. *Br J Clin Pharmacol* 2006;61:494–501.

14. Mangoni AA, Jackson SHD. The implications of a growing evidence base for drug use in elderly patients. Part 2. ACE inhibitors and angiotensin receptor blockers in heart failure and high cardiovascular risk patients. *Br J Clin Pharmacol* 2006;61:502–12.

15. Mangoni AA, Jackson SHD. The implications of a growing evidence base for drug use in elderly patients. Part 3. Beta-adrenoceptor blockers in heart failure and thrombolytics in acute myocardial infarction. *Br J Clin Pharmacol* 2006;61:513–20.

16. Dhesi JK, Allain TJ, Mangoni AA, Jackson SHD. The implications of a growing evidence base for drug use in elderly patients. Part 4. Vitamin D and bisphosphonates for fractures and osteoporosis. Review. *Br J Clin Pharmacol* 2006;61:521–8.

17. Royal S, Smeaton L, Avery AJ, Hurwitz B, Sheikh A. Interventions in primary care to reduce medication related adverse events and hospital admissions: systematic review and meta-analysis. *Qual Safety Healthcare* 2006;15:23–31.

Chapter 5

Cardiovascular disease

Stephanie Houlder, Tom Fahey, Khalid Ali,
and Chakravarthi Rajkumar

Introduction

Cardiovascular disease (CVD) is a leading cause of global morbidity and mortality, particularly among elderly people. This chapter will review common cardiovascular problems affecting elderly patients presenting to primary care including syncope, hypertension, heart failure, atrial fibrillation and ischaemic heart disease (IHD). This will be followed by an in-depth discussion of disease management and problems pertinent to the treatment of elderly patients.

Syncope

Epidemiology

Syncope is defined as 'the short-lived sudden loss of consciousness due to an interruption of adequate cerebral perfusion'. The majority of patients with a 'simple faint' never seek medical advice; hence the exact prevalence of syncope remains unknown. Syncope may present as falls in older people where co-morbidity, polypharmacy, amnesia, loss of consciousness, absence of a witness and cognitive impairment may make the diagnosis extremely difficult.[1]

Aetiology

There are several causes for syncope which can be broadly classified into those of neurological origin, cardiac origin, circulation and blood flow origin, metabolic and unexplained. It is very important to ascertain the circumstances of the syncopal episode by obtaining as detailed a history as possible, to examine the patient thoroughly, and to order the most relevant investigations based on the diagnostic possibilities. In the older population the commonest causes are vasovagal syncope, postural hypotension, and carotid sinus syndromes.[2]

Clinical Case

A woman aged 79 years presented to her general practitioner (GP) with a collapse while shopping the previous day. She fell to the floor with a preceding sense of dizziness and feeling generally unwell. She did not lose consciousness, and felt better when she lay on the floor. She had a 10 year history of hypertension and 2 weeks previously her GP had prescribed bendroflumethiazide 2.5 mg once daily. How would you investigate, diagnose and manage this patient?

Investigations and diagnosis

The investigations should aim at identifying the most likely cause for this woman's presentation and in her case an initial lying and standing blood pressure check is mandatory. She had a drop of

30 mmHg in systolic blood pressure on standing upright for 2 min; she had a regular pulse of 80/ min. This drop confirms a diagnosis of 'postural hypotension' as a cause for her syncope secondary to diuretic therapy.

The causes for syncope in an elderly population are multiple:

1) Polypharmacy: antihypertensive, antidepressants and antiarrhythmic medications are common culprits.[3] A careful review of medications is essential.

2) Common or 'simple' faint also referred to as 'vasovagal', 'vasomotor' or 'vasodepressor'. This is usually preceded by a triggering event such as prolonged standing, strong emotion, pain, fear. The patient describes a feeling of generalized weakness, sweating, nausea followed by fainting and a transient loss of consciousness. Patients regain their consciousness on the floor, colour returns to their face, blood pressure rises, and pulse increases. Here the history and presentation are typical, and a pulse, blood pressure check, and electrocardiogram (ECG) are adequate tests.

3) Cardiac causes of syncope are multiple and include rhythm abnormalities such as bradyarrhythmias, supraventricular and ventricular arrhythmias such as complete heart block (Stokes–Adams attacks), atrial fibrillation, and prolonged QT syndrome. To investigate these possibilities an ECG is needed. Patients may present with palpitations along with their syncopal episodes. If the symptoms of palpitations are infrequent a baseline ECG may not be diagnostic, and more prolonged ambulatory ECG monitoring may be needed. In some patients 48 h monitoring may still not capture any underlying arrhythmia, and in these cases a 'cardiac memo' or 'event monitor' is useful. These devices can detect up to 20% of patients with symptomatic arrhythmias.[4] Implantable loop recorders have been shown to improve the diagnostic yield with reduced syncopal episodes and improved quality of life.[5]

4) Structural cardiac abnormalities: some patients may have reduced cardiac output and poor cerebral perfusion causing syncope due to valvular lesions, left atrial myxomas, or hypertrophic obstructive cardiomyopathy (HOCM). Clinical examination may point towards one of these diagnoses and echocardiography is the investigation of choice.

5) Carotid sinus hypersensitivity: mainly older people; any slight pressure on the carotid sinus in the neck results in significant bradyarrhythmias and systemic hypotension due to reduced baroreflex sensitivity.[6] A tilt-table test where patients are tilted passively for 15–30 min with regular monitoring of pulse and blood pressure is diagnostic. A vasodepressor response (hypotension) or cardio-inhibitory responses (bradycardia) indicate a positive test.

Other diagnostic tests to help in the diagnosis of syncope may include ambulatory blood pressure monitoring, electroencephalogram if epilepsy is suspected, or computed tomography head scans, carotid Doppler ultrasonography when a transient ischaemic attack (TIA) is suspected.

Management

The management of syncope in the elderly population presents a challenge to physicians. It is important to identify the problem in primary care and to refer to the specialist 'falls' or 'syncope' clinic as necessary. It is important to get a detailed history, review medications, perform clinical examination and order relevant baseline investigations such as blood glucose, haemoglobin level, urea and electrolytes check, and an ECG. If drugs were thought to be the cause of syncope, they must be stopped. An ECG may reveal a cardiac cause, but in some patients more detailed investigations such as ambulatory ECG monitoring, implantable cardiac loop recorders or electrophysiological studies may be required. In all patients undergoing assessment for syncope, advice about driving should be provided by their GP. Specialist syncope clinics[7] in secondary care are needed for the diagnosis and management of patients with recurrent syncope.

Hypertension

Epidemiology

Hypertension is an independent risk factor for cardiovascular morbidity and mortality including IHD and cerebrovascular disease.[8] Fourteen per cent of people aged 75–84 years attend their GP with hypertension.[8]

Aetiology

The incidence of hypertension increases with age due to structural changes in the vessel wall which cause a reduction in vascular compliance.[9] Essential hypertension has a multifactorial aetiology with ethnicity, gender, alcohol, obesity and sedentary lifestyle being considered as major contributing factors. Secondary hypertension in which a specific aetiological factor can be identified affects 1–5% of the primary care population.[8]

Clinical Case

An man aged 80 years attends the general practice for a routine check-up. At the time of his visit his blood pressure is found to be 155/95 mmHg. He has a past medical history which includes type 2 diabetes mellitus and is a current smoker. How would you investigate, diagnose and manage this patient?

Investigations and diagnosis

Hypertension is usually asymptomatic and detected during routine clinical screening. National guidelines therefore recommend that all adults should have their blood pressure checked at five-yearly intervals.[10] The diagnosis of hypertension requires three elevated blood pressure measurements >140/90 mmHg to be obtained on three separate occasions.[11] Clinicians aiming to make a diagnosis of hypertension should be aware of white coat hypertension in which a transient elevation in blood pressure occurs during clinic visits. This has a prevalence of 18–60%.[12] The use of ambulatory monitoring is particularly useful for diagnosing hypertension in this group of patients.[8]

Management

Blood pressure reduction is beneficial in lowering cardiovascular risk with larger reductions in blood pressure having a more profound effect on morbidity and mortality.[8,13]

Non-pharmacological intervention

Non-pharmacological interventions targeting recognized risk factors can produce reductions in blood pressure (Table 5.1). These lifestyle modifications should be implemented following the initial diagnosis of hypertension (Figure 5.1).[11] These interventions are particularly important in the elderly population to reduce the need for multiple therapeutic agents.

When to initiate pharmacological intervention

The British Hypertension Society (BHS) and Scottish Intercollegiate Network have produced guidelines for the management of hypertension (Figure 5.2).[18] It is recommended that pharmacological intervention should be commenced for all patients with a sustained systolic blood pressure 160 mmHg or diastolic blood pressure 100 mmHg on three separate occasions. For blood pressures of 140–159/90–99 mmHg, the decision to treat depends on the additional presence of diabetes, end-organ damage and 10 year cardiovascular risk stratification.[10] End-organ damage includes CVD, renal impairment, hypertensive retinopathy and left ventricular hypertrophy.

Table 5.1 Effect of lifestyle modification on systolic blood pressure (BP)[a]

Intervention	Target	Approximate effect on systolic BP
Weight reduction	BMI <25 kg/m^2, 4–8% reduction in body weight	−3 mmHg[7]
Improved diet	Reduced saturated fat, five a day, oily fish	No meta-analysis data
Dietary sodium	<6 g/day for 4 weeks	−5 mmHg[8]
Physical activity	>30 min aerobic exercise >3 days per week	−4 mmHg[9]
Smoking	Cessation	No meta-analysis data
Alcohol	Males < 21 units and females <14 units	−3 mmHg[10]

[a] Based on information from References 14–18.
BMI, body mass index.

Cardiovascular risk stratification

Current UK recommendations are to assess cardiovascular risk using the Framingham risk function. This assessment tool was initially proposed in the early 1990s due to the unreliability of predicting CVD by single risk factor assessment alone.[19] Prognosis concerning future cardiovascular events such as stroke or myocardial infarction is quantified and estimated by means of multivariable

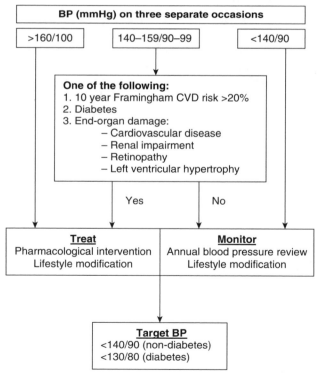

Fig. 5.1 Guidelines for the initiation of lifestyle and pharmacological intervention in hypertension (based on information from McManus et al.[18]). BP, blood pressure; CVD, cardiovascular disease.

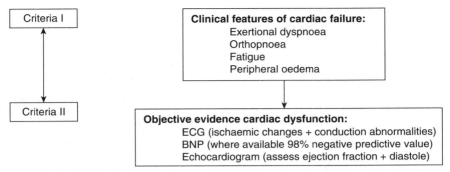

Fig. 5.2 Clinical and objective diagnostic tests required to make a formal diagnosis of heart failure (based on information from the European Society of Cardiology[31]). ECG, electrocardiogram; BNP, brain (B-type) natriuretic peptide.

risk assessment. This enables clinicians to combine risk factor information (based on age, gender, smoking status, presence of diabetes, lipid levels and blood pressure) and calculate the percentage risk that the patient will have a cardiovascular event within a specified time period.[20] A 10 year CVD risk of >20% should serve as a trigger for the initiation of antihypertensive medication. Additional measures to reduce cardiovascular risk should also be considered at the same time (e.g. stopping smoking, initiation of lipid-lowering medication and aspirin—see later section on primary and secondary prevention of CVD).

Risk stratification in elderly patients is important as the relative benefit of a risk-reducing treatment such as antihypertensive drugs is proportional to the absolute cardiovascular risk.[19] If the absolute risk of CVD is low, then the benefit from risk-reducing interventions will also be low and possible harms of medications may outweigh the small benefits.

There are concerns that the Framingham risk function overpredicts in the UK populations, increasing the hazard of inappropriate preventive therapy.[21] An alternative cardiovascular risk score, based on a UK general practice cohort, the CVD risk algorithm (QRISK), has been developed and appears to predict cardiovascular events more accurately in a UK population.[22,23]

Guidelines for pharmacological intervention

Following the decision to implement pharmacological management, the National Institute of Health and Clinical Excellence (NICE) and BHS guidelines should be followed. These advocate the 'ACD' approach to antihypertensive treatment which uses the division of hypertension into high and low renin states ('A': angiotensin-converting-enzyme inhibition or angiotensin receptor blockade; 'C': calcium channel blockade; or 'D': diuretics).[10] Hypertensive individuals aged >55 years tend to have lower levels of circulating renin. Thiazide diuretics, which exert their therapeutic effect independently of the renin–angiotensin–aldosterone system, are therefore recommended as first-line agents.[10,11]

An interval of four weeks should be allowed to assess the response to treatment.[10] If thiazides are ineffective, they should be combined with a second agent (either angiotensin-converting enzyme inhibitors (ACEIs) or calcium channel antagonists) until target blood pressure is reached.[10] Beta-blockers are no longer recommended in the early management of hypertension.[11] This is because they are inferior to other antihypertensive agents in reducing CVD and stroke, and they have also been associated with an increased risk of diabetes.[24,25]

Limitations of current guidelines in elderly people

NICE recommends that patients aged >80 years should receive the same treatment as those aged <80 years.[11] Unfortunately, most trials of antihypertensive agents do not include patients aged >80 years. Therefore, the clinical effectiveness of antihypertensives in this age group is less well understood. The Hypertension in the Very Elderly Trial (HYVET) has recently been published. This study found that the use of indapamide, either as a single agent or in combination with perindopril, significantly reduced stroke risk and all-cause mortality in patients aged >80 years, thus supporting the use of antihypertensive medication in elderly patients.[26]

Despite the positive findings from the HYVET study, it is important to remember that for elderly patients with multiple comorbidities prescribing strictly according to NICE guidance may be problematic. For example, thiazide diuretics which are recommended as first-line management have several recognized adverse effects including hypercholesterolaemia, impaired glucose tolerance, hyperuricaemia and hyponatraemia, which should be considered prior to initiation of treatment. ACEIs have renoprotective properties especially in diabetes and have been shown to reduce mortality in patients with heart failure.[8] Therefore, elderly patients may require a more tailored approach to management of hypertension which takes into account their comorbidities.[8]

Follow-up

All patients with hypertension should be reviewed on a 6-monthly basis.[10] Blood pressure targets are only achieved in 25–40% of patients receiving antihypertensive medications.[27] Common reasons for poor control include non-concordance with medication and recommended drug treatments not being implemented appropriately.[27] A large systematic review conducted in 2006 found that the most important factors in achieving blood pressure goals were patient recall, regular review and a stepped care approach to antihypertensive treatment.[27]

Heart failure

Epidemiology

Heart failure is defined as an inability of the heart to provide a cardiac output sufficient to meet the requirements of metabolizing tissues. It has an incidence of 11.6 per 1000 in those aged >85 years.[28]

Aetiology

The main causes of heart failure include IHD, chronic hypertension, dilated cardiomyopathy and valvular heart disease. Heart failure can be subdivided into systolic and diastolic dysfunction. Diastolic dysfunction arises secondary to impaired ventricular relaxation which impedes cardiac filling.[29] Systolic dysfunction arises due to an inability of the heart to eject blood.

Clinical Case

A woman aged 82 years presents to the general practice with a 3 month history of exertional dyspnoea, orthopnoea and ankle swelling. She has a past medical history of IHD, hypertension and is a current smoker of 30 pack-years. How would you diagnose heart failure and exclude other diagnoses? What would be your management?

Diagnosis

Clinical features of heart failure include fatigue, dyspnoea, orthopnoea and peripheral oedema. Unfortunately, symptoms such as dyspnoea and fatigue are not specific to CVD. In addition, elderly patients may present atypically with symptoms such as confusion. As a consequence, the rates of heart failure misdiagnosis can be as high as 50%.[30] The European Society of Cardiology (ESC) and NICE recommend that the diagnosis of heart failure should depend on a combination of clinical presentation and objective diagnostic tests such as echocardiogram (Figure 5.3).[31,32] It can be difficult to provide echocardiograms for all patients with suspected heart failure in primary care. Therefore, ECG and atrial naturitic peptides (where available) should form part of the initial investigation. Chest X-ray may also be useful to exclude other causes of dyspnoea. If these initial screening investigations are normal, the probability of heart failure is low.[33]

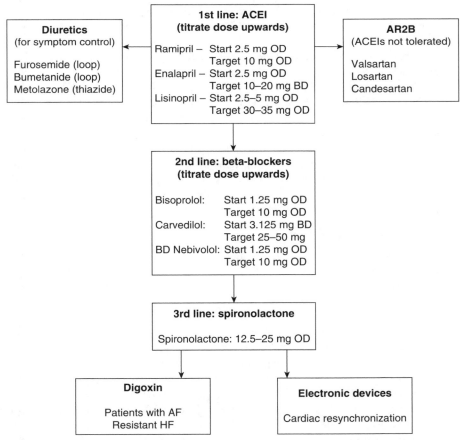

Fig. 5.3 Guidelines for the management of chronic systolic heart failure (based on information from NICE[32]). A2RB, angiotensin II receptor blocker; ACEI, angiotensin-converting enzyme inhibitor; OD, once per day; BD, twice per day; AF, atrial fibrillation; HF, heart failure.

Management

Heart failure has a poor prognosis with 50% of those affected dying within 4 years of diagnosis.[31] As such, early diagnosis and initiation of appropriate therapy is essential to reduce mortality and morbidity.

Non-pharmacological intervention

Several non-pharmacological interventions can be made following the initial diagnosis of heart failure. These include general education, weight reduction, smoking cessation, alcohol reduction and exercise-based rehabilitation programmes.[31,32] In more advanced heart failure, salt restriction and fluid restriction of 1.5–2 l/day is recommended.[31] Pneumococcal and influenza vaccinations are also advised.[32]

Pharmacological intervention

ACEIs should be used as first-line intervention for the management of heart failure (Figure 5.3). They exert their therapeutic effect through inhibiting the renin–angiotensin–aldosterone system. Several studies have shown ACEIs to improve mortality, functional capacity, and the risk of hospitalization.[34,35] Following initiation of ACEI, the dose should be increased at 2-weekly intervals until the optimal dose is achieved.[32] In addition, renal function should be monitored with each dose increase and at 3–6 month intervals.[31] Angiotensin receptor 2 blockers (AR2Bs) can be used if the patient experiences a problematic cough.

Beta-blockers should be used in all patients with stable heart failure following the initiation of ACEIs.[32] The combination of ACEIs and beta-blockers may reduce 2 year mortality from 34% to 14%.[36] Only bisoprolol, carvedilol and nebivolol are recommended for use in heart failure. The SENIORS trial has found nebivolol to be particularly effective in patients aged >70 years.[37]

Diuretics are used for symptomatic treatment. Loop diuretics such as furosemide and bumetanide reduce salt and water retention, providing relief from fluid overload and pulmonary congestion.[29] These agents have no effect on mortality.[29] Spironolactone, a potassium-sparing diuretic, is recommended for resistant heart failure. This agent is capable of reducing mortality by 30% when used in combination with ACEIs.[38]

Cardiac resynchronization

Resynchronization therapy using a biventricular pacemaker is indicated in patients with New York Heart Association (NYHA) stage III–IV heart failure, a left ventricular ejection fraction of <35% and ventricular dysynchrony indicated by a QRS complex duration of >120 ms.[31,32]

Difficulties of managing heart failure in elderly patients

A number of reports suggest that heart failure is poorly managed.[36] A recent large study in the primary care setting found that 50% of patients had inadequate symptomatic control.[36] This may be attributable to exaggerated concerns regarding the safety and tolerability of cardiac drugs, especially among frail individuals with multiple comorbidities and possible cognitive impairment.[30] Despite these concerns, ACEIs and beta-blockers are generally effective and well tolerated in this group.[31] However, the risk of hyperkalaemia is increased, especially if ACEIs and spironolactone are given in combination.[31] Electrolytes should therefore be monitored closely. In addition, beta-blockers should be avoided if the patient has a cardiac conduction defect.[31]

The incidence of diastolic heart failure increases with age and is thought to affect 40% of people aged >70 years.[39] There are limited trials regarding specific pharmacological interventions for diastolic heart failure.[40] However, ACEIs and beta-blockers are currently thought to be beneficial.[31]

Follow-up

Once the diagnosis of heart failure is established, severity can be monitored using functional limitation scores such as the NYHA. It is advised that patients should monitor and be aware of their optimal weight (the point at which they are euvolaemic and asymptomatic) to gauge control.[29] Weight gain of >2 kg in 3 days serves as a trigger for the patient to seek medical advice and organize adjustment of diuretic dose.[31]

Atrial fibrillation

Epidemiology

Atrial fibrillation (AF) is the commonest sustained tachyarrhythmia seen in clinical practice, affecting 5% of people aged >65 and 10% of those aged >80 years.[41,42] It represents a significant risk factor for thromboembolic diseases including stroke.[42]

Aetiology

Aetiological factors include increased age, hypertension, IHD, thyrotoxicosis, heart failure, valvular heart disease and excess alcohol consumption.[42]

Clinical Case

A 79-year-old man presents with a 2 week history of palpitations and intermittent shortness of breath. He has no other significant past medical history. On examination his pulse is irregular and ECG confirms AF. How would you manage this patient? Should this patient receive anticoagulation with warfarin?

Investigations and diagnosis

Atrial fibrillation can be asymptomatic or cause palpitations, dyspnoea, dizziness and syncope.[42] An ECG should be performed in all suspected cases to confirm the diagnosis.[43] In addition, individuals should undergo clinical investigations including routine bloods, thyroid function tests and chest X-ray to determine the aetiology.[42] An echocardiogram is indicated if there is evidence of structural heart disease.[43] Acute AF is defined as AF with a duration of >48 h.[42] Persistent AF lasts for several days but is amenable to cardioversion. Permanent AF is refractory to cardioversion or when cardioversion is contraindicated.[42]

Management

One of the main decisions required in the management of AF is whether to achieve rate or rhythm control. Rate and rhythm control are comparable in terms of cardiovascular morbidity and overall mortality.[41,44] Therefore, management should be influenced by the patient's age, symptoms, haemodynamic stability and the presence of comorbidities.[41]

Rate control

Rate control is achieved through the provision of pharmacological agents to maintain a resting heart rate of 60–90 bpm.[41] This reduces symptoms and maintains haemodynamic stability.[45] Rate control should be the preferred treatment for patients aged >65 years with a history of IHD or contraindications to the use of antiarrhythmic agents or cardioversion (Figure 5.4).[43]

Beta-blockers or rate-limiting calcium channel antagonists should be used as first-line agents to achieve rate control.[41,43] They delay conduction through the atrioventricular node and should be

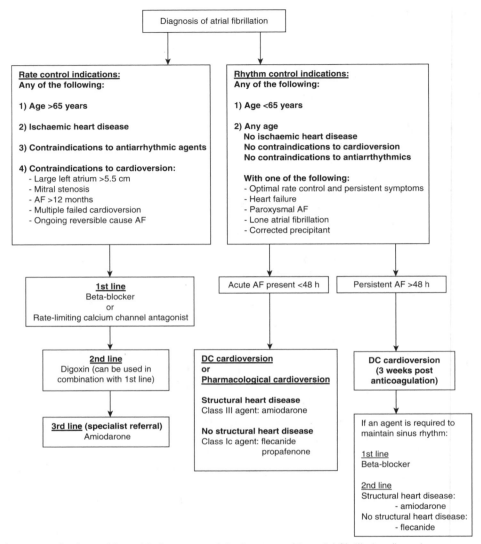

Fig. 5.4 Methods used for achieving rate and rhythm control in atrial fibrillation (based on information from NICE[43]). DC, direct current.

used cautiously in hypotension and heart failure.[45] If monotherapy is inadequate then digoxin can be added.[43] Digoxin is negatively chronotrophic but positively inotrophic.[45] It is therefore particularly useful for patients with AF and concomitant heart failure or hypotension.[45] Digoxin has limited efficacy as a rate-controlling agent following exercise and fever.[42] As a consequence, it should only be used as monotherapy in older sedentary patients.[43] Amiodarone is recommended if other drugs have failed (Figure 5.4).[41]

Rhythm control

The aim of rhythm control is to restore and maintain sinus rhythm. This can be achieved through the use of direct current (DC) cardioversion or pharmacological cardioversion.[41] Rhythm control is generally only indicated in elderly patients if they have persistent symptoms despite optimal rate control, or a concomitant diagnosis of cardiac failure (Figure 5.4).[42]

Rhythm control for acute atrial fibrillation

In acute AF (present for <48 h), pharmacological and DC cardioversion have similar effectiveness.[41] Pharmacological cardioversion is often preferred as it less invasive and easier to initiate.[41] In the absence of structural heart disease (coronary artery disease and left ventricular dysfunction), antiarrhythmic class Ic drugs such as flecanide or propafenone are the recommended first line.[43] These agents increase the tendency to develop other cardiac arrhythmias. Therefore, if structural heart disease is present, a class III agent such as amiodarone should be used (Figure 5.4).[43]

Rhythm control for persistent atrial fibrillation

Persistent AF (present for >48 h) should be treated with DC cardioversion. This has a success rate of up to 90%.[43,45] The patient should be anticoagulated for a minimum of 3 weeks prior to cardioversion.[43] If pharmacological agents are prescribed for the maintenance of sinus rhythm post cardioversion, beta-blockers are recommended as first line.[43]

Anticoagulation

Atrial fibrillation is associated with an increased risk of thromboembolic stroke.[45] The prevention of this complication in elderly patients represents a key target in the management of AF. Anticoagulation to prevent vascular events should be commenced at an early stage following the diagnosis of AF.[43] The main dilemma facing clinicians is which method of anticoagulation to use (warfarin or aspirin). This is particularly relevant for older people.

Stroke risk stratification

Although atrial fibrillation increases the possibility of thromboembolic stroke, the level of risk is dependent upon each individual's risk profile. Stroke risk should therefore be assessed in all patients to determine those most likely to benefit from warfarin therapy.[41]

One method for stroke risk stratification is the CHADS$_2$. This assesses a patient's risk of stroke based on that individual's number of stroke risk factors.[46] The patient's overall score indicates the most appropriate form of anticoagulation. A score of 1 represents low risk, thus advocating the use of aspirin. A score of ≥3 represents high risk and the need to consider warfarin therapy. The CHADS$_2$ score is limited by the lack of definitive guidance for anticoagulation in patients with moderate risk. An alternative risk stratification system is provided by NICE. This divides patients into low, moderate and high risk on the basis of age, comorbidities and previous stroke or TIA (Table 5.2).[43]

Warfarin

Meta-analysis of anticoagulation in AF has found that warfarin significantly reduces the risk of ischaemic stroke by up to 60% and is consistently superior to aspirin.[47] However, anticoagulation with warfarin is associated with an increased risk of intracranial haemorrhage.[47] As a consequence of this, clinicians can be reluctant to prescribe warfarin to elderly patients, especially those with a history of falls, bleeding and cognitive impairment.[42] Unfortunately, people in this group are most at risk of thrombosis and embolic events.[42]

The BAFTA study observed the effects of warfarin (target INR 2–3) and aspirin (75 mg) for stroke prevention specifically in an elderly population aged ≥75 years.[48] It found that there were fewer strokes in patients assigned to warfarin with no significant increase in the risk of major haemorrhage,[48] thus supporting the use of warfarin in an elderly population. This decision

Table 5.2 Risk stratification systems to guide anticoagulation strategies for atrial fibrillation[a]

Risk	Clinical features	Anticoagulant
Low	Age <65 years with no risk factors	Aspirin
Moderate	Age ≥65 years with no risk factors, or	Aspirin (consider warfarin)
	Age <75 years with hypertension, diabetes or vascular disease	
High	Previous TIA or ischaemic stroke, or	Warfarin
	Age ≥75 years with hypertension, diabetes or vascular disease, or	
	Clinical evidence of valvular heart disease or heart failure	

[a] Based on information from NICE.[43]
TIA, transient ischaemic attack.

should, however, be dependent on the likelihood of good compliance, the patient's lifestyle restrictions and risk of ischaemic stroke[42] (see Chapter 6).

Ischaemic heart disease

Primary prevention of ischaemic heart disease

For all elderly patients presenting to primary care it is important to identify those who are at risk of CVD and to implement appropriate preventive strategies. NICE has recently published a guideline for risk assessment and lipid modification for primary and secondary prevention of CVD. This guideline suggests that the 10 year CVD risk should be assessed in all patients using the Framingham risk function (described above). In addition, if the patient has a first-degree relative with premature coronary artery disease, this risk should be increased by 1.5.[49]

Primary prevention with a statin should be initiated for all people with a 10 year CVD risk of >20%. The drug of choice is simvastatin 40 mg. Following initiation of treatment, repeat lipid measurements are not indicated.[49] For secondary prevention, simvastatin 40 mg should be commenced with a target total cholesterol of <4 mmol/l and low density lipoprotein of <2 mmol/l.[49] If this is not achieved the statin dose can be increase to simvastatin 80 mg. Baseline liver function tests should be measured before commencement of statin therapy and at 3 and 12 months. Treatment should only be stopped if the liver function test levels reach three times the upper limit of normal. Patients should be advised to seek medical advice if they experience muscle pains.[49]

Secondary prevention of ischaemic heart disease

Epidemiology

It is estimated that in the UK 6–16% of men and 3–10% of women aged 65–74 years have experienced angina, a clinical syndrome characterized by discomfort in the chest, shoulder back, arm or jaw.[50] Unstable angina is distinguished from stable angina, acute myocardial infarction and non-cardiac chest pain by the pattern of symptoms (characteristic pain present at rest or on lower levels of activity), severity of symptoms (increased intensity, frequency or duration) and absence of persistent ST segment elevation on resting electrocardiogram.[51]

Aetiology

Stable angina is usually caused by coronary artery atherosclerotic disease. Rarer causes include valvular heart disease, hypertrophic cardiomyopathy, uncontrolled hypertension or vasospasm not related to atherosclerosis. The major risk factors for stable and unstable angina are the same as for other manifestations of IHD—older age, previous atheromatous disease, diabetes, smoking, hypertension, hypercholesterolaemia, male gender and a family history of IHD.[50,51]

Prognosis

Individuals with stable angina are two to five times more likely to develop other manifestations of coronary heart disease than those who do not have angina.[50] For those individuals with symptoms of unstable angina, 5–14% die within the year after diagnosis, with mortality risk greatest in the first month after diagnosis.[51] Therefore the purpose of diagnostic work-up is to improve symptoms, exercise capacity and quality of life in the short term and to prevent death and future cardiovascular events in the medium to long term. In addition, particularly in those with unstable angina, diagnostic work-up is important in identifying high risk individuals who benefit more from revascularization procedures.[50,51]

Investigations and diagnosis

Patients with suspected angina in primary care should have a detailed clinical assessment, including history and examination, blood pressure measurement, haemoglobin, thyroid function tests, cholesterol and blood glucose measurement.[52] Early referral should be considered for patients with new-onset symptoms and those with increasing chest pain. Ideally all patients with angina should be referred to a local chest pain clinic for exercise tolerance testing, but availability and access may vary according to local circumstances.[52]

Pharmacological management

Drug treatment should address symptom control and prevention of future cardiovascular events.[52] For symptom control, beta-blockers and sublingual nitrates are first-line agents; for patients intolerant of beta-blockers, alternatives include rate-limiting calcium channel blockers, long-acting nitrates or nicorandil. If symptoms persist, combination therapy with a beta-blocker and calcium channel blocker is indicated, but caution is required in terms of combing beta-blockers with rate-limiting calcium channel blockers.[52] In terms of prevention of future cardiovascular events, all patients should receive aspirin and a statin.[52]

Referral for revascularization

All patients with symptoms of deteriorating angina should be referred for urgent assessment to a chest pain clinic—anybody with chest pain at rest needs urgent admission. Patients with previous stable angina who have uncontrolled symptoms with a combination of a beta-blocker and calcium channel blocker should be considered for referral to a chest pain clinic.[52]

Psychological issues

In elderly people, the prevalence of depression is high, particularly in those who have suffered a myocardial infarction or who have undergone a revascularization procedure. Depression is an independent risk factor for future cardiovascular events, particularly in post-revascularization patients, so general practitioners should be aware of the higher risk of depression and implement treatments which can include medication, psychological therapies and cardiac rehabilitation.[52]

Shared decision-making

The implementation of long-term therapy for the prevention of CVD should involve a shared decision-making process in which the patient is given the opportunity to weigh up benefits and risks of treatment. This is particularly important for elderly patients as the pharmacokinetics of drugs are altered, increasing the risk of adverse effects.[53]

Evidence in both hypertension and atrial fibrillation suggests that actively involving patients in the decision-making process can improve knowledge about treatment options, make patients more realistic in their expectations and reduce decisional conflict.[54]

Conclusion

CVD is a major cause of morbidity and mortality, especially among elderly people. This chapter has highlighted the difficulties of diagnosing and managing common clinical conditions such as syncope, hypertension, atrial fibrillation, heart failure, and IHD in frail elderly patients with multiple comorbidities. It has also highlighted the importance of risk stratification and shared decision-making to ensure the appropriate level of intervention is achieved on a case-by-case basis.

References

1. Kenny RA. Syncope in the elderly: diagnosis, evaluation, and treatment. *J Cardiovasc Electrophysiol* 2003;14:S74–7.

2. Kenny RA. Neurally mediated syncope. *Clin Geriatr Med* 2002;18:191–210.

3. Verhaeverbeke I, Mets T. Drug-induced orthostatic hypotension in the elderly: avoiding its onset. *Drug Saf* 1997;17:105–18.

4. Linzer M, Pritchett ELC, Pontinen M, *et al*. Incremental diagnostic yield of loop electrocardiographic recorders in unexplained syncope. *Am J Cardiol* 1990;66:214–19.

5. Farwell DJ, Freemantle N, Sulke N. The clinical impact of implantable loop recorders in patients with syncope. *Eur Heart J* 2006;27:351–6.

6. Harrington F, Murray A, Ford GA. Relationship of baroreflex sensitivity and blood pressure in an older population. *J Hypertens* 2000;18:1629–33.

7. Martins JL, Fox KF, Wood DA, *et al*. Rapid access arrhythmia clinic for the diagnosis and management of new arrhythmias presenting in the community: a prospective, descriptive study. *Heart* 2004;90: 877–881.

8. Fahey T, Schroeder K: High blood pressure. In: Jones R, Hobbs R (eds), *Oxford Textbook of Primary Medical Care*, Volume 2, Section 1, Cardiovascular problems. Oxford: Oxford University Press; 2003.

9. Francesco US, Mattace-Raso MD, Tischa JM, *et al*. Arterial stiffness and risk of coronary heart disease and stroke: The Rotterdam Study. *Circulation* 2006;113:657–63.

10. Williams B, Poulter NR, Brown MJ, *et al*. British Hypertensive Society Guidelines for Hypertension Management (BHS IV): Summary. *Br Med J* 2004;328:634–40.

11. National Institute of Health and Clinical Excellence. *Hypertension: Management of Hypertension in Adults in Primary Care*. London: NICE; 2006.

12. MacDonald MB, Laing GP, Wilson MP, Wilson TW. Prevalence and predictors of white coat response in patients with treated hypertension. *Can Med Assoc J* 1999;16:265–9.

13. Blood Pressure Lowering Treatment Trialists Collaboration. Effects of different blood pressure lowering regimens on major cardiovascular events: results of prospectively designed overviews of randomised trials. *Lancet* 2003;362:1527–35.

14. Mulrow CD, Chiquette E, Angel L, *et al*. Dieting to reduce body weight for controlling hypertension in adults. *Cochrane Database Syst Rev* 1998;(4)CD000484.

15. He FJ, MacGregor GA. Effect of longer term modest salt reduction on blood pressure. *Cochrane Database Syst Rev* 2004;(1)CD004937.

16. Whelton SP, Chin A, Xin X, He J. Effect of aerobic exercise on blood pressure: a meta analysis of randomised controlled trials. *Ann Intern Med* 2002;136:493–503.

17. Xin X, He J, Maria G, Frontini LG. Effects of alcohol reduction on blood pressure: a meta-analysis of randomised controlled trials. *Hypertension* 2001;38:1112–1117.

18. McManus F, Freel EM, Connell JMC. Hypertension: educational review. *Scott Med J* 2007;52:36–42.

19. Jackson R, Barham P, Bills J, *et al.* Management of raised blood pressure in new zealand: a discussion document. *Br Med J* 1993;307:107–10.

20. Anderson KM, Odell PM, Wilson PWF, Kannel WB. Cardiovascular disease risk profiles. *Am Heart J* 1991;121:293–8.

21. Brindle P, Emberson J, Lampe F, *et al.* Predictive accuracy of the Framingham coronary risk score in British men: prospective cohort study. *Br Med J* 2003;327:1267–70.

22. Hippisley-Cox J, Coupland C, Vinogradova Y, *et al.* Derivation and validation of QRISK: a new cardiovascular disease risk score for the United Kingdom: prospective open cohort study. *Br Med J* 2007;335:136–48.

23. Hippisley-Cox J, Coupland C, Vinogradova Y, *et al.* The performance of the QRISK cardiovascular risk prediction algorithm in an external UK sample of patients from general practice: a validation study. *Heart* 2007;94:34–9.

24. Wiysonge CS, Bradley H, Mayosi BM, *et al.* Beta blockers for hypertension (Review). *Cochrane Database of Syst Rev* 2007;(1)CD002003.

25. Dahlof B, Sever PS, Poulter NR, *et al.* Prevention of cardiovascular events with an antihypertensive regimen of amlodipine adding perindopril as required versus atenolol adding bendroflumethiazide as required in the Anglo Scandinavian Cardiac Outcomes Trial Blood Pressure Lowering Arm (ASCOT-BPLA): a multicentre randomised controlled trial. *Lancet* 2005;366:895–906.

26. Beckett NS, Peters R, Fletcher AE, *et al.* Treatment of hypertension in patients 80 years of age or older. *N Engl J Med* 2008;358:1–12.

27. Fahey T, Schroeder K, Ebrahim S. Interventions used to improve control of blood pressure in patients with hypertension (Review). *Cochrane Database System Rev* 2006;(4):CD005182.

28. Cowie MR, Wood DA, Coats AJ, Thompson SG. Incidence and aetiology of heart failure; a population based study. *Eur Heart J* 1999;20:421–28.

29. Galin I, Baran DA. Congestive heart failure: guidelines for the primary care physician. *Mt Sinai J Med* 2003;70:251–264.

30. Hobbs FDR. Unmet need for diagnosis of heart failure: the view from primary care. *Heart* 2002;85(Suppl II):ii9–ii11.

31. Swedberg K. Guidelines for the diagnosis and treatment of chronic heart failure: executive summary. The Task Force for the Diagnosis and Treatment of Chronic Heart Failure of the European Society of Cardiology. *Eur Heart J* 2005;26:1115–40.

32. National Institute of Health and Clinical Excellence. *Chronic Heart Failure: Management of Chronic Heart Failure in Primary and Secondary Care.* London: NICE; 2003.

33. Fahey T, Jeyaseelan S, McCowan C, *et al.* Diagnosis of left ventricular systolic dysfunction (LVSD): development and validation of a clinical prediction rule in primary care. *Fam Pract* 2007;24:628–35.

34. The CONSENSUS Trial Study Group. Effect of enalapril on mortality in severe congestive heart failure. Results of the Cooperative North Scandinavian Enalapril Study Group (CONSENSUS). *N Engl J Med* 1987;316:1429–35.

35. SOLVD Investigators. Effect of enalapril on survival in patients with reduced left ventricular ejection fractions and congestive heart failure. *N Engl J Med* 1991;325:293–302.

36. Cleland JGF. Contemporary management of heart failure in clinical practice. *Heart* 2002;88 (Suppl II):ii5–ii8.

37. Flather MD, Shibata MC, Coats AJS, Van Veldhuisen. Randomised trial to determine the effect of nebivolol on mortality and cardiovascular hospital admission in elderly patients with heart failure (SENIORS). *Eur Heart J* 2005;26:215–25.

38. Pitt BB, Zannad F, Remme WJ, Cody R, *et al.* The effect of spironolactone on morbidity and mortality in patients with severe heart failure. *N Engl J Med* 1999;341:709–17.

39. Kumar A, Meyerrose G, Sood V, Roongsritong C. Diastolic heart failure in the elderly and the potential role of aldosterone antagonists. *Drugs Aging* 2006;23:299–308.

40. Brozena S, Jessup M. What every primary care physician should know. *Geriatrics* 2003;58:31–8.

41. Jenkins SM, Dunn FG. Key issues in the management of atrial fibrillation: protecting the patient and controlling the arrhythmia. *Scott Med J* 2007;52:27–35.

42. Watson T, Shanstila E, Lip G. Modern management of atrial fibrillation. *Clin Med* 2007;7:28–34.

43. National Institute of Health and Clinical Excellence. *The Management of Atrial Fibrillation*. London: NICE; 2006.

44. AFFIRM Investigators. Relationships between sinus rhythm, treatment and survival in the Atrial Fibrillation Follow Up Investigation of Rhythm Management (AFFIRM) Study. *Circulation* 2004;109:1509–13.

45. Lip G. Management of atrial fibrillation. *Lancet* 2007;370:604–18.

46. Brian F, Gage AD, Waterman WS. Validation of clinical classification schemes for predicting stroke: results from the National Registry of Atrial Fibrillation. *J Am Med Assoc* 2001;285:2864–70.

47. Hart RG, Lesly AP, Aguilar MI. Meta analysis: antithrombotic therapy to prevent stroke in patients who have nonvalvular atrial fibrillation. *Ann Intern Med* 2007;146:857–67.

48. Mant J, Hobbs R, Fletcher K, *et al*. Warfarin versus aspirin for stroke prevention in an elderly community population with atrial fibrillation (the Birmingham Atrial Fibrillation Treatment of the Aged Study, BAFTA): a randomised controlled trial. *Lancet* 2007;370:493–503.

49. Cooper A, O'Flynn N. Guidelines: risk assessment and lipid modification for primary and secondary prevention of cardiovascular disease. Summary of NICE guidance. *Br Med J* 2008;336(7655):1246–8.

50. O'Toole L. Angina (stable). *Br Med J Clin Evid* 2007;4:213.

51. Natarajan M. Angina (unstable). *Br Med J Clin Evid* 2005;10:209.

52. Anonymous. *SIGN 96. Management of stable angina, a national clinical guideline. Scottish Intercollegiate Guidelines Network*. Edinburgh: Quality Improvement Scotland; 2007.

53. Milton JC, Hill-Smith I, Jackson SHD. Prescribing for older people. *Br Med J* 2008;336:606–9.

54. Montgomery AA, Harding J, Fahey T. Shared decision making in hypertension: the impact of patient preferences on treatment choice. *Fam Pract* 2001;18:309–13.

Chapter 6

Stroke and transient ischaemic attack

Janice O'Connell, Michael Norton, and
Christopher Gray

Introduction

Stroke is a major cause of mortality and morbidity in the older population. Each year in England and Wales, 110 000 people suffer their first stroke and 30 000 individuals have a recurrent event. Most strokes occur in older people, with a peak incident age of >75 years. In the UK, cerebrovascular disease is the third major cause of death and the most important cause of severe adult disability in the community.[1] The spectrum of cerebrovascular disease ranges from reversible neurological symptoms and signs due to transient ischaemic attack (TIA) to permanent neurological deficit resulting from cerebral infarction or primary intracerebral haemorrhage. Furthermore, and of particular relevance in older people, cerebrovascular disease is a major cause of cognitive decline, not only due to vascular dementia but also as a contributor to Alzheimer's disease through a mixed vascular and Alzheimer's type pathology. Stroke is also the single most expensive medical disorder, consuming up to 6% of the total clinical budget.[2]

The high costs of both medical and social care for patients with stroke are well recognized by primary care practitioners. In addition, the major risk factors for cerebrovascular disease have been well defined and the management of modifiable risk factors outlined in national guidelines and service frameworks.[3,4] Until recently the burden of stroke on health and social services, patients and their carers has been relatively under-recognized in comparison with other long-term conditions such as cancer and coronary heart disease. However, with the publication of the Department of Health National Stroke Strategy in 2007 came greater recognition of the importance of stroke as a major cause of morbidity, disability and mortality in the UK.[5] As a result, major changes in the organization and delivery of both hospital and community stroke services in England and Wales will follow in the next decade.

From the general practice perspective, the inclusion of indicators for stroke and TIA in the Quality and Outcomes Framework as part of the General Medical Services (GMS) Contract for England and Wales has brought its own challenges for primary care including case recognition, disease registers and preventive strategies. In this chapter, we will explore some practical aspects of the prevention and management of stroke and TIA in older people in primary care and highlight recent advances in treatment.

Clinical presentation of TIA and stroke

Patients presenting to the primary care team with TIA

The World Health Organization diagnostic criteria make an arbitrary time distinction at 24 h from symptom onset between TIAs, where transient neurological dysfunction lasts <24 h, and the completed stroke, where symptoms and signs persist beyond this time.[6] However, more recent evidence shows that most TIAs resolve within 60 min, and TIA patients with symptoms lasting >6 h actually have radiological evidence of ischaemic change on magnetic resonance imaging (MRI) brain scan. A new definition for TIA has therefore been proposed: 'a brief episode of neurological dysfunction with symptoms lasting less than one hour and without evidence of acute infarction'.[7]

It needs to be recognised that a TIA is not a benign event. A UK primary-care-based study demonstrated that up to 12% of patients presenting with symptoms of transient focal neurological dysfunction (TIA) go on to develop a stroke within 7 days, with the risk greatest in the first 24 h.[8] Approximately 15% of all ischaemic strokes are heralded by a TIA that could have provided an opportunity to prevent a potentially devastating event. It is therefore important that patients with TIA are assessed and triaged rapidly in primary care, with appropriate immediate treatment and urgent referral for specialist assessment or admission in line with locally agreed guidelines.

Although many patients with TIA will present acutely to their general practitioner (GP) in the setting of an urgent surgery appointment or home visit, a significant number do not recognize the significance of transient neurological symptoms. Thus, there are a number of other ways in which such individuals may become known to the primary care team. These include opportunistic detection during a routine or non-urgent appointment with the GP or a member of the primary care nursing team and face-to-face or telephone encounter with the practice receptionist to request an appointment with the GP. Recognition of the symptoms of TIA by members of the public and non-clinical staff working in the primary care setting will be discussed in more detail later.

The clinical diagnosis of TIA is straightforward in many patients with sudden onset of focal neurological symptoms. In the absence of any focal disturbance in function, non-focal neurological symptoms such as light-headedness or faintness are unlikely to be due to a TIA. However, there are some focal symptoms that should probably not be considered as TIAs if they occur in isolation, e.g. dysphagia (Table 6.1). In addition to neurological history and examination, clinical assessment of the TIA patient in primary care should include pulse rate and rhythm, blood pressure and cardiovascular examination, particularly to detect cardiac murmurs and carotid bruits. Capillary blood glucose should be measured when the patient is first seen in order to exclude hypoglycaemia as a potentially reversible cause of the neurological deficit. If hypoglycaemia is diagnosed, this should be treated in accordance with local guidelines, with reassessment of the patient's neurological status following normalization of the plasma glucose level. Other investigations recommended in the patient presenting with TIA are listed in Table 6.2.

Given that most TIAs resolve in <1 h, many patients presenting to their GP will already have full resolution of symptoms. Patients who are still symptomatic and therefore more likely to have suffered a stroke should be referred to hospital by emergency ambulance. We will discuss further management of acute stroke later in the chapter. The details of local joint primary/secondary care guidelines for the management of TIA should be readily available to primary care teams. Such local protocols now need to reflect the recommendations of the recently published National Institute for Health and Clinical Excellence (NICE) guidelines for the diagnosis and initial management of acute stroke and TIA.[9] Furthermore, referral for specialist assessment should be prioritized, based on the individual's risk of subsequent stroke. The ABCD[2] scoring system is a widely used and validated method for assessment of stroke risk in TIA patients.[10,11] Age, blood pressure level, clinical features, duration of symptoms and presence of diabetes (see Table 6.3) allow a score out of 7 to be calculated. The higher the score, the higher is the risk of ischaemic stroke occurring within the next seven days. The new NICE guidelines place great emphasis on the importance of the ABCD[2] score in determining the most appropriate care pathway for the individual patient. In those with a score ≥4, referral for specialist assessment and investigation is recommended within 24 h of symptom onset. Patients with a score <4 should be seen by a stroke specialist within a week of the event (Figure 6.1). Any patient with crescendo TIAs (two or more

Table 6.1 Focal and non-focal neurological and ocular symptoms

Focal neurological/ocular symptoms	
Motor	Weakness or clumsiness of one side of the body, in whole or in part Simultaneous bilateral weakness[a] Difficulty in swallowing[a] Imbalance[a]
Speech and language	Difficulty in understanding or expressing spoken language Difficulty in reading or writing Difficulty in calculating Slurred speech[a]
Sensory	Altered feeling on one side of the body, in whole or in part
Visual	Loss of vision in one eye, in whole or in part Loss of vision in half or quarter of field Bilateral blindness Double vision[a]
Vestibular	A sensation of movement[a]
Behavioural or cognitive	Difficulty dressing, combing hair, cleaning teeth, geographical disorientation Forgetfulness[a]

Non-focal neurological symptoms
Generalized weakness or sensory disturbance Light-headedness Faintness Blackouts with altered or loss of consciousness or fainting Incontinence of urine or faeces Confusion Ringing in the ears

[a] As an isolated symptom, this does not necessarily indicate focal cerebral ischaemia unless there is an appropriately sited acute infarct or haemorrhage, or there are additional definite focal symptoms.
Adapted from Warlow et al., *Stroke: Practical Management*, 3rd edn. Oxford: Blackwell. p. 36.

Table 6.2 First-line investigations for transient ischaemic attack patients in primary care

Erythrocyte sedimentation rate	To exclude cranial arteritis or other inflammatory/vasculitic process
Full blood count	To check for anaemia or blood dyscrasia
Urea and electrolytes	To detect renal failure or electrolyte imbalance
Glucose	For diagnosis of hypo- or hyperglycaemia
Thyroid function tests	In patients with atrial fibrillation
Lipids	For diagnosis of hyperlipidaemia, monitoring of existing treatment
ECG	For cardiac rhythm, detection of myocardial infarction or ischaemia

Table 6.3 ABCD^2 score for risk stratification in patients presenting with transient ischaemic attack

A	Age >60 years	1
B	BP >140 and/or 90 mmHg	1
C	Clinical features	
	Unilateral weakness	2
	Speech disturbance without weakness	1
	Other	0
D	Duration:	
	>60 min	2
	10–59 min	1
	<10 min	0
D	Diabetes	1

BP, blood pressure.

events within a 7 day period) merits hospital referral regardless of ABCD^2 score. Patients with TIA involving the anterior circulation who are fit for and willing to consider potential endarterectomy require carotid imaging, which in most clinics will be initially by Doppler ultrasound. Carotid endarterectomy should be offered to individuals with 70–99% stenosis of the symptomatic internal carotid artery, since surgery in this group of patients results in a significant reduction in the risk of ipsilateral ischaemic stroke.[12] The benefit of carotid surgery declines with time from the initial cerebrovascular event, with endarterectomy ceasing to be of value at 12 weeks following TIA or minor stroke.[13] Hence, the recent NICE guidelines recommend that surgery should be performed within 2 weeks of the presenting symptoms in any patient with >70% carotid stenosis.[9] The intervention is purely preventive and patients must be expected to survive for >1 year after surgery to achieve benefit.[14] Age in itself is not a contraindication to carotid surgery, but in very elderly the presence of significant comorbidities that increase the risk of the procedure may negate any potential clinical benefits.

In real life, patients do not always seek early medical attention and the NICE guidelines recommend that such individuals should be treated as being at lower risk of stroke. The challenge for local healthcare providers in the UK is to provide a clinical pathway for all TIA patients that will meet in full the recommendations of the NICE guidelines in terms of timeliness of specialist assessment and investigation. In many areas, this will require considerable additional resources and presents a challenge for service commissioners and providers. Dialogue between local primary and secondary care services is essential in order to develop the most efficient and cost-effective referral pathways.

All patients with clinical symptoms suggestive of TIA should be commenced immediately on antiplatelet therapy, since there is powerful evidence for the benefits of its early use.[15] This should start with a loading dose of 300 mg aspirin orally, to be continued for 14 days and following which definitive long-term antiplatelet therapy should be given.[9] The most recent guidelines also recommend that best medical treatment of TIA patients should include control of blood pressure and hypercholesterolaemia, in addition to lifestyle measures such as smoking cessation and exercise. In many localities, TIA clinical pathways are not yet fully developed to reflect the NICE recommendations and lower risk patients may wait >1 week for specialist assessment. Thus, treatment with antihypertensive and cholesterol-lowering therapies may be commenced by the GP before assessment in secondary care has occurred. Rapid lowering of blood pressure in these lower risk TIA patients is not necessary and hypertension should be treated in line with the usual

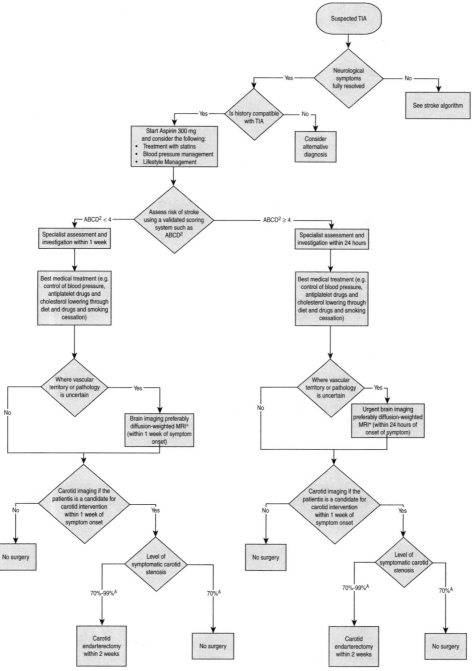

Fig. 6.1 Transient ischaemic attack (TIA) algorithm. Adapted from NICE guidelines.[9] [a]Except where contraindicated, in which case computed tomography should be used. [A]According to the European Carotid Surgery Trial criteria. MRI, magnetic resonance imaging.

guidelines. Precipitous reductions in blood pressure should be avoided in view of the theoretical risk of cerebral hypoperfusion in patients with undiagnosed severe bilateral carotid artery disease or aortic stenosis; however, in these patients there is often clinical evidence of the underlying lesion.

Despite the clear guidelines as to which patients with presumed TIA should be referred for a specialist opinion, management of a very frail older person with complex comorbidities can be difficult and often requires a more pragmatic approach by the primary care physician. Thus, in the case of an elderly bedbound nursing home resident with cognitive impairment presenting with short-lived focal neurological symptoms consistent with a TIA, it may be appropriate simply to commence aspirin therapy without the need for hospital referral. The diagnosis of TIA remains clinical and therefore in such patients advanced brain imaging is not always necessary.

Patients presenting to the primary care team with acute stroke

Patients presenting with a stroke should be admitted immediately to hospital, since there is clear evidence for the benefits of specialist stroke unit care.[16] If the clinical presentation is within 4.5 h of symptom onset, ambulance protocols should ensure that the patient is taken directly to a hyperacute centre with a thrombolysis service, where they can be assessed for suitability for treatment with recombinant tissue plasminogen activator (alteplase). Recent evidence has extended the potential time window for thrombolysis up to 4.5 h, although the current licensing indication for alteplase is within 3 h of stroke onset. In many patients presenting to hospital within the current time window, treatment cannot be considered because the onset time is unknown, e.g. patients waking with stroke symptoms, or those with language deficits for whom there is no witness. The current European approval from the European Medicines Evaluation Agency (EMEA) for the use of alteplase in acute ischaemic stroke restricts its use to patients aged <80 years. In order to further inform the safe use of thrombolysis in stroke, the EMEA required that outcomes following treatment with alteplase were monitored in a detailed post-marketing surveillance study, the Safe Implementation of Thrombolysis in Stroke Monitoring Study (SITS-MOST). Data from SITS-MOST confirmed that clinical outcomes such as mortality, functional recovery and intracerebral haemorrhage for patients treated in routine clinical practice were similar to those seen in randomized controlled trials.[17] More recent data both from a clinical trial and a SITS observational study suggest that alteplase may remain safe when given between 3 and 4.5 h following stroke onset.[18,19] These studies adhered to the European licensing requirements for the use of alteplase in stroke and thus patients aged >80 years were not included. There is limited evidence for the use of thrombolysis for ischaemic stroke in people aged >80 years, although the rate of intracerebral haemorrhage does not appear to be increased.[20] At a population level in North America and Europe, between 1% and 3% of all ischaemic strokes are currently treated with thrombolysis. The Department of Health's target is for 10% of all ischaemic strokes to receive thrombolytic therapy.[5] A formal extension of the European license for the use of alteplase up to 4.5 h after stroke may be granted by 2010. It is unclear if this extended treatment window will be accompanied by an increase in the age limit for treatment.

Even if and when the treatment window or upper age limit are extended, thrombolysis for acute ischaemic stroke is likely to remain a minority treatment. For the majority of patients, who will be predominantly older people, organized inpatient care on a specialist acute stroke unit provides the best outcomes in terms of avoidance of death or dependency.[16,21] There will be exceptions to the GP's decision to admit the patient to hospital, but these should only be where the diagnosis will not affect management, e.g. in some palliative care situations or where moving a frail older person from their usual place of residence would be inappropriate.

Pre-hospital recognition of TIA and stroke

It is clear from the preceding sections that early recognition of the symptoms of TIA and stroke is vital in order for patients to receive timely assessment and treatment. There is a general lack of public awareness of the symptoms of stroke and thus patients may delay seeking medical attention. The importance of public education regarding stroke and TIA is emphasized in recent guidelines and strategy documents.[5,9] Pre-hospital assessment tools have been developed to assist paramedics in the identification of patients with possible stroke. The Face Arm and Speech Test (FAST; Figure 6.2) is now an integral part of paramedic training programmes and has a 78% positive predictive value for stroke when used by ambulance staff.[22] The recent Act FAST public education campaign by the UK Stroke Association highlighted the importance of facial droop, speech disturbance and limb weakness as possible symptoms of stroke.[23] In primary care practices, the initial contact for patients with TIA or stroke may be with non-clinical staff such as receptionists and it is important to ensure that these individuals are aware that patients presenting with FAST symptoms need urgent medical review.

The accurate diagnosis of acute stroke in primary care and in the emergency department can be challenging, with important stroke mimics including sepsis, hypoglycaemia, delirium and functional disorders.[24] The Recognition of Stroke in the Emergency Room (ROSIER; Figure 6.3) scale has been validated for use in accident and emergency (A&E) departments, but not in the pre-hospital setting.[25] The ROSIER instrument is more detailed than the FAST test and has a superior positive predictive value for patients taken to A&E by ambulance (96% vs 88%). The ROSIER scale recognizes the need to exclude stroke mimics such as seizure or syncope and also includes visual field assessment and measurement of blood glucose. However, this tool has not been validated for use by primary care practitioners. Thus, patients presenting outside hospital with sudden onset of neurological symptoms should be screened for a diagnosis of TIA or stroke using the FAST test. Whereas the FAST test has good sensitivity and specificity (88% and 97% respectively) for the detection of anterior circulation syndromes, it is less reliable in the detection of lesions affecting the posterior circulation that cause other focal symptoms such as diplopia and vertigo (see Table 6.2). This should be borne in mind in the clinical assessment of the patient. Furthermore, in any patient presenting with focal neurological symptoms, blood glucose should be measured to exclude hypoglycaemia before referral to hospital.

Primary care management of patients with previous stroke and TIA

General management

The assessment and management of patients presenting with a history of previous TIA and stroke is of great importance. This group of patients has an increased risk of further TIA, stroke (30–43% risk within 5 years) and other cardiovascular events including myocardial infarction. National stroke guidelines in the UK suggest that all patients should have an individualized strategy for

Facial palsy	Yes	No
Affected side	L	R
Arm weakness	Yes	No
Affected side	L	R
Speech impairment	Yes	No

Fig. 6.2 Face, Arm and Speech Test for initial assessment of patients with possible stroke. Adapted from North East Ambulance Service NHS Trust paramedic assessment sheet.

ROSIER Scale
Stroke Assessment

The aim of this assessment tool is to enable medical and nursing staff to differentiate patients with stroke and stroke mimics.

Assessment Date ☐☐☐☐☐☐ Time ☐☐☐☐

Symptom onset Date ☐☐☐☐☐☐ Time ☐☐☐☐

GCS E=☐ M=☐ V=☐ BP ☐☐ *BM ☐

If BM < 3.5 mmol/l treat urgently and reassess once blood glucose normal

Has there been loss of consciousness or syncope?
Y (−1)☐ N (0) ☐

Has there been seizure activity?
Y (−1)☐ N (0) ☐

Is there a <u>NEW ACUTE</u> onset (or on awakening from sleep)?

I.   Asymmetric facial weakness   Y (+1)☐ N (0) ☐

II. Asymmetric arm weakness   Y (+1)☐ N (0) ☐

III. Asymmetric leg weakness   Y (+1)☐ N (0) ☐

IV. Speech disturbance   Y (+1)☐ N (0) ☐

V.   Visual field defect   Y (+1)☐ N (0) ☐

*Total Score_____(−2 to +5)

Provisional diagnosis: ☐Stroke ☐Non-Stroke (specify)_____

* Stroke is likely if total scores are > 0. Scores of </=0 have a low possibility of stroke but not completely excluded.

Fig. 6.3 The Recognition of Stroke in the Emergency Room (ROSIER) scale for the assessment of patients with possible stroke. Reproduced with permission from Nor et al.[25] (downloaded from http://www.newcastle-hospitals.org/downloads/clinical-guidelines).

stroke prevention implemented within a maximum of 7 days of acute stroke or TIA.[4] It should therefore be anticipated that patients who have had a recent assessment by specialist secondary care services should be receiving appropriate secondary preventive treatment. The primary care team needs to clarify this and to ensure that patients and, if appropriate, their carers understand the various aspects of this secondary prevention plan, including lifestyle advice such as smoking cessation. For patients with residual disability, it is important to ensure that other aspects of the ongoing rehabilitation and care requirements are reviewed and refined as appropriate. This will include any requirements for physiotherapy, speech and language therapy and occupational therapy input and any required adaptations to the home. Issues such as planned return to work and driving status will also need consideration. Good communication between primary and secondary services, community stroke teams and other agencies such as social care is essential in the transition from hospital to community.

Patients may also present to their GP with a distant history of cerebrovascular disease and it should be ascertained if all necessary assessments and investigations have already been performed. For all such patients, appropriate lifestyle advice should be provided and cardiovascular risks will need to be assessed on a regular basis, with treatment to reduce such risk factors, according to national and local guidelines. All patients with a history of cerebrovascular disease should be included on the practice's stroke register. Many primary care practices arrange for previous stroke and TIA patients to be followed up in a cardiovascular secondary prevention clinic within the practice, with routine follow-up at least annually.

Drug therapy for secondary stroke prevention

In terms of medication, all patients who have had an ischaemic stroke or TIA should be commenced on antithrombotic therapy. Combination therapy with low dose aspirin (50–300 mg) and modified release dipyridamole 200 mg twice per day is recommended for these patients and has been shown to be more effective than aspirin alone in the prevention of recurrent stroke and other occlusive vascular events.[26,27] The combination of treatment with aspirin and dipyridamole should be continued for 2 years following the presenting event.[26] Clopidogrel is sometimes used as an alternative, although recent evidence suggests equivalence with the combination of aspirin and dipyridamole rather than superiority in the secondary prevention of stroke.[28] The use of clopidogrel as a single antiplatelet agent should thus be reserved for patients who are truly aspirin allergic or intolerant.[4] There is no evidence for the use of aspirin plus clopidogrel after ischaemic stroke and indeed the combination has been shown in clinical trials to increase the risk of haemorrhagic complications.[29] Warfarin therapy is of proven efficacy in the secondary prevention of cerebrovascular disease in non-valvular atrial fibrillation.[30] Anticoagulation should be started in patients with atrial fibrillation but not until brain imaging has excluded haemorrhage and, in view of the risks of haemorrhagic transformation of the infarct, may be delayed for up to 14 days after the ischaemic event in patients with disabling stroke. Secondary care specialists will usually make decisions regarding the initiation of warfarin therapy in patients with atrial fibrillation who have had a stroke or TIA. However, since many of these patients are elderly, frail and have complex comorbidities, the GP is well placed to advise on the suitability of long-term anticoagulation therapy. There may be issues such as poor concordance with medication, risk of falls or cognitive impairment that alter the risk:benefit ratio for warfarin therapy in very elderly people. In such cases, antiplatelet therapy should be prescribed. Anticoagulant therapy should not be given to patients with ischaemic stroke who are in sinus rhythm unless a source of cardiogenic embolism has been identified.

In addition to antithrombotic therapy, long-term secondary preventive therapy following stroke or TIA should include appropriate management of other vascular risk factors such as hypertension, diabetes mellitus and hypercholesterolaemia. Management of hypertension is important following TIA, haemorrhagic and ischaemic stroke and requires a tailored approach, see Chapter 5. The choice of drugs for an older patient will be influenced by pre-existing cardiovascular and non-cardiovascular comorbidities. However, there is evidence for the beneficial effect of angiotensin-converting enzyme inhibitors (ACEIs) in reducing risk of recurrent stroke, even in patients who are not hypertensive. The PROGRESS trial recruited 6105 hypertensive and normotensive patients with a history of cerebrovascular disease.[31] The maximum beneficial effect was seen in patients on combined therapy with perindopril plus the diuretic, indapamide. Mean blood pressure lowering on combined therapy was 12/5 mmHg compared with perindopril monotherapy (mean: 5/3 mmHg). Treatment with perindopril plus indapamide resulted in a relative risk reduction for recurrent stroke of 43%, compared with a non-significant 5% decrease with perindopril alone. Further evidence to support the use of ACEIs after stroke comes from the HOPE study, in which 9297 high risk vascular patients aged ≥55 years received treatment with the ACEI ramipril or placebo, irrespective of initial blood pressure.[32] Ramipril resulted in modest reductions in office blood pressure compared with placebo (3.8/2.8 mmHg). Nevertheless, overall results confirmed that the relative risk of any stroke or fatal stroke was decreased by 32% and

61% respectively. These studies suggest that the use of ACEIs should be considered as part of the overall secondary preventive strategy for TIA and stroke patients.

Treatment of hyperlipidaemia is outlined in Chapter 5. Current stroke guidelines recommend that all patients with TIA or ischaemic stroke should be treated with a statin if they have a total cholesterol >3.5 mmol/l or low density lipoprotein cholesterol >2.5 mmol/l.[4] For older patients with type 2 diabetes mellitus, good glycaemic control is obviously important in order to decrease the risk of further cardiovascular events. However, very tight control should probably be avoided as recent clinical trials in type 2 diabetes suggest that mortality may be increased when blood glucose concentrations are lowered below current recommended levels.[33]

Primary stroke prevention

Primary prevention of cardiovascular disease by detection and management of vascular risk factors such as hypertension, diabetes and hyperlipidaemia is addressed in Chapters 5, 10, and 14. In many cases, the demarcation between primary and secondary prevention of cardiovascular disease is arbitrary, since risk factor modification undertaken following myocardial infarction should result in a reduction of the individual's likelihood of future ischaemic stroke.

The prevalence of non-valvular atrial fibrillation increases with age and is an important risk factor for ischaemic stroke in older people. Stroke risk stratification schemes for patients with atrial fibrillation have been outlined in Chapter 5. Primary care teams have an important role to play in the opportunistic detection of atrial fibrillation. Palpation for an irregular pulse should be performed during any clinical encounter with an older person, since this has been shown to be an effective screening method for the arrhythmia.[34] Indeed, previous work done in our department suggested that older people themselves are able to detect an irregular radial pulse with minimal instruction from health care professionals.[35]

Conclusion

The next decade is likely to witness major changes in the organization and delivery of stroke services in the UK as a result of the publication of national guidelines coupled with advances in clinical practice. Primary care teams have an essential function to perform in the early identification, assessment and specialist referral of patients with symptoms of TIA and stroke. Furthermore, primary care services will continue to play a vital role not only in the primary prevention of stroke as part of their overall cardiovascular risk reduction strategies, but also in the secondary preventive and ongoing care of patients with known cerebrovascular disease.

References

1. Isarol PA, Forbes JF. The cost of stroke to the National Health Service in Scotland. *Cerebrovasc Dis* 1992;1:47–50.
2. MacDonald BK, Cockerell OC, Sander JW, Shorvon SD. The incidence and lifetime prevalence of neurological disorders in a prospective community-based study in the UK. *Brain* 2000; 123(Pt 4):665–76.
3. Department of Health. *National Service Framework for Older People*. London: Department of Health; 2001.
4. Intercollegiate Working Party for Stroke. *National Clinical Guidelines for Stroke*, 3rd edn. London: Royal College of Physicians; 2008.
5. Department of Health (2007) *National Stroke Strategy*. London: Department of Health.
6. World Health Organization. Cerebrovascular diseases: prevention, treatment and rehabilitation. Report of a WHO meeting. *WHO Tech Rep Ser* 1971;469:1–57.

7. Albers GW, Caplan LR, Easton JD, *et al*. Transient ischemic attack—proposal for a new definition. *N Engl J Med* 2002;347:1713–6.

8. Coull AJ, Lovett JK, Rothwell PM. Population based study of early risk of stroke after transient ischaemic attack or minor stroke: implications for public education and organisation of services. *Br Med J* 2004;328:326.

9. National Institute for Health and Clinical Excellence. *Stroke: National Clinical Guidelines for Diagnosis and Initial Management of Acute Stroke and Transient Ischaemic Attack*. London: NICE; 2008.

10. Rothwell PM, Giles MF, Flossmann E, *et al*. A simple score (ABCD) to identify individuals at high early risk of stroke after transient ischaemic attack. *Lancet* 2005;366:29–36.

11. Johnston SC, Rothwell PM, Nguyen-Huynh MN, *et al*. Validation and refinement of scores to predict very early stroke risk after transient ischaemic attack. *Lancet* 2007;369:283–92.

12. European Carotid Surgery Trialists' Collaborative Group Randomised trial of endarterectomy for recently symptomatic carotid stenosis: final results of the MRC European Carotid Surgery Trial (ECST). *Lancet* 1998;351:1379–87.

13. Rothwell PM, Eliasziw M, Gutnikov SA, Warlow CP, Barnett HJ. Endarterectomy for symptomatic carotid stenosis in relation to clinical subgroups and timing of surgery. *Lancet* 2004;363:915–24.

14. Rothwell PM, Warlow CP. Prediction of benefit from carotid endarterectomy in individual patients: a risk modelling study. European Carotid Surgery Trialists' Collaborative Group. *Lancet* 1999;353:2105–10.

15. Rothwell PM, Giles MF, Chandratheva A, *et al*. Effect of urgent treatment of transient ischaemic attack and minor stroke on early recurrent stroke (EXPRESS study): a prospective population-based sequential comparison. *Lancet* 2007;370:1432–42.

16. Stroke Unit Trialists' Collaboration. Collaborative systematic review of the randomised trials of organised inpatient (stroke unit) care after stroke. *Br Med J* 1997;314:1151–9.

17. Wahlgren N, Ahmed N, Davalos A, *et al*. Thrombolysis with alteplase for acute ischaemic stroke in the Safe Implementation of Thrombolysis in Stroke-Monitoring Study (SITS-MOST): an observational study. *Lancet* 2007;69:275–82.

18. Hacke W, Kaste M, Bluhmki E, *et al*. Thrombolysis with alteplase 3 to 4.5 hours after acute ischemic stroke. *N Engl J Med* 2008;359:1317–29.

19. Wahlgren N, Ahmed N, Davalos A, *et al*., SITS investigators. Thrombolysis with alteplase 3–4.5 h after acute ischaemic stroke (SITS-ISTR): an observational study. *Lancet* 2008;372:1303–9.

20. De Keyser J, Gdovinova Z, Uyttenboogaart M, Vroomen PC, Luijckx GJ. Intravenous alteplase for stroke: beyond the guidelines and in particular clinical situations. *Stroke* 2007;38:2612–8.

21. Seenan P, Long M, Langhorne P. Stroke units in their natural habitat: systematic review of observational studies. *Stroke* 2007;38:1886–92.

22. Harbison J, Hossain O, Jenkinson D, Davis J, Louw SJ, Ford GA. Diagnostic accuracy of stroke referrals from primary care, emergency room physicians, and ambulance staff using the face arm speech test. *Stroke* 2003;34:71–6.

23. Stroke Association. *Suspect a stroke? Act FAST*. Available at: http://www.stroke.org.uk.

24. McNeil A. How accurate are primary care referral letters for presumed acute stroke? *Scott Med J* 2008;53:11–12.

25. Nor AM, Davis J, Sen B, *et al*. The Recognition of Stroke in the Emergency Room (ROSIER) scale: development and validation of a stroke recognition instrument. *Lancet Neurol* 2005;4:727–34.

26. National Institute for Health and Clinical Excellence. *Technology Appraisal 90. Clopidogrel and modified release dipyridamole in the prevention of occlusive vascular events*. London: NICE; 2005.

27. Halkes PH, Van Gijn J, Kappelle LJ, Koudstaal PJ, Algra A. Aspirin plus dipyridamole versus aspirin alone after cerebral ischaemia of arterial origin (ESPRIT): randomised controlled trial. *Lancet* 2006;367:1665–73.

28. Sacco RL, Diener HC, Yusuf S, *et al*. Aspirin and extended-release dipyridamole versus clopidogrel for recurrent stroke. *N Engl J Med* 2008;359:1238–51.

29. Diener HC, Bogousslavsky J, Brass LM, *et al.* Aspirin and clopidogrel compared with clopidogrel alone after recent ischaemic stroke or transient ischaemic attack in high-risk patients (MATCH): randomised, double-blind, placebo-controlled trial. *Lancet* 2004;364:331–7.

30. European Atrial Fibrillation Trial (EAFT) Study Group. Secondary prevention in non-rheumatic atrial fibrillation after transient ischaemic attack or minor stroke. *Lancet* 1993;342:1255–62.

31. Progress Collaborative Group. Randomised trial of a perindopril-based blood-pressure-lowering regimen among 6,105 individuals with previous stroke or transient ischaemic attack. *Lancet* 2001;358;1033–41.

32. Yusuf S, Sleight P, Pogue J, Bosch J, Davies R, Dagenais G. Effects of an angiotensin-converting enzyme inhibitor ramipril on cardiovascular events in high risk patients. The Heart Outcomes Prevention Evaluation Study Investigators. *N Engl J Med* 2000;342:145–53.

33. Action to Control Cardiovascular Risk in Diabetes Study Group, Gerstein HC, Miller ME, Byington RP, *et al.* Effects of intensive glucose lowering in type 2 diabetes. *N Engl J Med* 2008;358:2545–59.

34. Sudlow M, Thomson R, Thwaites B, Rodgers H, Kenny R. Prevalance of atrial fibrillation and eligibility for anticoagulants in the community. *Lancet* 1998;352:1167–71.

35. Baxter AJ, Crabtree L, Hildreth AJ, Gray CS, O'Connell JE. Self-screening for atrial fibrillation. *Lancet* 1998;352:1858.

Chapter 7

Neurological problems

John Hindle and Catherine Hindle

Introduction

Minor neurological symptoms are common in primary care but serious neurological disorders are rare. The challenge for the general practitioner (GP) is to separate the large number of somatic and non-specific neurological symptoms from those representing significant underlying disease.

Fatigue, dizziness, headache, back pain, insomnia and numbness are among the ten most common presenting symptoms in primary care, but only a small proportion of these are due to an underlying organic cause.[1] The most common presentations are non-specific neurological symptoms followed by back syndromes and headaches with the most common neurological disorders being cerebrovascular disease, shingles and diabetic polyneuropathy.[2]

Presentations and management of stroke and transient ischaemic attacks (TIAs) are dealt with separately in Chapter 6.

Neurological history

The key to good assessment of a neurological problem is a detailed and relevant history which is often the only diagnostic tool available to the clinician. GPs are in a good position to gain the history because they are aware of each individual's background, circumstances and previous history, and are also aware of any recent change in symptoms. The history obtained from the patient should be supplemented, if possible, by an account from someone who knows them well, especially if a patient suffers from mental impairment or if the presentation includes loss of consciousness.

Neurological examination

It is possible to conduct a brief and relevant neurological screening examination in the surgery to exclude significant underlying disease. In older people, assessment of cognitive function is important. During the consultation one can observe the behaviour, movement and facial expression of the patient. Brief cranial nerve testing could include an assessment of facial movements, eye movements and pupils. Motor examination is more objective than sensory examination; therefore, unless specific sensory symptoms are a presenting feature, an assessment of strength in the major muscle groups is more important. Deep tendon and plantar reflexes should be checked although these can be open to interpretation. An assessment of coordination using rapid alternating movements is easily performed. An assessment of tremor should include observation of the tremor at rest, with outstretched hands and on holding objects. It is important to assess walking to look for slowness of movement, stiffness and gait pattern.

Headaches

Background

Fifteen per cent of adults have migraine and 80% of the population will, at some stage, have episodic tension headache. Forty-five per cent of headaches presenting to the GP are of tension type, 30% migraine and the rest are due to other causes although it is often difficult to define the precise diagnosis.[4]

Headaches can be divided into primary and secondary.[5] Primary are those due to migraine, tension headaches and cluster headaches, and secondary are due to an underlying identifiable cause such as sinusitis, subarachnoid haemorrhage, brain tumour or temporal arteritis. A more practical approach is to separate those headaches that are potentially serious, which are more likely to have been of recent onset, from those that are not serious, which are often chronic and recurrent (Figure 7.1). Guidelines for the management of headache in adults are available from the British Association for the Study of Headaches (BASH)[5] but need special consideration in older patients.[6]

Headache history

A clear history is the most useful tool in making a diagnosis of the cause of a headache. It is important to understand the timing, frequency, duration, severity, character, site, precipitating and relieving factors, and associated features of headaches.[4] The best way to help with the differential diagnosis is to ask the patient to keep a diary of the headaches.

Recent-onset headaches

New onset of migraine is relatively uncommon in older people and other causes of headache should be considered.[6] There may be evidence of sinus or ear infection or dental problems. A recent history of viral illness with coryza and cough may be associated with headache secondary to viraemia. If there is any evidence of meningism in the form of neck stiffness, photophobia, change in level of consciousness or focal neurological signs, then subarachnoid haemorrhage, meningitis or encephalitis should be considered. Subarachnoid haemorrhage presents with an acute severe headache in the back of the neck or occiput coming on in a matter of seconds. This may lead to acute deterioration and prostration although occasionally patients are able to remain active. Acute subarachnoid haemorrhage may be preceded by a warning bleed. Primary intracerebral haemorrhage usually presents acutely with stroke symptoms. A low grade background headache combined with variable confusion, fluctuation in neurological signs and consciousness may be due to an underlying subdural haematoma. Chronic subdural haematoma may be more difficult to diagnose and may present with further bleeding into the chronic subdural. Somatic symptoms in those aged >50 years may point towards temporal arteritis. This may be associated with symptoms of polymyalgia with shoulder girdle aching. Only a small proportion of patients have temporal artery tenderness but the presence of jaw claudication is highly suggestive. Symptoms of a progressive headache, particularly if associated with nausea or vomiting, early morning headache, headache worse on straining or bending and any suggestion of focal neurological symptoms suggests the possibility of an intracranial space occupying lesion. Patients with recent-onset severe headache, especially if the history contains red flags, should be referred (Table 7.1).[1,6]

Chronic recurrent or less serious headaches

Tension type headaches

Although the prevalence of tension type headache peaks around the age of 40–49 years in both sexes, they are still very common in older people. Tension type headache is characterized

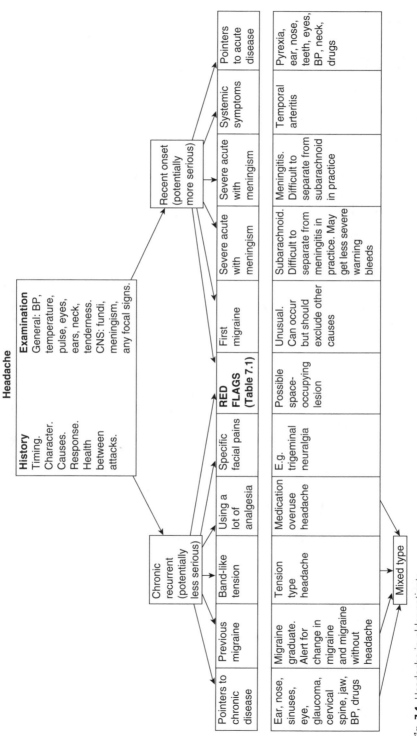

Fig. 7.1 Headache in older patients.

BP, blood pressure; CNS, central nervous system.

Table 7.1 Neurological red flags and their possible causes

Red flag symptoms	Possible cause
New-onset severe headache: the single and the worst	Subarachnoid haemorrhage
Significant change in 'normal' chronic headache	Possible raised intracranial pressure, tumour
Headache worse on coughing, straining, or early in the morning	Possible raised intracranial pressure, tumour
Any symptoms or signs suggestive of meningism	Subarachnoid, meningitis
New-onset focal neurological symptoms or signs	Stroke, tumour
Fluctuating consciousness	Tumour, subdural haematoma
Fluctuating neurological symptoms or signs	Tumour, subdural haematoma
Visual field defect or blindness	Stroke, tumour
New onset of confusion	Delirium (see Chapter 22), infection, medication
Focal progressive weakness	Tumour, progressive stroke, radiculopathy, cord compression, myelopathy
Generalized progressive weakness	Guillain–Barré, Myasthenia
Weakness with sphincter disturbance	Cauda equina compression
Nagging spinal pain/band-like pain progressing to limb weakness	Malignant spinal cord compression
Loss of consciousness with features suggestive of seizure	Epilepsy: structural brain disease

by recurrent episodes of mild-to-moderate headache without associated symptoms of nausea, vomiting, photophobia or phonophobia. The headache is a bilateral, diffuse, dull, aching and band-like pain, with a pressing, tightening, non-pulsating quality sometimes worse on touching the scalp and aggravated by noise. It can be episodic or chronic. Tension type headache may be due to activation of hyperexcitable neurons from the head and neck muscles associated with tenderness. Patients may have had recurrent headaches for years prior to presentation. Although the headache can be associated with anxiety and general tension, it is not clear how emotional triggers activate the mechanisms of head pain. There is no association with personality disorder or neurosis.[1,7]

Management Management of tension type headache should be focused on preventive measures. General wellbeing, fitness and exercise are important, but may be difficult in older patients. Reducing stressful situations, relaxation therapy and cognitive behavioural strategies may help reduce tension and stress. The intermittent use of analgesics may be appropriate, but combinations including codeine and dihydrocodeine should be avoided since this may precipitate medication overuse headaches.[7] Non-steroidal anti-inflammatory drugs (NSAIDs) are advocated in adults but may be poorly tolerated in older patients. Evidence for prophylactic treatment is limited to the use of amitriptyline, which may not be tolerated by older people because of the anticholinergic and cardiovascular side-effects.

Migraine

Most migraine sufferers are between the ages of 30 and 40 years, and there is a decline in the frequency of migraine in the fifth or sixth decade of life.[6] Where migraine persists into old age its characteristics may change, including the development of migraine without headache. New-onset migrainous type headache in old age, particularly if severe, warrants the exclusion of other causes of severe headache.[6] The history is the most important tool in the diagnosis of migraine. Migraine can occur with or without aura. Aura characteristically occurs between 5 and 60 min prior to the onset of headache and may include transient visual, sensory and speech disturbances with visual symptoms being the most common, consisting of flickering lights, spots, lines or blind spots. Migraine with aura may be associated with increased risk of vascular disease. The headache can last from 4 to 72 h. It has a unilateral location, pulsatile quality and moderate or severe pain intensity. During the headache, there is usually nausea, vomiting or photophobia.[8]

Management Management includes non-drug treatment such as relaxation or massage and avoidance of factors such as food triggers, stress or poor sleep pattern. In adults, pharmacological treatment is stepwise, only moving to the next step after three treatment failures on the present step.[5,8] The recommended initial treatment in younger adults is aspirin or ibuprofen, but not codeine, dihydrocodeine or paracetamol, with nausea treated acutely with prochlorperazine, metoclopramide or domperidone.[5,8] Older patients are more prone to gastric side-effects with aspirin and NSAIDs and the extrapyramidal effects of prochlorperazine and metoclopramide.[6,9] Treatments need to be considered carefully and adapted to the individual bearing in mind their comorbidity. In older patients, paracetamol is the safest and best-tolerated acute treatment.[6,9] For headache uncontrolled by simple analgesics, regular prophylaxis may be required. The first choice in younger adults is a triptan, but these are not recommended in older patients. Other prophylactic treatments include antidepressants, β-adrenoceptor antagonists, calcium channel antagonists, ACE inhibitors and antiepileptics. Selection of a drug from one of these classes should be dictated by the patient's comorbidities. Efficacy data for all these treatments in older patients is lacking.[9]

Other recurrent headaches

Chronic daily headache is defined by the frequency of headache, which has a characteristic different from migraine, and may be related to cervical pathology, depression, medication overuse or chronic tension headache.[4,5]

Chronic headache can result from overuse of medications used to treat migraine. These headaches are often worse on wakening and may be increased after physical exertion. Medication might be taken pre-emptively to try to prevent headache but pain can also result from withdrawal or reduction in dosage of opiates.[4,5] Codeine withdrawal headache is self-limiting. Management should include counselling as to the appropriate use of medications.

The pain of cervicogenic headache may radiate laterally, over the occiput or to the vertex. Although musculoskeletal abnormalities including the entrapment of 2nd and 3rd cervical nerve roots have been postulated as causes, the exact aetiology is unclear and there is no clear association with cervical spondylosis. Treatment of the headache should be with simple analgesics. There is no evidence for the use of neck braces/supports or occipital nerve block. Physiotherapy is the treatment of choice for musculoskeletal symptoms.

A non-specific headache can be a symptom of primary angle closure glaucoma.[5] This does not occur before middle age and risk factors include a family history, female gender and hypermetropia. Most often the headache and eye pain are episodic and mild.

Cluster headaches usually occur in younger people and are extremely rare in old age.

It is common for older patients to have a mixed aetiology for recurrent headaches. This may include a tension type headache superimposed on other causes such as cervicogenic pain.

Suspected brain tumour

Many patients presenting with headache are concerned about the possibility of an underlying brain tumour. Less than 1% of headaches referred to outpatients have an intracranial lesion.

Brain tumours are more likely to present with progressive neurological deficit, particularly weakness of the limbs, speech defect or seizure, than with a headache. Nevertheless, headaches of recent onset accompanied by features of raised intracranial pressure, focal or non-focal neurological symptoms, unexplained cognitive impairment or a change in behaviour or personality should have an urgent referral (Table 7.1).[4,5]

Neurological causes of collapse

Background

Transient loss of consciousness is a common problem in older people. It affects 50% of the population at some stage during life and it accounts for ~3% of attendances at accident and emergency departments and 1% of hospital admissions. The three main causes of transient loss of consciousness are cardiovascular causes (syncope), dysfunction of the nervous system (most commonly epilepsy) and psychogenic causes (Figure 7.2).

Epilepsy

The incidence of epilepsy is high in childhood, decreases in adulthood and then rises again in older people. The prevalence of epilepsy in older people aged >60 years is 1180 per 100 000, with an annual incidence in those aged >60 years of 117 per 100 000. GPs with a list size of 2000 patients will have between 10 and 20 people who are on treatment with antiepileptic drugs and will see one or two new cases of epilepsy per year.[10,11]

Epilepsy is a sign of underlying brain disorder with the manifestation of epilepsy depending on which part of the brain is affected, how it spreads through the brain, the underlying cause and the age of the individual. Seizures can be generalized or focal. Primary generalized seizures, which include generalized tonic/clonic seizures, typical absences and myoclonus, usually have an onset earlier in life. Seizures in old age are usually focal in origin and may include temporal lobe epilepsy, frontal lobe epilepsy or occipital epilepsy. Generalized tonic/clonic seizures seen in older people are usually secondary generalized seizures from a focal origin. Sixty per cent of people with epilepsy have convulsive seizures, the majority of which are secondary generalized tonic/clonic seizures. Among older subjects the proportion of patients with an underlying identifiable cause is higher than in patients of younger age groups, 49% being due to vascular disease and 11% due to tumours.[10,11] Other possible precipitants of seizures include alcohol withdrawal, drug intoxication, cerebral infection and inflammation, head injury or intracerebral haemorrhage.

The diagnosis of collapse is based on the history and, if possible, an eyewitness account (Figure 7.2). The history should include a review of past medical history including cerebral insults, head injury and psychiatric disturbances. Useful discriminators of seizure are the presence of cyanosis, a lateral tongue bite, incontinence during the episode and post-ictal confusion.[12] Syncope often has a precipitant with a prodromal period of symptoms. Psychogenic seizures may be associated with panic and hyperventilation.

Neurological examination is often normal unless there is focal deficit related to a focal origin of the seizure. Cardiovascular examination and an electrocardiogram are essential, particularly in older patients with a differential diagnosis of syncope.

An electroencephalogram may not be helpful in the diagnosis of seizures in older people since there may be significant abnormalities in vascular disease and non-epileptic causes of blackout, but one may be requested by a specialist in difficult cases. Patients should have brain imaging since the origin of the seizures is likely to be focal.[12]

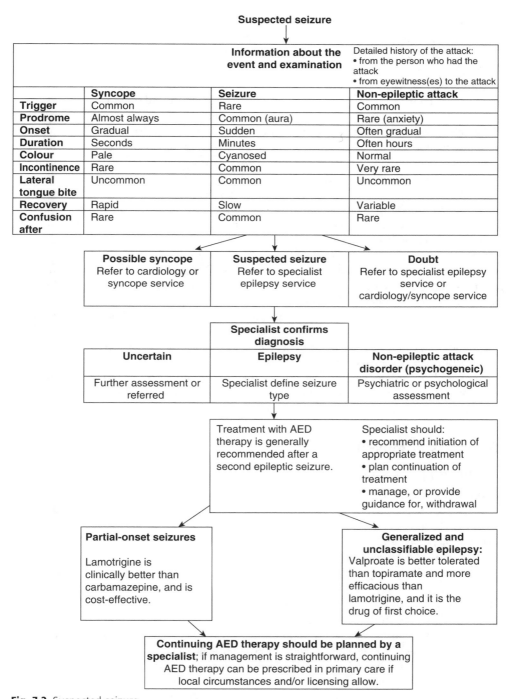

Fig. 7.2 Suspected seizure.
Adapted from Hadjikoutis and Smith[12] and NICE.[13] AED, antiepileptic drug therapy

Management

All individuals with a recent suspected seizure should be referred urgently to ensure early diagnosis. The specialist should determine the seizure type, aetiology and comorbidity.[13]

Usually, treatment will be initiated only after more than one unprovoked seizure unless there is a neurological deficit or a structural lesion on scanning.[13,14] In a provoked seizure, long-term treatment is not usually required. The National Institute of Health and Clinical Excellence guidelines in the UK recommend carbamazepine, lamotrigine, oxcarbazepine, sodium valproate or topiramate first line for partial seizures, and carbamazepine, lamotrigine, sodium valproate or topiramate first line for generalized tonic clonic seizures.[13] The SANAD study showed that lamotrigine was clinically better than carbamazepine in partial seizures and that sodium valproate was the drug of choice for seizures with generalized or uncertain onset.[15,16] Phenytoin is not recommended as a first-line anticonvulsant in older patients. Treatment should be as monotherapy, taking doses up to the recommended maxima before considering alternative treatments. There are complex interactions between all anticonvulsant drugs, some of which are unpredictable, reducing efficacy or increasing toxicity of one or both drugs. Comorbidities need to be considered when choosing treatment since some anticonvulsants have cardiovascular toxicity, and sodium valproate can exacerbate parkinsonism. Once treatment is stabilized, changing formulations or brands is not recommended owing to differing bioavailability. There is a small risk of sudden unexpected death in epilepsy which should be minimized by optimizing seizure control.

Patients with epilepsy should have a comprehensive care plan with treatment tailored to their individual circumstances and needs. All patients should have a regular structured review. Initially the monitoring and review should be done in conjunction with secondary care but, once stable, patients can be reviewed in primary care on an annual basis.

Status epilepticus is an emergency because prolonged seizures can lead to hypoxia and brain damage. Any patient with very frequent seizures, or who fails to recover between seizures, requires urgent admission to a hospital which has intensive care facilities.

Disorders of movement

Parkinson's disease

Parkinson's disease (PD) is the second commonest cause of chronic neurological disability after stroke. The prevalence of PD increases with increasing age and the prevalence in the UK is ~150 per 100 000 population with incidence of 10.8 cases of PD and 16.6 cases of parkinsonism per 100 000 population. The mean age of onset of PD is in the seventies.[17,18]

The diagnosis is based on a good history. Patients with tremor may present to the GP earlier than patients with akinesia and slowness. The tremor is mainly present at rest rather than on action. Patients may complain of a feeling of slowing down or stiffness, with difficulty getting in and out of bed, turning over in bed or getting in and out of a car. They may have slowing of gait, freezing in doorways, and shuffling. Fine tasks may be difficult, including doing up buttons, and writing, which becomes small. There may be mild slurring and quietness of speech and dribbling on the pillow at night. At onset, there should be no confusion, hallucinosis or cognitive impairment. Patients with PD onset in older age are less likely to have a family history.

Examination may show reduction of facial expression and spontaneous movements, quiet speech or dribbling. Eye movements should be normal. The limbs should show *asymmetrical* increased tone, most easily detectable at the wrist with 'cog-wheeling'. There should be slowness of movement, called bradykinesia, associated with fatigability and reduced amplitude. Not all patients have tremor, but when it is present it is a rest tremor disappearing on action. There can be diagnostic difficulty because some patients with PD have a mild postural tremor. Patients may also demonstrate increased tone and reduced agility in the legs with a shortened stride length, extra steps to turn and reduced arm swing on the side which is most affected. Examination of the glabellar tap is of no help in diagnosing PD (Figure 7.3).

Neurological signs that would exclude PD include the presence of spasticity, brisk reflexes, extensor plantar responses, and the presence of cerebellar signs.

The most common differential diagnosis of PD in patients with tremor is essential tremor (ET) (Figure 7.4).[19] Cerebrovascular disease can present with parkinsonism which is usually more symmetrical, often affecting the legs more than the arms and giving rise to small steps (*marche à petit pas*). Similar gait disturbance can be found with normal pressure hydrocephalus. The differential diagnosis includes other multisystem degenerations which have a more complex clinical picture and a less good prognosis. Multiple system atrophy (MSA) can present with parkinsonism and autonomic disturbance including urinary symptoms, erectile dysfunction and dizziness due to postural hypotension. The age of onset for patients with MSA tends to be younger than for PD, in the fifties and sixties. Progressive supranuclear palsy (PSP) can present with parkinsonism, early falls and gaze palsy. PSP has an earlier average age of onset and a more rapidly progressive course than PD. Spontaneous hallucinosis, cognitive impairment and sensitivity to neuroleptics may be present in dementia with Lewy bodies. Drug-induced parkinsonism is more symmetrical, usually with less tremor. A history of the use of neuroleptic agents and antiemetics (metoclopramide and prochlorperazine) is often missed on referral.[18,20]

Management

Where PD is suspected, patients should be referred *untreated* to a specialist in a movement disorder or PD clinic. Treatment prior to referral can lead to diagnostic confusion. The patient will benefit from access to a specialist nurse, occupational therapist, physiotherapist and speech and language therapist at diagnosis.[17,21] Most GPs will manage PD under the guidance of a specialist team but may be more directly involved in managing comorbid conditions which are common in older people.[22]

There is no evidence to support the use of any particular drug treatment in early or late PD. Treatment should be individualized and adjusted according to the patients' own circumstances and comorbidities. Treatment options include levodopa, dopamine agonists and monoamine-oxidase B-inhibitors. Anticholinergics are not a treatment of choice for older people because of side-effects and the propensity to cause confusion.[17]

Patients should not wait for substantial disability before starting medication. The specialist may advise starting with a treatment which delays the requirement for levodopa, such as a monoamine-oxidase B-inhibitor (selegiline 5–10 mg or rasagiline 1 mg) or a dopamine agonist. Dopamine agonists that are ergotamine derivatives have significant fibrotic side-effects and are no longer recommended (pergolide, cabergoline). The choice of oral dopamine agonist is between pramipexole and ropinirole. Pramipexole is taken three times daily and ropinirole can be prescribed either three times daily or as a once daily modified release combination. Both require dose titration. Domperidone may be needed for nausea, which is usually transient. The slow release rotigotine skin patch is an alternative to oral preparations.

Levodopa is still the 'gold standard' treatment and is prescribed in a fixed dose combination with a dopamine decarboxylase enzyme inhibitor which improves efficacy (levodopa plus carbidopa as Sinemet™ or co-careldopa; levodopa plus benserazide as Madopar™ or co-beneldopa). In older people there is less risk of developing long-term dyskinesia and on/off fluctuations associated with levodopa. The dose is usually titrated from 62.5 mg three times daily to 125 mg three times daily after 2–4 weeks for older people. The 110 mg combination is no longer used.

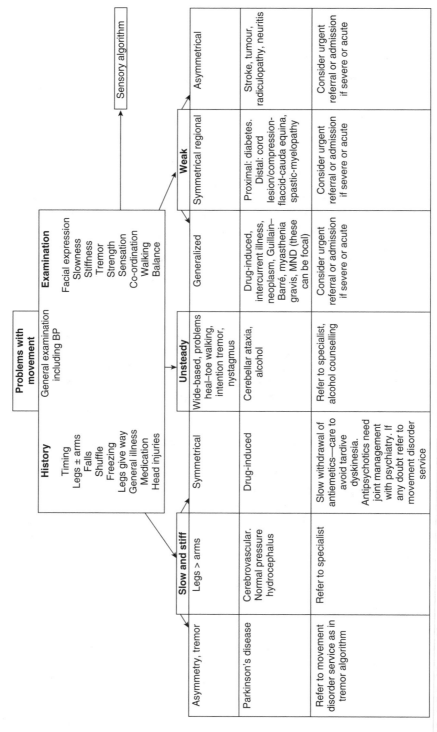

Problems with movement

	History	Examination
	Timing Legs ± arms Falls Shuffle Freezing Legs give way General illness Medication Head injuries	General examination including BP
		Facial expression Slowness Stiffness Tremor Strength Sensation Co-ordination Walking Balance → Sensory algorithm

Slow and stiff

Asymmetry, tremor	Symmetrical Legs > arms
Parkinson's disease	Cerebrovascular. Normal pressure hydrocephalus
Refer to movement disorder service as in tremor algorithm	Refer to specialist

Unsteady

Wide-based, problems heal–toe walking, intention tremor, nystagmus	Slow withdrawal of antiemetics—care to avoid tardive dyskinesia. Antipsychotics need joint management with psychiatry. If any doubt refer to movement disorder service
Cerebellar ataxia, alcohol	Drug-induced
Refer to specialist, alcohol counselling	

Weak

Generalized	Symmetrical regional	Asymmetrical
Drug-induced, intercurrent illness, neoplasm, Guillain– Barré, myasthenia gravis, MND (these can be focal)	Proximal: diabetes. Distal: cord lesion/compression- flaccid-cauda equina, spastic-myelopathy	Stroke, tumour, radiculopathy, neuritis
Consider urgent referral or admission if severe or acute	Consider urgent referral or admission if severe or acute	Consider urgent referral or admission if severe or acute

Fig. 7.3 Problems with movement.
BP, blood pressure.

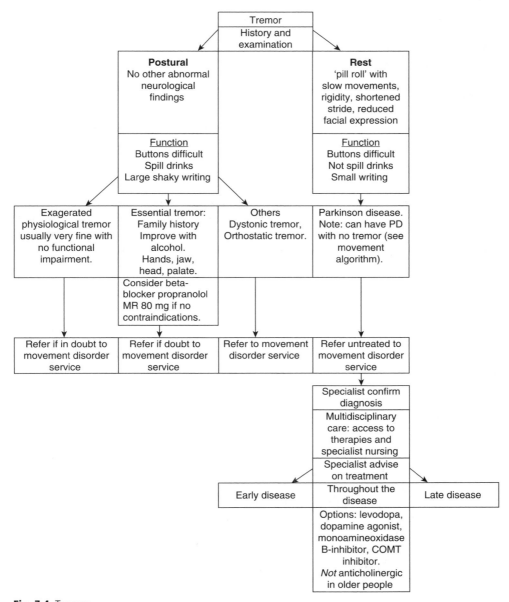

Fig. 7.4 Tremor.
PD, Parkinson disease; MR, modified release; COMT, catechol-*O*-methyl transferase.

Levodopa-based therapy can be augmented by adding entacapone, a catechol-*O*-methyl transferase (COMT) enzyme inhibitor, either as an additional tablet given with each dose of levodopa or as the fixed dose combination Stalevo™. Treatments for severe PD include apomorphine (subcutaneous injections or infusion), Duodopa™ (intraduodenal infusion) or neurosurgery. Neurosurgery is not normally considered in older patients due to increased morbidity. There is little current experience with the use of Duodopa in older patients. Apomorphine can be used and well tolerated in selected patients and is most often used as a continuous subcutaneous infusion.

As the disease progresses, patients can develop additional problems including cognitive impairment, visual hallucinosis, psychosis, falls, incontinence, dribbling and immobility. All these will require individual specialized treatment and liaison with the multidisciplinary team and the secondary care specialist.[17,21]

Management of mental health problems in Parkinson's disease

As PD progresses, cognitive impairment will occur in >80% of patients and it is more common in older people.[23] Cognitive impairment with onset >1 year following the diagnosis of PD is called PD dementia. If there is very early dementia associated with parkinsonism, this is dementia with Lewy bodies. In PD, the pattern of cognitive impairment affects planning processes more than memory. Patients may respond to acetylcholinesterase inhibitors which may be used under specialist advice, often through a shared care agreement. Currently, rivastigmine has a licence in the UK for the treatment of PD dementia but patients may also be prescribed donepezil.

Depression may occur in up to 40% of patients with PD and may be a presenting feature.[23] Decisions regarding treatment of depression are best taken in conjunction with the specialist. Treatment options include cognitive therapy, selective serotonin reuptake inhibitor (SSRI) antidepressants or combined inhibitors such as mirtazepine. Tricyclic antidepressants are not recommended owing to their side-effects.

After 5 years, 30% of patients with PD will have hallucinosis.[23] This starts with vivid dreams and illusions and may progress to stereotypical visual hallucinations of people or animals which are more common in the evening and overnight. The specialist may opt for a reduction of medications to try to alleviate the hallucinosis. Hallucinosis in older patients is often associated with cognitive impairment and such cases may be considered for acetylcholinesterase inhibitors. Traditional neuroleptics should not be used. Atypical antipsychotics may be considered, starting with small doses of quetiapine or clozapine (which requires a specialist prescription and haematological testing). See Chapter 22.

Essential tremor

Essential tremor (ET) is common in older age and is sometimes described as familial tremor when there is a strong family history. ET is usually a benign condition, rarely causing significant disability and social embarrassment. The core criterion for a diagnosis of ET is bilateral tremor of the hands and forearms without rest tremor. Supportive criteria include a long duration (>3 years), positive family history and a characteristic improvement of the tremor with alcohol. The tremor is postural and can also affect the jaw, tongue, head, palate, pharynx, respiratory muscles and legs. There should be no extrapyramidal signs of slowness, rigidity or loss of postural reflexes and no gait disturbance. Writing is much larger, irregular and shaky compared with PD. Patients may have an isolated head tremor (Figure 7.4).

Red flags raising doubt about the diagnosis are unilateral tremor, leg tremor, parkinsonism, gait disturbance, focal tremor, isolated head tremor with abnormal posture and drug treatment which could cause tremor.[24] The differential diagnosis includes PD and enhanced physiological tremor, which usually has a tremor of lower amplitude and higher frequency than ET. Medications which can cause tremor include neuroleptics, antiemetics, lithium, bronchodilators, steroids, anticonvulsants, calcitonin, thyroid hormones, cytotoxics and antiarrhythmics such as amiodarone. Other differentials include cerebellar tremor, dystonia, orthostatic tremor and psychogenic tremor.[24]

Management

Many patients are reassured by the diagnosis of ET since they are concerned that they may have PD. Most patients do not require treatment. Referral should be considered in cases of diagnostic doubt or for advice on treatment. Fifty to sixty per cent of patients may get some benefit from beta-blockers such as propranolol. This can be used in carefully selected patients but avoided if there is poor peripheral circulation, low blood pressure, heart failure, airways obstruction or asthma. Other treatments include anticonvulsants and benzodiazepines. Primidone may be tried but is often poorly tolerated in older people because of sleepiness and confusion. It has to be given in small doses, starting with 62.5 mg (one-quarter of a 250 mg tablet) increased on a weekly basis according to response. Clonazepam (0.5 mg) may have some benefit particularly if there is sleep disturbance.[24]

Restless leg syndrome

Restless leg syndrome (RLS) is a common disorder although only a small percentage of people experience any impairment or disability. Restless leg can be associated with neurodegenerative disorders including PD. RLS may be related to abnormalities of spinal conduction and iron metabolism in the basal ganglia and may be familial.[25]

RLS consists of an irresistible urge to move the legs because of discomfort. This is much worse at rest and relieved by moving the legs or walking. It is worse in the evening or at night and usually improves after 4–6 a.m. It may be associated with jumping of the legs in the evening and over-night. The disturbance of sleep can lead to tiredness the following day and can interrupt the sleep of the partner.

Examination does not reveal any specific neurological abnormality unless RLS is associated with another neurological disorder.

Management

RLS may improve with lifestyle changes. Patients should reduce tea, coffee or alcohol consumption later in the day. They may consider retiring to bed earlier, getting a better pattern of sleep. Serum ferritin should be checked and oral iron given even if it is in the normal range but <50 ng/ml. Dopaminergic therapy may be considered for patients with significant interference in their life, particularly associated with periodic limb movement in sleep, using small doses of a dopamine agonist, pramipexole or ropinirole.[25] Many GPs may prefer specialist advice prior to prescribing these drugs.

Normal pressure hydrocephalus

Idiopathic normal pressure hydrocephalus normally presents in older people. The incidence is reported between 1.8 per 100 000 and 2.2 per million, with a prevalence of 4 in 100 000 people. It is one of the potentially treatable causes of dementia and gait impairment. Patients may present with a combination of gait disorder, cognitive impairment, dementia and urinary symptoms.

Management

Patients presenting with a combination of these problems should be referred. Assessment will include brain imaging and possibly a lumbar infusion test or a high volume spinal tap to look at response to cerebrospinal fluid (CSF) reduction.[26] Patients who have good response, particularly gait improvement, may be considered for ventriculorperitoneal shunting.

Ataxia

Eight-five per cent of people have normal gait at age 60 years but this decreases to 18% by 85. For normal gait function there needs to be an intact interaction between systems including vestibular, visual sensory and higher cortical functions; basal ganglia, brain stem and cerebellum; spinal cord, nerve roots and peripheral nerves; muscles, bones, joints and ligaments, supported by the cardiovascular system. Non-neurological disorders may be the commonest cause of gait impairment. In terms of neurological disorder, the commonest causes are sensory ataxia, myelopathy, multiple strokes and parkinsonism (Figure 7.3). Cognitive factors play an important role in gait which may be impaired in dementia.[27]

Ataxia is a common presentation in older people and may be due to disorder of cerebellar function.[27] Damage to the mid-line structures, the vermis of the cerebellum, results in a central ataxia with disturbance of equilibrium and unsteadiness on standing, walking or even sitting. Damage to the hemisphere structures of the cerebellum produces signs on the same side as the lesion. The signs of cerebellar dysfunction include difficulty controlling fine movements, inaccuracy of movement, difficulty judging distance (dysmetria), difficulty performing rapid alternating movements (dysdiadochokinesia), intention tremor, pendular reflexes and reduced tone. Nystagmus results from disease affecting the cerebellar connections with the vestibular nuclei. Patients may have disturbances of speech with a scanning or explosive speech.

Gradually progressive ataxia may be due to a degenerative cause. More rapid development of ataxia may be due to neoplastic lesion such as cerebello-pontine angle tumours and infections. Cerebellar dysfunction occurs in degenerative conditions including idiopathic cerebellar degeneration, multiple system atrophy and hereditary spino-cerebellar ataxias some of which can present in older age. Tumours affecting the cerebellum and tumours elsewhere causing paraneoplastic subacute cerebellar degeneration can present with ataxia.[28] Other causes of ataxia include alcohol abuse, vitamin B_1 or B_{12} deficiency, myxoedema, and hypoglycaemia. Ataxia can be drug-induced, particularly by the anticonvulsants carbamazepine, phenytoin and primidone, major tranquillizers, other sedatives or hypnotics. Other drugs may have ataxia as a rare side-effect, including amiodarone.[29]

Management

A drug history and alcohol history should be taken and implicated drugs stopped. Routine blood tests should include blood count, blood sugar, electrolytes, liver functions, thyroid functions, B_{12} and folate levels.

Patients with ataxia should be referred for assessment. In many elderly patients, the cause of ataxia is unknown despite extensive investigation.

Spinal conditions

The spinal canal is a rigid structure, so any expanding disease process or lesion within the canal, or extrinsic to the canal, will eventually produce cord or root compression. Common causes include cervical myelopathy, tumours, infection, disc degeneration, haematomas and cystic lesions.

Cervical spondylotic myelopathy

Cervical spondylotic myelopathy is the most common cause of spinal cord compression in older adults.[30] Advanced age-related degeneration of the cervical spine can cause cervical cord compression and compress nerve roots, causing radiculopathy. Symptoms may be insidious and can include neck stiffness and pain, limb pain and weakness. Common signs include wasting of the small muscles of the hands, hyper-reflexia, Lhermitte's sign (tingling down back following neck flexion) and sensory changes. The differential diagnosis includes any condition causing myelopathy such as multiple sclerosis and motor neuron disease (MND), although both are less common in older people. MND is usually associated with wasting and fasciculation of the arms and legs, not found in cervical spondylosis.

Management

Management includes exclusion of diabetes-related amyotrophy and vitamin B_{12} deficiency. Plain cervical spine X-rays are of no value and should not be requested. Patients with significant symptoms should be referred for assessment and diagnosis. This assessment should include magnetic resonance imaging (MRI) of the spine. In patients who are mildly affected, a watchful waiting may be adopted. Non-surgical therapies have been tried but evidence for efficacy is lacking. Suitable patients with significant compression may require surgical treatment.[30] It is important for patients to understand that intervention may only arrest progression.

Other spinal cord disease

Malignant deposits in the vertebral body growing posteriorly and expanding within the epidural space may cause cord compression. This can present with nagging pain, which may be localized or develop into a band-like pain. Patients may develop subtle sensory and motor changes which can sometimes be difficult to elicit. Occasionally, patients can present with pseudo-ataxia due to very mild weakness. Compression of the pyramidal tracts should produce an upper motor neuron lesion with brisk reflexes although initially patients can have reduced reflexes and tone. Neurological signs vary depending upon the level of compression of the cord and whether there is a lateral compressive lesion, a partial unilateral cord lesion or a central cord lesion. There can be false localizing neurological signs suggestive of a lesion at a different level. Lesions above L1 will compress the cord but lesions below this level will compress the conus or cauda equina, leading to lower motor neuron signs in the legs and loss of bladder control.

Vascular lesions of the cord present acutely and can be indistinguishable from compression.

Management

Any suggestion of possible cord compression or acute spinal lesion should lead to urgent referral because there may be a sudden catastrophic deterioration in the patient's condition.

Weakness and sensory disturbances

Neuropathy

Neuropathy is a common disorder in older people with a prevalence of up to 8000 per 100 000 population.[31] It can be caused by damage to the nerve axon itself or damage to the myelin covering of nerve fibres. Diabetes is the commonest cause in the UK.

Peripheral neuropathy can be divided into acute, subacute and chronic symmetrical polyneuropathies, and multiple mononeuropathies.[31] Acute neuropathy is a diagnostic emergency.

Neuropathy may present with altered sensation, pain, weakness or autonomic symptoms. Features can be variable, resembling other neurological disorders including radiculopathy, myelopathy and neuromuscular diseases (Figures 7.3 and 7.5).

Acute inflammatory post-infectious polyneuropathy, Guillain–Barré syndrome, affects 2 per 100 000 per year and can be fatal. Respiratory or gastrointestinal infection may be followed by paraesthesia and proximal or distal weakness. Most characteristically, the reflexes are all diminished. Early diagnosis can sometimes be difficult, particularly if the reflexes are retained. Suspicion of Guillain–Barré requires urgent hospital admission.

Chronic inflammatory demyelinating polyneuropathy (CIDP) is similar to Guillain–Barré but has a slower course. It more commonly affects younger people in whom it has a fluctuating course, whereas in older people it tends to be progressive.

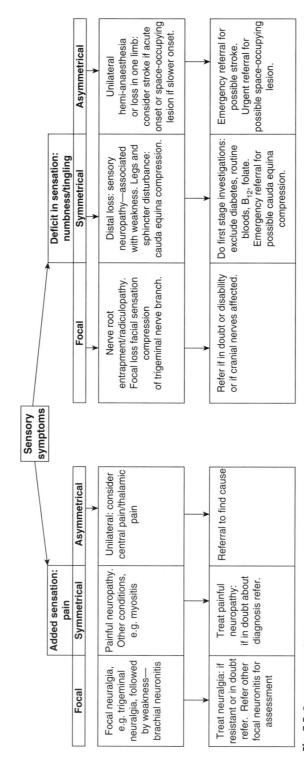

Fig. 7.5 Sensory symptoms.

The figure shows a flowchart beginning with **Sensory symptoms**, which branches into two categories: **Added sensation: pain** and **Deficit in sensation: numbness/tingling**.

Added sensation: pain divides into **Focal**, **Symmetrical**, and **Asymmetrical**:

Focal	Symmetrical	Asymmetrical
Focal neuralgia, e.g. trigeminal neuralgia, followed by weakness—brachial neuronitis	Painful neuropathy. Other conditions, e.g. myositis	Unilateral: consider central pain/thalamic pain
Treat neuralgia: if resistant or in doubt refer. Refer other focal neuronitis for assessment	Treat painful neuropathy: if in doubt about diagnosis refer.	Referral to find cause

Deficit in sensation: numbness/tingling divides into **Focal**, **Symmetrical**, and **Asymmetrical**:

Focal	Symmetrical	Asymmetrical
Nerve root entrapment/radiculopathy. Focal loss facial sensation compression of trigeminal nerve branch.	Distal loss: sensory neuropathy—associated with weakness. Legs and sphincter disturbance: cauda equina compression.	Unilateral hemi-anaesthesia or loss in one limb: consider stroke if acute onset or space-occupying lesion if slower onset.
Refer if in doubt or disability or if cranial nerves affected.	Do first stage investigations: exclude diabetes, routine bloods, B$_{12}$, folate. Emergency referral for possible cauda equina compression.	Emergency referral for possible stroke. Urgent referral for possible space-occupying lesion.

Most peripheral neuropathies, particularly in older people, are chronic symmetrical poly-neuropathies and develop over several months or years.[31] There are many possible causes of polyneuropathy including nutritional deficiency (vitamin B_{12}), drugs, alcohol, malignancies, connective tissue disorders, metabolic disorders and amyloidosis. A history of previous exposure to alcohol, toxins and drugs (e.g. metronidazole) that may cause neuropathy, and of symptoms suggestive of underlying disease, should be obtained. Hereditary neuropathies usually present in juveniles or early adulthood. Full physical examination should be undertaken, particularly to exclude underlying tumours.

Management

There are three stages to investigation of chronic peripheral neuropathy.[31] Stage I can be under-taken in general practice and includes examination of the urine for glucose and protein, haemato-logical tests for full blood count, erythrocyte sedimentation rate, vitamin B_{12} and folate levels, and biochemistry for fasting glucose, renal function, liver function and thyroid function. If no cause is found on basic investigation, referral is appropriate. Second stage investigations include electro-myogram (EMG) and nerve conduction studies, further biochemical testing, immunological tests and appropriate imaging. The third stage of investigation includes more detailed biochemical testing, CSF examination, detailed immunological tests, more detailed imaging for underlying tumours, possible nerve biopsy and a molecular genetic test, particularly in younger patients.

Diabetic neuropathy/painful neuropathy

Diabetic neuropathy is the most common cause of painful neuropathy. It is more common in insulin-dependent diabetics in older age and in poorly controlled diabetes.[32] It is probably due to vascular disease. It may present as a peripheral polyneuropathy, autonomic neuropathy, cranial nerve palsies or amyotrophy with pain and weakness in the legs.

The clinical features of neuropathic pain are of a burning cold pain. This may be associated with sensory symptoms such as paraesthesia, numbness and itching. The pain may be paroxysmal with stabbing electric shock-like sensations. Pain might be provoked by stimuli that do not normally produce pain or there may be a raised sensory threshold (Figure 7.5).

Management

The most important aspect of treatment is improving the control of diabetes. Systematic reviews have shown that tricyclic antidepressants, anticonvulsants and opiates are effective treatments for neuropathic pain in diabetes.[33] Details of management of neuropathic pain can be found in Chapter 25.

Mononeuropathies and plexus syndromes

Disease affecting a single cranial or peripheral nerve is called a mononeuropathy. This can affect a number of nerves one by one, in which case it is called mononeuritis multiplex. Where damage does not restrict itself to one particular nerve but affects a number of branches of the brachial or lumbar plexus, producing widespread weakness of a limb, this is called a plexopathy. Illnesses predisposing to mononeuropathies include diabetes, sarcoidosis, and vasculitis. Mononeuropathy can also be caused by nerve entrapment, particularly at the wrist, the risk being increased in conditions such as myxoedema or acromegaly. Multiple mononeuropathy is an acute neuropathy which is a neurological emergency. The commonest cause is vasculitis, but other causes include underlying carcinomas and lymphomas. Consideration should be given to referral of patients with neuropathy for specialist assessment.

Brachial neuronitis (neuralgic amyotrophy)

Brachial neuronitis is an uncommon condition of unknown aetiology.[34] The onset is most often in the age group 20–60 years but it can occur in older age when it is often misdiagnosed as cervical spondylitic radiculopathy. It can occur following viral illness or inoculation. The history is of acute severe burning pain over the shoulder, with weakness of shoulder and/or arm muscles which occurs days or even weeks later.

Management

Diagnosis is best made by specialist referral and assessment using EMG or MRI. Treatment is supportive and improvement usually occurs over months. The lumbar plexus can be affected in a similar manner.

Herpes zoster (shingles/post-herpetic neuralgia)

Shingles is caused by reactivation of the varicella zoster DNA herpes virus. Following primary infection, the virus remains dormant for many years in the dorsal root ganglia of the spinal cord or in the ganglia of the cranial nerves. Patients are usually aged >50 years. It may also occur in younger patients who are immunocompromised. There is a vesicular rash associated with a painful burning sensation. Motor weakness can occur in 20% of patients due to damage of the anterior horn cell. Post-herpetic neuralgia occurs in 10% of patients but the incidence increases with age. Patients may be left with a chronic burning pain. The pathogenesis of post-herpetic neuralgia is unknown.[35]

Management

Antivirals (acyclovir, valaciclovir, famciclovir) may help speed the resolution of the acute eruption and are indicated in immunocompromised patients, patients with ophthalmic zoster and in older patients. The treatment of neuralgia is the same as for other painful neuropathies using anticonvulsants and antidepressants.[35]

Trigeminal neuralgia

Trigeminal neuralgia is a clinical diagnosis based purely on the history. The incidence is 27 per 100 000 and increases with increasing age, afflicting twice as many women as men.[36] The key feature is a severe, brief, sharp facial pain which may last from seconds to minutes. It has a typical distribution in the sensory divisions of the trigeminal nerve, most particularly affecting the maxillary or mandibular branches. Pain may be evoked by touching areas of the face called trigger zones. Attacks of pain are stereotyped in individual patients. The symptoms cannot be attributed to any other underlying neurological deficit and there is no clinically evident neurological deficit on examination. Occasionally the pain can be so severe that patients have difficulty eating or drinking. Some patients get a background ache described as a mixed or atypical neuralgia. Investigations may be needed to clarify the differential diagnosis and investigate possible identifiable causes. Five to ten per cent of cases are secondary to other conditions and some are due to compression of the entry of the nerve root either by myelin deposits or vascular compression. The differential diagnosis includes dental infections, temporo-mandibular joint pain, atypical facial pain, migraine and temporal arteritis.[36]

Management

Referral should be considered in patients who are younger, have atypical features, focal neurological signs or who do not respond to medical treatment.

Carbamazepine is the drug of choice although many older patients develop adverse side-effects. The dose of carbamazepine required varies from 400 mg to 2400 mg daily. Oxcarbazepine may be considered for patients who experience side-effects on carbamazepine. The dose escalation of carbamazepine commences with 100 mg twice daily increasing by 100 mg every three days to a maximum of 1200 mg daily; the equivalent dose of oxcarbazepine is 150 mg twice a day, with dose escalation by 300 mg every three days to a maximum dose 1800 mg.[36,37]

Failure of treatment should prompt review of the diagnosis and referral. Other treatments include gabapentin, lamotrigine, baclofen, phenytoin, clonazepam, sodium valproate or topiramate. When rapid control of pain is required, local anaesthetic nerve blocks and subcutaneous sumatriptan have been tried. Neurosurgical procedures can be undertaken including microvascular decompression, ablative treatments or radiofrequency lesioning of the nerve.[36,37]

Facial nerve palsy (Bell's palsy)

Bell's palsy is the commonest cause of acute facial weakness. In this lower motor neuron facial nerve palsy, there is a characteristic weakness of both the lower and upper quadrants of the face, which includes difficulty closing the eye. On attempting to close the eye and show the teeth, the eye on the affected side does not close and the eyeball rotates upwards and outwards (Bell's phenomenon). The palsy results from damage or inflammation of the facial nerve in the internal auditory canal, possibly caused by viruses. One-third of patients with acute lower motor neurone-facial palsy have an attributable cause such as diabetes, trauma, and inflammatory conditions including sarcoid, parotid tumours and herpes zoster infection. The latter can affect the ganglion near the external auditory meatus, so patients with facial palsy should have otoscopy.[38]

Management

Referral should be considered with any abnormal presentation or atypical signs. Eight-five per cent of adults improve within the first three weeks. About one in six patients can be left with some facial weakness, and if this is significant it can cause eye problems and disfigurement.

Patients should be treated with oral prednisolone 50 mg daily for 10 days. This should be started within 72 h of onset and will make the recovery more likely. There is no evidence to support the use of antivirals.[38]

Other disorders

Multiple sclerosis

Multiple sclerosis (MS) is a condition affecting young adults with a peak age incidence of 20–40 years. It is characterized by signs and symptoms of widespread white matter disease in the brain and spinal cord with a relapsing and remitting or progressive course. It is rare to have an onset age >60 years, and only ~1% of cases have onset in old age. Older patients should continue to have access to specialist MS services which may work in collaboration with rehabilitation services for older people. Patients should graduate into older age already on treatment, or with a treatment plan devised and supervised by specialist services.[39]

Motor neurone disease

Motor neurone disease (MND) and amyotrophic lateral sclerosis (ALS) describe the same condition, with progressive degeneration of both upper and lower motor neurones. The mean age of onset is 55 years but it can present in old age. It has an incidence of 2 per 100 000 per year and a prevalence of 6 per 100 000. MND can cause progressive muscular atrophy, a frontal dementia, pseudobulbar palsy or bulbar palsy. The median survival is ~2–3 years. The aetiology of MND is unknown although a small proportion of cases have a genetic origin. Seventy-five per cent of patients present with asymmetrical wasting and weakness of the muscles, with 25% presenting with bulbar and/or pseudobulbar palsy which may be mistaken for stroke in older patients.

Management

Suspicion of MND requires specialist referral and appropriate investigation. This will include EMG and nerve conduction studies, and brain and spinal cord imaging as appropriate.

Treatment includes consideration of support for feeding and respiration. Drug therapy with riluzole may be considered and may prolong the survival by a few months.[40]

Myasthenia gravis

Myasthenia gravis is disorder of neuromuscular transmission which is characterized by weakness and fatigue of some or all muscle groups or sometimes just extraocular muscles. The weakness is worse in the arms after sustained and repeated exertion. This occurs particularly at the end of the day and is relieved by rest. Although up to 90% present in early adult life (age <40 years), a small number may present in older age. Any patient with suspected myasthenia should be referred for specialist assessment. This will include antibody tests, a Tensilon™ (edrophonium) test, and computed tomography of the chest to exclude thymoma. Treatment is with cholinomimetics and by immunosuppression with steroids.

Meningitis

The assessment and management of acute meningitis in older people is similar to that in all age groups. Meningitis can present in a more cryptic fashion in older people. Older patients are more likely to have pneumococcal meningitis or unusual organisms including *E. coli*.

Driving and neurological disorder

Management of neurological disorders should include maintaining independence through driving. The Driver and Vehicle Licensing Authority (DVLA) has specific regulations relating to a number of neurological disorders.[41]

Epileptic attacks are the most frequent medical cause of collapse at the wheel. Patients are not permitted to drive for ≥1 year from the date of the last attack if the seizure occurred while awake. If the patient remains seizure-free for ≥7 years since the last attack, a 3 year licence will be issued up to the age of 70 years. There are specific regulations for the withdrawal of antiepileptic medication.

Following a simple faint there are no driving restrictions.

Following loss of consciousness with a low risk of recurrence, the patient can drive 4 weeks after the event. If there is a high risk of recurrence, the patient can only drive 4 weeks after the event if the cause has been identified and treatment undertaken.

It is patients' own responsibility to inform the DVLA and their insurance company of their neurological disorder. Most patients with chronic disorders are able to continue safe driving. The DVLA will contact the specialist, and the medical advisor may decide on suspension or a 1, 2 or 3 year licence depending on the circumstances.

Summary

Attention to detail in history-taking, undertaking a focused neurological examination and aware-ness of how common neurological disorders present should lead to improved confidence in diagnosing, managing and referring older people presenting with neurological symptoms in primary care.

References

1. Mayou R, Farmer A. Functional somatic symptoms and syndromes. *Br Med J* 2002;325:265–8.

2. MacDonald BK, Cockerell OC, Sander JWAS, Shorvon SD. The incidence and lifetime prevalence of neurological disorders in a prospective community based study in the UK. *Brain* 2000;123:665–76.

3. Fleming DM, Cross KW, Barley MA. Recent changes in the prevalence of diseases presenting for health care. *Br J Gen Pract* 2005;55:589–95.

4. Fuller G, Kaye C. Headaches. *Br Med J* 2007;334:254–6.

5. British Association for the Study of Headache. *Guidelines for All Healthcare Professionals in the Diagnosis and Management of Migraine, Tension-Type, Cluster and Medication-Overuse Headache.* Hull: Department of Neurology, Hull Royal Infirmary; 2007. Available at: http://www.bash.org.uk http://216.25.100.131/upload/NS_BASH/BASH_guidelines_2007.pdf

6. Haan J, Hollander J, Ferrari MD. Migraine in the elderly: a review. *Cephalalgia* 2006;27:97–106.

7. Loder E, Rizolli P. Tension-type headache. *Br Med J* 2008;336:88–92.

8. Goadsby P. Recent advances in the diagnosis and management of migraine. *Br Med J* 2006;332:25–9.

9. Sarchielli P, Mancini ML, Calabresi P. Practical considerations for the treatment of elderly patients with migraine. *Drugs Aging* 2006;23:461–89.

10. Stokes T, Shaw EJ, Juarez-Garcia A, Camosso-Stefinovic J, Baker R. *Clinical Guidelines and Evidence Review for the Epilepsies: Diagnosis and Management in Adults and Children in Primary and Secondary Care.* London: Royal College of General Practitioners; 2004. Available at: http://www.nice.org.uk/nicemedia/pdf/CG020fullguideline.pdf

11. Velez L, Selwa LM. Seizure disorders in the elderly. *Am Fam Physcn* 2003;67:325–32.

12. Hadjikoutis S, Smith PEM. Approach to the patient with epilepsy in the outpatient department. *Postgrad Med J* 2005;81:442–7.

13. National Institute for Health and Clinical Excellence. *The Epilepsies—The Diagnosis and Management of the Epilepsies in Adults and Children in Primary and Secondary Care. Clinical Guideline 020.* London: NICE; October 2004. Available at: http://www.nice.org.uk/nicemedia/pdf/CG020NICEguideline.pdf

14. Myint PK, Staufenberg EFA, Sabanathan K. Post-stroke seizure and post-stroke epilepsy. *Postgrad Med J* 2006;82:568–72.

15. Marson AG, Al-kharusi AM, Alwaidh M, *et al.* The SANAD study of effectiveness of carbamazepine, gabapentin, lamotrigine, oxcarbazepine, or topiramate for treatment of partial epilepsy: an unblinded randomised controlled trial. *Lancet* 2007;369(9566):1000–15.

16. Marson AG, Al-kharusi AM, Alwaidh M, *et al.* The SANAD study of effectiveness of valproate, lamotrigine, or topiramate for generalised and unclassifiable epilepsy: an unblinded randomised controlled trial. *Lancet* 2007;369(9566):1016–26.

17. National Institute for Health and Clinical Excellence. *Parkinson's Disease—Diagnosis and Management in Primary and Secondary Care. Clinical Guideline 035.* London: NICE; June 2006. Available at: http://www.nice.org.uk/nicemedia/pdf/cg035niceguideline.pdf

18. Clarke C. Parkinson's disease. *Br Med J* 2007;335:441–5.

19. Meara J, Bhomick BK, Hobson P. Accuracy of diagnosis in patients with presumed Parkinson's. *Age Ageing* 1999;28:99–103.

20. Macphee G. Diagnosis and differential diagnosis of Parkinson's disease. In: Playfer J, Hindle J (eds), *Parkinson's Disease in the Older Patient.* Oxford: Radcliffe; 2008.

21. Parkinson's Disease Society of the United Kingdom. *The Professional's Guide to Parkinson's Disease.* November 2007. Available at: http://www.parkinsons.org.uk/PDF/PubProfessionalGuideNov07.pdf

22. Hindle JV, Hindle CM, Hobson P. Co-morbidity and the frequency of general practitioner consultations in Parkinson's disease in the United Kingdom. *Mov Disord* 2007;22:1054–5.

23. Hindle JV. Neuropsychiatry. In: Playfer J, Hindle J (eds), *Parkinson's Disease in the Older Patient*. Oxford: Radcliffe; 2008.

24. Nahab F, Peckhan E, Hallett M. Essential tremor, deceptively simple …. *Pract Neurol* 2007;7:222–33.

25. Chaudhuri K R. *Management of Restless Leg Syndrome in Primary Care. UK Guidelines.* Available at: http://www.restlesslegs.org.uk/RLSUK_guideline.pdf

26. National Institue for Health and Clinical Excellence. *Lumbar Infusion Test for the Investigation of Normal Pressure Hydrocephalus. Interventional Procedure Guidance 263.* London: NICE; June 2008. Available at: http://www.nice.org.uk/nicemedia/pdf/IPG263Guidance.pdf

27. Snijders AH, van de Warrenberg BP, Giladi N, Bloem BR. Neurological gait disorders in elderly people: clinical approach and classification. *Lancet Neurol* 2007;6:63–74.

28. Vincent A, Bien CG. Paraneoplastic neurological diseases. ACNR 2007;7:6-8 Available at: http://www.acnr.co.uk/ND07/ACNRND07_paraneo.pdf

29. Hindle JV, Ibrahim A, Ramaraj R. Ataxia caused by amiodarone in older people. *Age Ageing* 2008;37:347–8.

30. Young WF. Cervical spondylotic myelopathy: a common cause of spinal cord dysfunction in older persons. *Am Fam Physcn* 2000;62:1064–70.

31. Hughes RAC. Peripheral neuropathy. *Br Med J* 2002;324:466–9.

32. Hall GC, Carroll D, McQuay HJ. Primary care incidence and treatment of four neuropathic pain conditions: a descriptive study 2002–2005. *BMC Fam Pract* 2008;9:26.

33. Wong M, Chung JWY, Wong TKS. Effects of treatments for symptoms of painful diabetic neuropathy: systematic review. *Br Med J* 2007;335:87.

34. Miller JD, Pruitt S, McDonald TJ. Acute brachial plexus neuritis: an uncommon cause of shoulder pain. *Am Fam Physcn* 2000;62:2067–72.

35. Opstelten W, Eekhof J, Neven AK, Verheij T. Treatment of herpes zoster. *Can Fam Physcn* 2008;54:373–7.

36. Bennetto L, Patel NK, Fuller G. Trigeminal neuralgia and its management. *Br Med J* 2007;334;201–5.

37. Chong MS, Hester J. Medical treatment of trigeminal neuralgia. *Adv Clin Neurosci Rehab* 2007;7:19–21. Available at: http://www.acnr.co.uk/SO07/ACNR_SO07_medical.pdf

38. Update on managing Bell's palsy. *Drug Ther Bull* 2008;46:53–4.

39. National Institute for Health and Clinical Excellence. *Management of Multiple Sclerosis in Primary and Secondary Care. Clinical Guideline 008.* London: NICE; 2003. Available at: http://www.nice.org.uk/nicemedia/pdf/cg008guidance.pdf

40. National Institute for Health and Clinical Excellence. *Guidance of the Use of Riluzole (Rilutek) for the Treatment of Motor Neurone Disease.* London: NICE; 2001. Available at: http://www.nice.org.uk/nicemedia/pdf/RILUZOLE_full_guidance.pdf

41. Driver and Vehicle Licensing Centre. *At a Glance Guide to the Current Medical Standards of Fitness to Drive. Drivers Medical Group.* Swansea: DVLA; 2008. Available at: http://www.dvla.gov.uk/media/pdf/medical/aagv1.pdf

Chapter 8

Respiratory problems

Stephen Allen and Patrick White

Introduction

Respiratory conditions account for ≥15% of primary care consultations in people aged ≥65 years. A third of these consultations (which also include all upper respiratory infections) are due to obstructive lung disease, split in a ratio of 3:2 between chronic obstructive pulmonary disease (COPD) and asthma. Asthma is a rare cause of death in this age group, in contrast with COPD deaths. Obstructive lung disease is therefore the main subject of this chapter, but we also highlight pneumonia, lung malignancy, and tuberculosis, which present life-threatening challenges and can be very demanding of primary care teams.

We will use a number of case examples to illustrate these problems and to give the primary care clinician some pointers as to how elderly people with respiratory illnesses can be assessed and managed to try to improve function, symptoms and outcomes. We also focus on the need for high quality organization of services. Organized care is the key to successful management of asthma and COPD in a primary care setting where the majority of people with these conditions are managed. Effective organization demands up-to-date disease registers, the capacity to conduct lung function testing, and arrangements to review patients at regular intervals. It gives the opportunity to prioritize care of patients at particular risk. Good organization of the care of asthma and COPD has the potential to revolutionize the outcome of these diseases.

The diagnosis and management of respiratory problems in older patients, particularly the very aged, is characterized by a number of complicating factors that are rarely seen in younger adults and children. These include:

1) Elderly people are less able to sense a rise in airflow resistance, so they are less likely to report spontaneously, or take early action to alleviate, a deterioration in their asthma or COPD.

2) The mode of presentation of respiratory disease is often atypical, and can be dominated by the functional failure that occurs as a result of hypoxia, dehydration or hyponatraemia. An elderly patient with an exacerbation of asthma can therefore present with acute confusion, falls, immobility, incontinence or a combination of two or more of these, and might not always mention breathlessness, cough or wheezing.

3) The physical signs of disease in the respiratory tract are less clear as a result of the ageing changes that occur in the lung parenchyma, airways, chest wall and dorsal spine. For example, it is not uncommon to find medium-pitched crackles at the lung bases in elderly subjects at rest, which sometimes, but not invariably, clear with coughing or deep breathing. A kyphoscoliotic chest often has asymmetrical breath sounds. Some patients with pneumonia remain afebrile or have low-grade fevers that are easily missed or of uncertain significance.

4) Elderly patients with cognitive impairment, for example with a Mini-Mental State Examination (MMSE) score of <24 or an Abbreviated Mental Test Score (AMTS) <7, are rarely able to perform full spirometry or other lung function tests that require cooperation and coordination. It is more difficult to obtain objective evidence of airways disease in this group.

5) The normal ranges commonly presented by modern hand-held spirometers are not based on populations which adequately represent normal people aged >65 years. The relevant predicted equations are available, but unless they are specifically used care should be taken to avoid overdiagnosis of airflow obstruction in old age.

6) Treatment is often made difficult by diagnostic uncertainty, co-morbidities, memory disorders and inability to self-administer drug regimens. Pressurized metered dose inhalers (pMDIs) are difficult to use at any age, and should only be prescribed routinely in the elderly with a spacer or in the form of a breath-actuated inhaler. Powder devices are generally simpler and more reliable to demonstrate and use.

7) Most people with cognitive impairment (MMSE <24 or AMTS <7) are unable to learn consistently to use any inhaler device. These patients will depend on drug administration by a carer.

8) Multiple comorbidities are common and symptoms may be the result of two or more pathologies. A patient with COPD who becomes hypoxic may suffer a worsening of heart failure at the same time, which together may lead to hypotension or falls.

Theme 1: airways disease

Case 1

A woman aged 84 years was found wandering in her back garden by her daughter. She was disoriented, anxious, and had passed urine into her clothes, but did not spontaneously complain of any respiratory symptoms. The daughter was able to explain to the visiting general practitioner (GP) that the patient was normally fully *compos mentis*, self-caring and continent, and took no medication. She had never smoked and had had no serious illnesses other than a tendency to be wheezy in hot weather in her youth. The daughter had noticed that her mother seemed to be unusually short of breath when she was escorted back into her house. On examination the GP confirmed the disorientation in place and time, noted wheezy breathing, and found a respiratory rate of 24 per minute, pulse rate of 112 and expiratory rhonchi with a prolonged expiratory phase and slight asymmetry of air entry at the lung bases. The finger oxygen saturation was 91% on air. The patient was unable to perform a peak expiratory flow.

The history and physical signs suggested asthma. The GP had to decide whether to send the patient to the general hospital, a community hospital, or treat her at home.

Factors in favour of admitting the patient to the general hospital included:

1) She was acutely confused, probably because of the hypoxia.

2) The illness was a substantial worsening of her lifelong tendency to mild asthma.

3) The patient lived alone.

4) The asymmetrical air entry might have been due to a pneumothorax, lobar collapse, basal pneumonia or a pleural effusion, so a chest radiograph was needed.

5) She had a number of features of potentially life-threatening asthma (confusion, hypoxia, tachycardia, raised respiratory rate).

6) She was observed to be short of breath on minimal exertion and at rest.

An elderly patient with an attack of asthma might be suitable for management at home, in a care home or community hospital if:

The attack is part of a familiar pattern that usually responds quickly to first-line treatments.

1) There is competent supervision by family or care staff and the GP is able to provide or arrange the necessary medical review.

2) There are no symptoms or physical signs of severe asthma.

3) There are no signs of possible pneumothorax or other important differential diagnoses, such as left heart failure, lower respiratory tract infection, inhaled foreign body or upper airway obstruction.

4) Bronchodilator drugs in adequate doses can be given by spacer, and the patient is able to take oral medications and drink sufficient fluids.

5) The patient prefers to stay at home and has the mental capacity to make that choice.

6) The patient is terminally ill with another pathology and a decision has been made to give palliative treatments only.

Case 2

A man aged 78 years with a 60 pack-year smoking history presented to his GP's surgery with progressively declining exercise tolerance due to exertional breathlessness, persistent productive cough and ankle swelling. At his last visit spirometry had revealed a greatly reduced FEV_1 (35% of predicted forced expiratory volume in 1 s) and an FEV_1:FVC (forced vital capacity) ratio of 43%, indicating moderately severe airflow obstruction. The working diagnosis was COPD. He continued to smoke. He took an ipratropium metered-dose inhaler intermittently. The patient complained of orthopnoea and had recently started to sleep in a chair. On examination he was *compos mentis* (MMSE 28/30) and not breathless at rest. His pulse rate was 88, blood pressure (BP) 125/85 mmHg, jugular venous pressure not raised and cardiac apex normal and not displaced. His chest had signs of hyperinflation (loss of hepatic and cardiac dullness, use of accessory muscles of respiration and poor expansion), a few sparse medium-pitched rhonchi at end-expiration but was otherwise normal on auscultation. There was mild pitting leg oedema below both knees. The finger oxygen saturation at rest was 94%.

The GP had to decide the reason for the patient's worsening breathlessness. The main differential diagnoses in this case were:

1) Progression of the COPD.

2) Left heart failure.

3) Pulmonary embolism.

4) New lung pathology such as pulmonary fibrosis or carcinoma of the bronchus.

5) Another factor contributing to breathlessness, such as anaemia.

A chest radiograph was arranged that showed hyperinflated lung fields, a normal cardiothoracic ratio (CTR) and no other abnormalities. His haemoglobin was 14 g/dl and renal function normal. Therefore, anaemia was ruled out, new lung pathology was unlikely (though still a possibility) and the normal CTR reduced the likelihood of heart failure. The ankle oedema was probably gravitational from sleeping in a chair. While pulmonary emboli remained a possibility the GP decided to work with the probability that the symptoms were due to the COPD and decided to try to optimize treatment in accordance with the National Institute for Health and Clinical Excellence (NICE) COPD guidelines[1] as follows:

1) Try again to persuade the patient to stop smoking.

2) Obtain new baseline spirometry to monitor the response to treatment (this was realistic in this elderly man because he had no evidence of dementia and had performed spirometry previously).

3) Prescribe regular combination inhaled long-acting beta-agonist and inhaled steroids, and long-acting antimuscarinic bronchodilators (tiotropium). There is a choice of devices with both of these options.

4) Arrange for him to attend the local pulmonary rehabilitation group.

5) Influenza and pneumococcal immunization.

6) Review with repeat spirometry and a report on his exercise tolerance (e.g. Medical Research Council (MRC) dyspnoea scale).

If he responds adequately to this approach, no further investigation is indicated. If he worsens he should be referred for further investigation, including echocardiography, and possibly high resolution computed tomography (CT) scanning to rule out fibrosis and recurrent pulmonary emboli.

Airway disease or obstructive lung disease always has a chronic component even if it only presents as asthma following an acute upper respiratory infection. The key to effective prevention of acute severe episodes is in the identification of patients at higher risk, the ability to review inhaler use and the recovery of lung function, and the provision of a long-term personal plan for secondary prevention and intervention in the event of an exacerbation.

The key elements of chronic disease management in obstructive lung disease are the disease register and the system for active recall and review. In asthma care, treatment should be determined according to the steps of the BTS/SIGN guidelines.[2] In COPD the dominant themes should be smoking cessation, pulmonary rehabilitation, and the optimization of drug treatment.

Lung function testing in frail older people

The secure diagnosis of obstructive or restrictive lung diseases demands spirometry to support the history and physical signs. Because older people are more likely to be forgetful of symptoms it can be argued that spirometry is diagnostically even more important in that age group. While cognitive impairment reduces the likelihood of performing reliable full spirometry, most elderly patients can manage it, but there are some useful alternatives that can be tried. In a primary care setting there are two additional challenges in providing spirometry—ensuring the test is done reliably and to an acceptable standard and making an accurate interpretation. Primary care spirometry can be as good as the best in a specialist setting, but it is sometimes unacceptably poor. A reasonable approach in primary care is as follows:

1) For people aged >65 years, minor degrees of apparent obstruction and slightly less than predicted FEV_1 and FVC values can lead to false-positive conclusions. They must always be interpreted carefully within the overall clinical context. Where possible, predictive values should be based on equations derived from normal populations of appropriate age and ethnicity.

2) Peak expiratory flow (PEF) can be performed independently by many people with normal cognitive function. Those with mildly impaired cognition (MMSE 20–24) can often do PEF if attended and encouraged by a skilled helper. However, as with spirometry, obtaining a meaningful PEF depends on the patient instantly generating sufficient expiratory pressure to reach the true value.

3) Some patients with mild cognitive impairment can reliably perform the earlier parts of forced spirometry, particularly FEV_1. This can still be useful even if the FVC cannot be obtained.

An FEV_1 in the predicted normal range indicates that there is unlikely to be a clinically substantial lung volume defect.

4) If there is still doubt and more sophisticated assessment (such as by CT scanning) might be needed, the patient can be referred to a specialist department.

Long-term treatment of asthma and COPD in old age

The BTS/SIGN guidelines for the diagnosis and treatment of asthma and the NICE guidelines for the treatment of COPD should be used. These are likely to be replaced in due course by international guidelines – the GINA guidelines for asthma[3] and the GOLD guidelines for COPD.[4] They are based on current evidence and are largely applicable in old age despite the poor recruitment of frail elderly patients into trials. A detailed rehearsal of the guidelines is beyond the scope of this chapter. There are some important pointers for the primary care doctor that can improve the maintenance management of asthma and COPD in old age. These are:

1) Use the published guidelines as the ideal starting point for diagnostic and treatment decisions.

2) Be careful not to miss the new onset of asthma in old age; wheezy old people do not all have COPD; use the diagnostic criteria and look for reversibility of airflow obstruction and steroid responsiveness.

3) It is never too late to benefit from stopping smoking.

4) Choice of inhaler is of even greater importance in elderly patients who should demonstrate their competence and confidence in their inhaler use at every attendance.

5) For patients unable to manage an inhaler even with assistance, the provision of an air pump and nebulizer set can be very effective, though help will be needed with timing and dosage.

6) Because some elderly patients cannot sense early deterioration in their airflow resistance, step 2 of the asthma guideline (regular inhaled steroid and fast-acting bronchodilator when needed) may not be suitable in old age. Evidence is accumulating to suggest that step 2 for all elderly patients should be regular combination inhaled steroid and inhaled bronchodilators.

7) One of the chief risks for elderly patients with obstructive airways disease is that they become increasingly housebound and effectively disappear from regular surveillance until they suffer from an acute exacerbation. Primary care teams hold the key to the effective management of these patients because they have disease registers. However, it may become necessary to establish community-based specialist teams that are integrated between primary and secondary care in order to maximize the management and support of these vulnerable patients.

Indicators for admission to hospital during an exacerbation of COPD in an elderly patient suitable for escalated treatment include:

◆ worsening symptoms despite treatment

◆ severe or worsening oxygen desaturation (≤92%)

◆ potential need for closely monitored oxygen supplementation

◆ signs of ventilatory failure, particularly carbon dioxide retention

◆ history of previous need for ventilatory support

◆ functional failure, such as confusion, particularly in people without close and competent home support

◆ unusual or asymmetrical auscultatory signs

◆ signs of heart failure or circulatory collapse

◆ features of systemic sepsis such as high fever, hypotension

- other acute comorbidities that might need treatment in hospital
- complex palliative needs that cannot be arranged at short notice in the community.

Theme 2: pneumonia

Case 1

A man aged 88 years, who lived with his daughter and her family and was normally functionally independent, became short of breath, disoriented in time and place and complained of a sharp pain in the left side of his chest when breathing deeply or coughing. His GP assessed him at home and found him to have a tympanic membrane temperature of 38.5°C, respiratory rate of 22 per minute, heart rate of 104, BP of 115/65 mmHg (lower than his usual BP) and finger oxygen saturation of 90% on air. There were signs of consolidation at the left lung base. The patient was known to have renal impairment with a stable serum creatinine of ~190 μmol/l. The working diagnosis was left lower lobe pneumonia with pleurisy.

This patient had several markers of severity and features associated with a high risk of mortality from pneumonia. These were:

1) Advanced age.
2) Acute confusion.
3) Renal impairment.
4) Hypotension.
5) Hypoxia.

Urgent admission for inpatient treatment as a severe community-acquired pneumonia was the preferred approach in this case. On the other hand, a well-supported elderly patient with clear clinical signs of pneumonia but with few or none of these features could be safely given treatment in the community, provided that the following precautions are taken:

1) An appropriate antibiotic (using a current local protocol) should be given without delay.
2) Adequate fluid intake.
3) Resident competent attendant.
4) Medical review within 24 h or sooner if the patient worsens.
5) Refer to hospital if the patient's condition has not improved at review, or deteriorates at any stage of the treatment.

The presentation of pneumonia in frail elderly patients is often obscured by comorbidities, lack of typical features and functional failure. Occasionally, patients with radiologically positive pneumonia have little or no febrile response, low amplitude or no leukocytosis, atypical physical signs and absence of breathlessness and cough. Some present with acute 'geriatric' problems, such as falls or confusion and minimal signs, such as sparse crackles at a lung base. A chest radiograph is very helpful under these circumstances, though it is reasonable to make a diagnosis on clinical grounds, particularly if the latest episode is part of a pattern in that individual. There has been growing interest in prognostic prediction tools in pneumonia. In the UK, the CURB65 score, which is derived from the British Thoracic Society pneumonia guidelines, is gaining wide acceptance for both hospital and community use. This allocates one point for each of the following:

- confusion (AMTS <8/10)
- urea >7.0 mmol/l

◆ respiratory rate >30/min

◆ systolic BP <90 mmHg or diastolic BP <60 mmHg

◆ age >64 years.

A patient with a score of 2 usually needs inpatient treatment, and a score of ≥3 indicates severe pneumonia with a high 30 day mortality.

Alternatively, the clinician can use a severity prediction tool developed by Bont *et al.* in The Netherlands for elderly patients (aged >65 years) with respiratory tract infection in the community setting.[5] This rule allocates one point for each of: age >79 years, previous hospitalization, heart failure, diabetes, use of oral corticosteroids, previous use of antibiotics for the episode, a diagnosis of pneumonia, and exacerbation of COPD.

The risk of 30 day hospitalization or death rises with the score. Patients with scores of ≤2 have a risk of ~3% and can generally be managed out of hospital. Those with a score of ≥7 have a >30% risk and will almost always need to be admitted to hospital. Those in the 3–6 range have a risk of ~10% and their need for hospital admission will vary with the circumstances of the individual patient.

Lower respiratory tract bacterial infections, including lobar and patchy (broncho-)pneumonias are common in older people. Reasons for this include:

1) Accumulation of chronic respiratory tract damage, such as is seen in patients with chronic bronchitis and emphysema.

2) Other comorbid conditions that predispose to lower respiratory infection, such as chronic heart failure, bronchogenic carcinoma and bronchiectasis.

3) Aspiration of oropharyngeal secretions into the airways due to age-related changes in the integrity of swallowing, cerebrovascular disease, extrapyramidal conditions and other disease processes that interfere with safe swallowing.

4) There is some evidence that waning cell-mediated and humoral immunity might play a part.

In primary care the risk of contracting pneumonia can be reduced by immunizing against influenza and pneumococcal infection. Steps taken to reduce aspiration into the airways have been shown to be effective. These include upright positioning before eating or drinking and thickening fluids for patients with impaired swallowing. Other measures do not have a strong evidence base, but stopping smoking is probably helpful (and of course has other major benefits), as is good control of chronic heart failure and COPD.

Theme 3: lung malignancy

For the purpose of this chapter we will concentrate on bronchogenic carcinoma as the model for lung cancer in old age because that is the commonest primary malignant lung tumour encountered. There are, however, some observations that can be made that lay a platform for further discussion. Evidence from epidemiological and case ascertainment research shows that:

1) The diagnosis of lung cancer in old age (≥75 years) is more likely to be delayed when compared with younger patients. While some of the reasons for this are related to lack of clarity of the presenting symptoms and signs, as described above, there is evidence that under-use of plain chest radiography from primary care is a factor. Chest radiography is inexpensive, safe and widely available. It is easy for the patient to take part and it has a high diagnostic yield in unwell elderly people (not only for malignancy, of course). Further, because the prognosis for carcinoma of the bronchus is so poor, there might be a spillover of nihilism onto all aspects of pulmonary neoplastic disease.

2) Most elderly people with good cognitive function can cooperate with bronchoscopy and tolerate the procedure well.

3) Some elderly people with bronchogenic carcinoma have well-preserved functional and physiological indices and are suitable for surgical treatment.

4) Not all lung tumours have a uniformly poor prognosis. For example, intrathoracic lymphoma often responds well to treatment. Therefore, whenever possible, an accurate diagnosis should be used as the basis for clinical decisions.

Case 1

A man aged 83 years consulted his GP because he had taken several weeks to recover from an apparent chest infection. His cough had not settled and he started to have daily episodes of haemoptysis. He was a current light smoker but had a 55 pack-year total exposure. His exercise tolerance was less than half a mile on level ground and spirometry a few months earlier had shown an FEV_1 45% of predicted, FVC 65% of predicted and an FEV_1:FVC ratio of 52% indicating moderately severe airflow obstruction. His MMSE was 29/30 and he expressed a wish to know why his health was deteriorating. He was sent for a chest radiograph that showed a mass at the right lung hilum that was suggestive of a primary tumour. He was referred to hospital for assessment and had a bronchoscopy that confirmed the presence of a neoplasm in the right main bronchus, and biopsy confirmed a squamous carcinoma. The tumour was inoperable.

This patient's GP was right to take steps to secure the diagnosis despite the fact that the patient had reduced pulmonary reserve. The benefits for the patient were:

1) He could be given a correct diagnosis and a well-informed prognosis.

2) He could be confident that a treatable condition had not been missed.

3) The patient and his family could work with the GP and palliative care services to plan his ongoing care, anticipate problems and receive information about help available in the later stages of the disease for symptoms such as pain, nausea, breathlessness, weakness and dysphagia.

For some very frail patients, for example those with advanced dementia or severe stroke living in a nursing home, it is often not appropriate to pursue a definitive diagnosis if a lung malignancy is suspected. Under these circumstances it is reasonable to make a working clinical diagnosis and take account of any symptoms arising from a tumour when deciding the overall management plan.

In older patients, the modes of presentation that might prompt a search for lung malignancy include:

1) Any deterioration in general health in a smoker, ex-smoker or patient with known exposure to asbestos. This includes rapid decline in functional status, such as falls or immobility, and uncharacteristic low mood.

2) Persistent cough that is out of the patient's usual pattern.

3) Haemoptysis, particularly if it occurs or continues outside the context of a chest infection.

4) Breathlessness, weakness, reduced appetite, weight loss and chest pain, particularly when there is no other explanation.

5) Any physical sign that might be caused by lung malignancy, for example, asymmetrical breath sounds, signs of lung consolidation, collapse or pleural effusion, stridor, dysphonia, bovine cough, finger clubbing, cervical lymphadenopathy or the effects of metastases. This list is not

exhaustive and occasionally the presentation will be with one of the rare paraneoplastic skin or neurological conditions.

6) Recurrent chest infections or slow, incomplete resolution of pneumonia.

In patients with an established diagnosis of lung cancer, radiotherapy may have an important role in relieving symptoms and improving prognosis. Indications for specialist assessment for palliative radiotherapy include haemoptysis, increasing breathlessness, and bone pain.

Theme 4: diagnoses not to be missed

Tuberculosis

Tuberculosis (TB) is not rare in the UK, and there is a rise in incidence in old age in the indigenous population and in migrants from areas of high prevalence, such as South Asia, sub-Saharan Africa and some parts of Eastern Europe. Some of these cases are new infections and some are the result of reactivation of dormant TB as cell-mediated immunity wanes in old age. TB is usually treatable, and the outcomes in elderly patients are good if the diagnosis is made early enough. If pulmonary TB is suspected (cough, haemoptysis, weight loss, fever, poor appetite, weakness (the presentation is very similar to lung cancer)) the next step is to arrange a chest radiograph without delay and with a low threshold. If TB is suspected the patient must always be referred to a specialist department. If the first radiograph is normal or equivocal it should be repeated after a short interval.

Pulmonary embolus

Pulmonary embolus is the hidden and frequently forgotten alternative diagnosis in patients who present with acute breathlessness, and it more likely to be missed if it is not accompanied by pleuritic chest pain. It is a diagnosis which is easy to ignore in the absence of a history of trauma, surgery, air travel, pregnancy, and leg swelling. If pulmonary embolus is suspected, urgent hospital assessment is always required (unless the patient is terminally ill with an established pathology) so that the diagnosis can be confirmed by ventilation-perfusion isotope scanning or CT pulmonary angiography. Treatment should be started if indicated and a search for predisposing pathology undertaken.

References

1. National Institute of Health and Clinical Excellence. Chronic obstructive pulmonary disease treatment guideline. http://www.nice.org.uk/nicemedia/pdf/CG012_niceguideline.pdf
2. British Thoracic Society/Scottish Intercollegiate Guidelines Network. Asthma guideline. http://www.sign.ac.uk/guidelines/fulltext/63/index.html
3. GINA Asthma guideline. http://www.ginasthma.org
4. GOLD COPD guideline. http://www.goldcopd.com/
5. Bont J, Hak E, Hoes AW, Schipper M, Schellevis FG, Verheij TJ. A prediction rule for elderly primary-care patients with lower respiratory tract infections. *Eur Respir J* 2007;29:969–75.

Further reading

ATS/ERS spirometry standards. http://www.thoracic.org/sections/publications/statements/pages/pfet/pft2.html

National Institute of Health and Clinical Excellence. Lung cancer guideline. http://www.nice.org.uk/CG024

Chapter 9

Gastroenterology

Willie Hamilton and Keith Bodger

Introduction

Despite the complex anatomy of the gastrointestinal (GI) tract, disorders of it produce a relatively small number of symptoms. These fall into three main groups: symptoms referable to the upper GI tract; abdominal pain; and symptoms of disordered bowel habit. To this list should be added the 'alarm', or 'red flag', symptoms of loss of weight and overt or occult GI bleeding (haematemesis, melaena, rectal bleeding, iron deficiency anaemia) which may occur alone or alongside common GI symptoms. Loss of weight frequently arises from non-GI disease. Anaemia is again not specific to the GI tract, but iron deficiency anaemia is such a cardinal feature of occult GI malignancy (particularly colorectal cancer), it is worthy of discussion here.

All of these symptoms are relatively commonly presented by elderly people to general practitioners (GPs). That makes them tricky for the clinician, as benign explanations for the symptom are the norm, yet the doctor must remain alert to the possibility of serious disease. General practice always has an element of risk management or 'tolerance of uncertainty'—no more so than with GI complaints. However, new symptoms or those accompanied by alarm features require special care.

Consultations referable to the GI tract become more common with age. Around one person in ten aged 60–64 years will consult their GP each year with a GI problem; this rises to one in seven aged 70–74 years and one in five aged 80–84 years.[1] There is little difference between genders in consultation rates for GI disease. Within these consultations the commonest complaint is dyspepsia (with nearly 2% of the elderly population consulting each year for this). Constipation, non-specific abdominal pain and heartburn are also common complaints, with constipation in particular increasing dramatically in incidence with age.

As patients present with symptoms, as opposed to presenting with diseases, we have structured this chapter by considering symptoms first (providing diagnostic guidance and a view on when to consider further investigation) and have then focused on selected specific diagnoses. In the real world of primary care, this clear distinction between symptoms and diseases becomes blurred—many symptoms are treated perfectly adequately without a precise diagnosis. It may be that empirical symptom-based management can allow formal investigation to be deferred until the patient re-attends, either with a recurrence of the disorder, or with a failure of treatment. The knack of general practice is in knowing when investigation can be deferred, and how much to share the (small) possibility of serious disease with the patient.

Symptoms of gastrointestinal disease

Upper gastrointestinal symptoms

'Dyspepsia' and 'reflux'

The terminology used for upper gut symptoms is controversial and this can make interpretation of guidelines and individual clinical trials problematic. In its broadest definition, dyspepsia is a term encompassing 'symptoms referral to the proximal portion of the GI tract'[2] and includes epigastric pain and discomfort, heartburn, regurgitation, and assorted other foregut symptoms such as nausea, eructation, early satiety and bloating.[2] This contrasts with the rigid definition of dyspepsia applied in therapeutic clinical trials which focuses on epigastric pain *per se* and specifically excludes the typical symptoms of gastro-oesophageal reflux disease (GORD). However, the broader definition is generally used—particularly in the setting of primary care.[2,3] The label of 'gastritis' is often used synonymously with dyspepsia, but it is a vague term—the presence or absence of 'gastritis' endoscopically or histologically has limited correlation with symptoms. The term 'functional' or 'non-ulcer' dyspepsia is preferable when describing a dyspeptic patient with normal or minor findings at gastroscopy.

Taking the broad definition of dyspepsia, the key organic causes are peptic ulceration, GORD (including both 'endoscopy-negative' reflux and oesophagitis) and malignancy, although gallstones also fall within the differential diagnosis of epigastric pain. The majority of patients with dyspepsia lack a serious organic underlying diagnosis ('functional' or 'non-ulcer' dyspepsia) but symptom-based diagnosis of the underlying cause of upper abdominal discomfort is unreliable and the prevalence of organic lesions rises with age.[4] Whereas the emphasis in younger dyspeptics is on empirical treatment, the approach in older people is to consider early investigation in cases of new-onset dyspepsia. In the UK, investigation of patients aged >55 years presenting with recent onset and persistent dyspepsia is advocated,[2] with alarm features triggering rapid referral at any age. This is discussed further in the section on oesophageal and gastric cancer.

The potential role of *Helicobacter pylori* infection in dyspeptic conditions is an important consideration in the elderly population. The prevalence of infection rises with age in Western populations and may be as high as 80% in the very elderly group.[5] *H. pylori* infection is recognized as the leading cause of peptic ulceration worldwide. In the elderly population there is also a significant contribution from non-steroidal anti-inflammatory drugs (NSAIDs) and a higher incidence of *H. pylori*-negative ulcers.[6] The availability of non-invasive tests for *H. pylori* (serology, urea breath tests or faecal antigen testing) has enabled a 'test-and-treat' approach to be adopted in younger dyspeptic patients but this approach is not applicable in the older undiagnosed dyspeptic patient in whom there is a higher chance of sinister pathology. The approach to identification and treatment of *H. pylori* infection in those who have an established endoscopic diagnosis is discussed in the later section on specific diseases associated with the infection.

The prevalence of reflux disease, or GORD, rises with advancing age.[7] The classical clinical presentation is with heartburn and/or regurgitation and the response to empirical acid suppression is generally good. However, GORD may present in atypical ways in older individuals and symptoms of chest pain, regurgitation, vomiting and dysphagia are more common than simple heartburn.[7] Complications of reflux, including peptic strictures, bleeding and respiratory complications (e.g. aspiration) are also more common modes of presentation in older subjects. Elderly subjects are more likely to receive bisphosphonates for osteoporosis and/or NSAIDs for osteoarthritis, and these agents are increasingly recognized as risk factors for oesophagitis.

Dysphagia

Dysphagia is a common complaint in older people. Surveys have revealed that up to 10% of people aged >50 years have experienced troublesome dysphagia.[8] It has prognostic importance in a nursing home setting—6-month mortality in residents with dysphagia is significantly higher than in those without.[9] In this age group, the role of oropharyngeal defects ('swallowing disorders') is an important consideration in addition to the common oesophageal pathologies. Difficulty or delay in the initiation of swallowing may be distinguishable from oesophageal dysphagia by a careful history and observation of the patient swallowing. There may be local (e.g. dysarthria) or general neurological features (e.g. signs of Parkinson's disease or cerebrovascular disease—see Chapter 7). Elderly subjects with cognitive–perceptive and/or neurological disease are at particular risk of oropharyngeal dysphagia.[8]

Oesophageal causes of dysphagia include GORD, particularly in the presence of more severe grades of oesophagitis or a complicating peptic structure. However, it is also a cardinal symptom of oesophageal malignancy and an 'alarm feature' meriting early investigation. Indeed, dysphagia had the strongest predictive value for upper GI cancer of any of the so-called alarm features in a large study of people aged >55 years referred for fast-track investigation.[10] Gastroscopy is the key investigation for excluding organic obstructive lesions but oropharyngeal functional disorders may require video-fluoroscopy, specialist speech and language therapy, and neurological assessments. Primary motility disorders of the oesophagus, such as achalasia, are uncommon and require referral for formal physiological studies to confirm the diagnosis.

Abdominal pain

Abdominal pain is one of the commonest symptoms in primary care, reported by 2–5% of patients each year.[11] It is the commonest symptom in adults requesting out-of-hours care, or attending casualty departments;[12] admissions for patients with abdominal pain total around half a million days in hospital each year.[11] In some patients, there is a clear diagnosis—often non-GI—such as a urine infection.

However, the differential diagnosis is wide, ranging from the minor through the more serious (e.g. biliary colic) to the life-threatening (e.g. cancer). Initial treatment is often given on a provisional diagnosis, based on the localization of pain and presence of any associated upper or lower GI symptoms. A definite diagnosis is rarely established at the first consultation, and patients return (often repeatedly) until a diagnosis is mode. At least a quarter of those with chronic abdominal pain remain undiagnosed.[13] Furthermore, diagnostic errors are relatively common, in that 10% of colorectal cancers are erroneously diagnosed with irritable bowel syndrome (IBS) in the year before their cancer is identified;[14] 40% of patients with coeliac disease have pain for >5 years before diagnosis.[15] GPs need to be alert for alarm features that should trigger prompt investigation.

The frequency of the underlying diagnoses is largely unknown. One study of new presentations of abdominal pain in a large UK electronic database identified formal diagnoses in only 10% of patients. Dyspepsia, IBS and gallbladder disease were the commonest diagnoses.[11] However, this study examined only patients where GPs had recorded the code for unspecified abdominal pain, so excluded all those in whom an initial diagnosis had already been made. It was also unable to identify characteristics of the pain, or concurrent symptoms, that may have been diagnostically valuable.

Predictive values for underlying diseases have been estimated in only one study—of colorectal cancer.[16] That study estimated a positive predictive value of 2% for patients presenting to primary care with abdominal pain for colorectal cancer in patients aged >70 years.[17] Furthermore, older patients with colorectal cancer are more likely to present with non-specific symptoms such as abdominal pain than younger patients.[18]

Primary care investigation of abdominal pain may not be necessary, as the history and physical examination may reveal the diagnosis. If not apparent at the first consultation, the picture may become clearer on review. Thus most patients will not be investigated, and will receive reassurance, advice, or treatment on a clinical diagnosis. If a working diagnosis cannot be made, initial investigation will be simple, with a full blood count and urinalysis being most GPs' choices. Only with continuing pain and non-contributory initial results would further investigation (ultrasound, upper GI endoscopy, or colonoscopy) be required. This simple sequence of investigations would be changed if additional features suggested a particular diagnosis, such as rectal bleeding, or weight loss.

Change in bowel habit: 'diarrhoea' and 'constipation'

Complaints relating to defecation increase in frequency considerably with age and patients may apply the terms 'constipation' or 'diarrhoea' to a wide range of specific symptoms. Constipation may imply reduced stool frequency, altered stool form (harder, larger or lumpy stools), straining, difficulties initiating a bowel movement, a sense of incomplete evacuation, a need to spend a prolonged time on the toilet; or the term may be used by patients to indicate symptoms of pain or bloating. Similarly, diarrhoea may imply increased stool frequency, passage of softer or liquid stools, passage of mucus, urgency or incontinence (see Chapter 19).

Over a quarter of the UK population aged >65 years describe that they have to strain to pass a stool, with 14% describing themselves as constipated.[19] Some 23% describe urgency of defecation, and 10% have loose stools frequently. However, only 9% of the population describe a recent change in bowel habit,[19] and only 1.5% describe a change which they regard as significant enough to report to primary care.[20]

The differential diagnosis for both constipation and diarrhoea is wide, but the relative frequencies of individual causes in older subjects are largely unknown. Drugs and diet feature high on the list for both diarrhoea and constipation, but infections are probably the commonest cause of acute diarrhoea. They may also be a feature of other morbidities, such as constipation with Parkinson's disease, and diarrhoea with hyperthyroidism or inflammatory bowel disease. Both symptoms may occur with IBS, although this is a rare diagnosis to occur for the first time in older people.

A good dietary history is needed and the patient's list of drugs will need to be reviewed (one problem is that almost any drug can cause constipation or diarrhoea, and the *British National Formulary* is of limited help in this regard). Although the focus of diagnostic effort is generally exclusion of colorectal cancer, it must be remembered that only a very small percentage of elderly sufferers with either symptom will have an underlying cancer. Perhaps because the risk of cancer is relatively low, it is these symptoms (and anaemia), which are most associated with delay in diagnosis, and have a worse prognosis.[21,22] Diarrhoea, either increased loosening or increased frequency of the stools, is more predictive of cancer than constipation.[23] The risk of a cancer with these symptoms has been estimated for patients aged >70 years:[17,24] for patients presenting to general practice, the risk with diarrhoea is 1.7%, and for constipation 1.3%. Nevertheless, the association of altered bowel habit with any alarm symptom merits prompt investigation and persisting symptoms of recent onset are best investigated.

Faecal incontinence refers to the involuntary loss of formed stool. This can be a devastating symptom for patients and their carers. The prevalence in elderly people is high with multiple possible causes, including advancing age, previous obstetric trauma, diabetes, faecal impaction, stroke, and dementia. Faecal impaction can be identified by rectal examination, supplemented if necessary by simple plain radiography, and it is an eminently treatable cause of loss of continence (see Chapter 19).[25]

'Alarm' symptoms

Weight loss

Loss of weight is a feature of almost any serious illness, but is also a common feature of healthy ageing. However, weight loss serious enough to be reported by the elderly patient has to be investigated, and the chance of a malignancy approaches 10%, with a clear relationship between the amount of weight lost and the chance of cancer.[25] As always in general practice, a good history, including diet, will help to refine the differential diagnosis. Indeed, isolated weight loss is very rare, and thorough investigation of such patients is often unrewarding where other symptomatic clues are completely lacking.[26]

Anaemia

In the general population, anaemia becomes more common with increasing age. A large prevalence study was reported from the USA in 2004, with anaemia defined as a haemoglobin <13.0 g/dl in men and <12.0 g/dl in women.[27] In the age group 65–74 years, 7.8% of men and 8.3% of women were anaemic; the percentage with anaemia increased progressively with each age band up to ≥85 years, when 26% of men and 20% of women were anaemic. Around 20% of elderly patients with anaemia have iron deficiency, and 10% either folate or vitamin B_{12} deficiency. A further 30% have anaemia of chronic illness, most usually renal impairment (see Chapter 11).[27]

As measurement of haemoglobin is so common in primary care, patients are often found to be anaemic, without a particular underlying cause having been considered. Whatever the reason for the blood test, it is mandatory to investigate anaemic patients, at least with a ferritin, B_{12} and folate. A faecal occult blood test will be helpful if positive, but cannot be relied upon if negative—in that 60% of patients with cancer in the pilot study of the UK national colorectal cancer screening programme had negative occult bloods.[28] Current guidance for urgent investigation of anaemia misses some patients with a moderate risk of cancer, particularly men. For men aged >60 years with a haemoglobin <11g/dl and features of iron deficiency, the risk of cancer is 13% and for women with a haemoglobin <10 g/dl and iron deficiency it is 7.7%.[29]

GI bleeding

Symptoms of overt GI bleeding clearly demand appropriate investigation with immediate hospital assessment required for the vast majority of those reporting haematemesis or melaena. Advanced age is a strong predictor of mortality in upper GI bleeding and inpatient management is the rule. Rectal bleeding in elderly people requires investigation to distinguish the common ano-rectal conditions (e.g. haemorrhoids or fissure) from more serious organic causes, particularly cancer. As already indicated, dysphagia is an alarm feature meriting active exclusion of oesophagogastric malignancy. Vomiting is an extremely common symptom in primary care but when persistent or occurring in the context of new-onset dyspepsia it demands referral for investigation.

Specific GI diagnoses

For the most part, management of GI disorders in an elderly population proceeds in the same way as for younger adults. What follows is an overview of selected problems which are either more common or merit particular consideration in older individuals.

H. pylori infection and associated conditions

Eradication of *H. pylori* is indicated in patients with an established diagnosis of peptic ulcer disease. It leads to ulcer healing and effective cure for most patients.[5] Older patients should not be denied the benefits of this treatment. This includes targeting patients with a new diagnosis established at gastroscopy but also includes those in whom the diagnosis of peptic ulcer disease was proven in the past. Symptom-free patients receiving long-term acid suppressants for peptic ulcer disease should be tested and treated where appropriate. This may allow treatment to be stopped. Serology for *H. pylori* is simple and widely available. A positive *H. pylori* serology result is a reasonable basis for treatment in a patient who has never been offered eradication therapy before. Serology is not an appropriate test in patients who have received eradication therapy in the past. Antibodies to

H. pylori may remain for some years even after successful clearance of the infection. The [^{13}C]urea breath test is preferred for monitoring success of treatment and a positive result indicates current infection. It can be prescribed on an FP10, comes with full instructions and the procedure can be carried out easily in primary care. Although it is unnecessary to check the success of eradication therapy routinely if symptoms have resolved, it is wise to be cautious in those with a history of complicated peptic ulcer (e.g. haemorrhage) and to verify clearance of the organism by a breath test. Studies of faecal antigen testing are promising, but accuracy may be better in younger than in older subjects.[30]

The symptomatic benefits of eradicating *H. pylori* infection in non-ulcer (functional) dyspepsia are disappointing (the number needed to treat for one symptomatic cure is ~14 patients) but it is nevertheless worthwhile offering treatment.[31] That said, it is inappropriate to embark on repeated attempts at clearing the infection in those without an established history of peptic ulceration.

There is no evidence to suggest modifying the choice of eradication regimen in elderly patients.[32] Drug interactions may become a consideration in those with multiple comorbidities and concomitant polypharmacy. Triple therapy appears well tolerated in elderly subjects, but specific data on the side-effect profiles and success rates of individual drug regimens in older subjects is not available.

Gastro-oesophageal reflux disease

Reflux is managed along standard lines in the older subject with lifestyle advice, antacids and acid suppressants titrated to achieve symptom control. Although on-demand, step-up and step-down approaches apply equally well to older subjects, continuous therapy with a proton pump inhibitor (PPI) is indicated in patients with complicated GORD. This is particularly important in those in whom a peptic stricture has required endoscopic dilation, since continued treatment reduces the frequency and severity of recurrence.[7] There is some evidence to suggest that older subjects may require a higher level of acid suppression to achieve control of reflux than younger subjects and hence PPIs are preferable to H_2-antagonists in this group.[7] There is increasing evidence for an association between long-term acid suppression and infections, particularly *Clostridium difficile* and campylobacter.[33] Although this association is unquestioned, it is not that strong inasmuch as long-term PPIs approximately double the risk of infection. This association has been used to encourage GPs to minimise use of PPIs, but given the relative rarity of these infections, it is likely the benefits from treatment outweigh the risks. The advent of laparoscopic surgery means that fundoplication has become an accepted alternative to drug treatment and results of surgery in the fit elderly individual are excellent.

Functional disorders

A large proportion of elderly subjects with GI symptoms will have a diagnosis of a functional disorder, following investigations showing no serious structural disease. Functional dyspeptic symptoms are treated with reassurance, lifestyle advice, a review of medications and empirical treatment with antacids, acid suppressants, *H. pylori* eradication and antiemetic (prokinetic) agents. Difficult functional pains may respond to low dose tricyclic antidepressants. IBS is generally a longstanding problem and there are no special considerations in older people. However, functional constipation deserves special mention as it is both common and challenging to treat. The causes of simple constipation in elderly subjects are multiple and include relative inactivity due to declining mobility, poor hydration or diet, side-effects of drug treatment and systemic illness (e.g. diabetes mellitus, hypothyroidism, Parkinson's disease, etc.). Empirical treatment with a range of laxatives is the norm but there is little good evidence to support choice of agent in older subjects.

Coeliac disease

There is increased awareness that coeliac disease is underdiagnosed in elderly patients.[34] Around 2–10% of adult cases are diagnosed after the age of 70 years. Symptoms can be absent and the condition may come to light after identifying anaemia, iron or folic acid deficiency either 'incidentally' or following consultation with non-specific systemic symptoms. Clinical presentation varies markedly but severe malabsorption with wasting and steatorrhoea is rare in older patients. Symptomatic patients, whose symptoms may include diarrhoea or constipation, often experience substantial delay in diagnosis—in one study the mean diagnostic delay for people aged >65 years was 17 years (range: 0–58 years).[34] The availability of serological tests, including anti-endomysial and anti-tissue transglutaminase antibodies, makes accurate non-invasive screening straightforward but duodenal biopsy is required to confirm villous atrophy. Adopting a gluten-free diet in later life is clearly challenging and newly diagnosed patients require considerable dietetic support.

Gastrointestinal cancer

Cancer is a disease of older age, and GI cancers are no exception. Younger patients may develop any of the GI cancers, especially if they have a genetic predisposition, but the main burden is borne by the elderly population. Men aged 83 years have an annual incidence of colorectal cancer six times higher than men aged 53 years (who, incidentally, are the ones invited to partake in the UK national screening programme). Similar—or more extreme—numbers pertain for oesophageal, stomach or pancreatic cancers.

These four main GI cancers—colorectal, stomach, oesophagus and pancreas—account for nearly a quarter of all new cancer diagnoses in the UK. The commonest in terms of incidence is colorectal cancer, with >36 000 new diagnoses in the UK each year, or 13% of new cancer diagnoses. At the level of the individual GP, this equates to about one new diagnosis per full-time doctor per year. The incidence of colorectal cancer is changing very little over time. The three other relatively common cancers have similar incidences: stomach 8000 new diagnoses per year, oesophagus 7800 and pancreas 7600, so each accounts for ~3% of new cancer diagnoses. However, this similarity hides a dramatic secular change, with stomach cancer halving in incidence over the last 30 years—and with no sign that the decline is levelling off. Conversely, oesophagus cancer is rapidly increasing, primarily in males. It is likely that oesophagus, and then pancreas, will overtake stomach cancer in incidence in the next few years. All four of these cancers are more common in males, though the difference is relatively small in colorectal cancer. Although there are a few familial syndromes including colorectal cancer, these almost invariably affect younger patients.

Mortality figures are dismal for the three rarer cancers, with three-quarters of patients with stomach cancer dying early from their disease, and nearly all patients with pancreas or oesophageal cancers dying rapidly from their disease. By contrast, survival is good in colorectal cancer, so patients aged 60–69 years have a 5 year survival of >45%, and even patients aged 80–89 years have a 35% survival. Thus, there are more deaths from oesophagus, stomach and pancreas combined, than there are from colorectal cancer.

Diagnosis of GI cancer

Colorectal cancer

For the most part, there are few differences in symptoms of colorectal cancer in elderly compared with younger patients.[18] Thus, around a quarter present as an emergency,[35] with emergency presentations no more common in elderly than in younger patients.[36] The remaining three-quarters present with symptoms, usually to their GP. The risk of a cancer with these symptoms is

Table 9.1 The risk of colorectal cancer in patients presenting symptoms to their general practitioner

Symptom	PPV for consulting population (%)	
	40–69 years	≥70 years
Rectal bleeding	1.4	4.8
Loss of weight	0.74	2.5
Abdominal pain	0.65	2.0
Diarrhoea	0.63	1.7
Constipation	0.2	1.3

Reproduced in part from Reference 17.
PPV, positive predictive value.

shown in Table 9.1. Clearly, risks are higher for each symptom in the older age group, but this simply reflects the increased incidence in older people, rather than a higher proportion of cases having a particular symptom. However, even in older individuals, the risk of colorectal cancer for all of the common symptoms is relatively low, making the decision whether to refer for investigation difficult. This is particularly so as the main investigation for suspected colorectal cancer is colonoscopy, with its need for bowel preparation, its discomfort, and its small—but real—risk of perforation. In the frail, investigation may be by barium enema, but this still has the disadvantage of bowel preparation and does not give a tissue diagnosis.

The national guidance for colorectal cancer diagnosis is of limited value in the elderly population. It suggests referral of patients aged >60 years, with any of the following:

+ rectal bleeding with a change in bowel habit to looser stools and/or increased stool frequency persisting for ≥6 weeks
+ rectal bleeding without anal symptoms (such as soreness, discomfort, itching, lumps or prolapse) persisting for ≥6 weeks
+ change of bowel habit to looser stools and/or increased stool frequency, without rectal bleeding and persisting for ≥6 weeks
+ a right lower abdominal mass or a rectal mass
+ unexplained iron deficiency anaemia in men (Hb <11 g/dl) or women (Hb <10 g/dl).

The problem with the first three of these recommendations is that rectal bleeding is experienced by only ~40% of elderly people with cancer, with a similar percentage having diarrhoea. Many of these are the same people, so that these recommendations only capture the minority of patients harbouring a cancer. Much research in this field is aimed at finding an intermediate test for use in general practice—one that can identify patients with a low-risk but not no-risk symptom of colorectal cancer who truly have a risk high enough to warrant investigation. Until such a test is found, elderly patients and their GPs have two choices: either to increase the number of referrals of patients with low risk symptoms, or to continue with a quarter of patients presenting as emergencies.

However, GPs do not just assemble a list of symptoms and refer based on the assessment of risk. General practice is much more subtle than that, and there is quite good evidence in the cancer diagnostic field that GPs can identify at least some of those at higher risk. GPs may have to suffer the wrath of the rapid investigation clinic in referring patients who do not fit the relatively non-evidence-based referral criteria, but it is wiser to trust your feeling that 'something isn't right' than to blindly follow guidance.

Oesophageal and stomach cancers

Although the symptom profiles of these cancers have been published from secondary care case series, there are almost no data on the symptoms as presented to the GP. As noted earlier, dysphagia is a sinister symptom, carrying a risk of oesophageal cancer of almost 10% in men aged >65 years, and ~4% in women in the same age group.[37] Weight loss and symptoms of gastro-oesophageal reflux are the other two common symptoms of oesophageal cancer.[38] Unfortunately, reflux symptoms are almost ubiquitous within the elderly population, and the identification of individual patients with cancer from the many who present with similar symptoms, but in whom the diagnosis is not cancer, is difficult.

The National Institute of Health and Clinical Excellence (NICE) referral guidelines for upper GI cancer are shown in Boxes 9.1 and 9.2.

There has been considerable argument about the merit of this guidance. Surgical case series reports have shown that delays may be long and associated with a worse prognosis.[39] However, the alarm features of oesophageal cancer were present in 85% of cases in a recent endoscopy series (the remaining 15% having dyspepsia alone), suggesting that for oesophageal cancer, the guidance works reasonably well.[40] Like many cancers, there is a complex relationship between the duration of symptoms and survival from oesophageal cancer, with no clear benefit seen from speedy diagnosis. Thus, considerable effort has gone into surveillance of Barrett's oesophagus.

Barrett's oesophagus refers to the finding of metaplastic (intestinalized) epithelium in the distal oesophagus, a finding reported in up to 10–15% of patients investigated for chronic GORD.[41] A pathway from Barrett's oesophagus through grades of dysplasia to established adenocarcinoma is well-established but the annual risk of progression is low—at ~0.5% of patients per annum in reported series.[42] Screening endoscopy and multiple biopsy is recommended every 2 years in the UK. There is no consensus as to the age-threshold for offering ongoing surveillance. Elderly patients tolerate gastroscopy well, but in those with serious comorbidity or limited life expectancy surveillance will become inappropriate. Progress in endoluminal therapies (e.g. argon plasma coagulation, photodynamic therapy) for high grade dysplasia or localized disease means that fitness for oesophagectomy is no longer the only consideration for patients remaining in surveillance programmes, albeit this form of treatment remains the only proven curative treatment for the minority of cases progressing to oesophageal cancer.

Box 9.1 The NICE referral guidelines for upper gastrointestinal (GI) cancer

Patients of any age with dyspepsia who present with any of the following:

- chronic GI bleeding
- dysphagia
- progressive unintentional weight loss
- persistent vomiting
- iron deficiency anaemia
- epigastric mass
- suspicious barium meal result.

Patients aged ≥55 years with unexplained and persistent recent-onset dyspepsia alone.

Box 9.2 UK guidelines (2005 version) for urgent referral for further investigation of possible upper gastrointestinal cancer

Patients with unexplained worsening of their dyspepsia, and known to have any of the following risk factors:

◆ Barrett's oesophagus

◆ dysplasia, atrophic gastritis or intestinal metaplasia

◆ Peptic ulcer surgery >20 years ago

◆ unexplained weight loss or iron deficiency anaemia in the absence of dyspepsia

◆ persistent vomiting and weight loss in the absence of dyspepsia.

Identification of patients at high risk of stomach cancer is easy if they have weight loss, GI bleeding or a mass. The much more difficult group is those with dyspepsia. One concern is that treatment with an acid-reducing agent, such as a PPI, may delay diagnosis and worsen the prognosis. In fact it seems to do the former of these, but not the latter.[43] Patients using antisecretory drugs are diagnosed on average 4 months later, but have a similar staging and prognosis.

Pancreatic cancer

It seems almost inevitable that this cancer is diagnosed late and has a dismal prognosis. Fewer than 20% have surgically resectable disease at diagnosis. The classic presentation is with obstructive jaundice and weight loss.[44] This may be preceded by more vague symptoms of fullness, bloating and pain. Indeed, pain is experienced by almost all patients. A minority also go on to develop diabetes. By the time demonstrable physical signs, such as a mass, have developed, the prognosis is dire.

The simplest investigation is abdominal ultrasound—and this is recommended in NICE guidance for obstructive jaundice. However, it can be difficult to tease out the site of a possible malignancy in patients with epigastric pain and weight loss, so choosing between urgent ultrasound or gastroscopy may be difficult. Ultrasound investigation is not wholly reliable either, in that a small percentage of those shown to have a pancreatic cancer have negative scans. Magnetic resonance (MR) imaging, and MR-cholangiography in particular, and computed tomography have important roles in diagnosis and staging of proven tumours. Endoscopic retrograde cholangiopancreatography can identify small tumours situated near the ampulla of Vater, and histological or cytological samples can be taken, but this invasive technique is reserved for patients with proven biliary obstruction in whom therapy is anticipated. Stenting is now a standard approach for palliation in unresectable tumours. Endoscopic ultrasound has an increasing role in diagnosis and staging.

References

1. Anonymous. *Morbidity Statistics from General Practice.* Fourth national study 1991–2. London: HMSO; 1995.

2. Bodger K, Eastwood P, Manning S, Daly M, Heatley R. Dyspepsia workload in urban general practice and implications of the British Society of Gastroenterology Dyspepsia guidelines (1996). *Aliment Pharmacol Ther* 2000;14:413–20.

3. Delaney B, Ford A, Forman D, Moayyedi P, Qume M. Initial management strategies for dyspepsia. *Cochrane Database Syst Rev* 2005;(19):CD001961.

4. Talley NJ, McNeil D, Piper D. Discriminant value of dyspeptic symptoms: a study of the clinical presentation of 221 patients with dyspepsia of unknown cause, peptic ulceration, and cholelithiasis. *Gut* 1987;28:40–6.

5. Marshall B. *Helicobacter pylori. Am J Gastroenterology* 1994;89:S116–128.

6. Lee M, Feldman M. The ageing stomach: implications for NSAID gastropathy. *Gut* 1997;41:422–424.

7. Tack J, Vantrappen G. The aging oesophagus. *Gut* 1997;41:422–424.

8. Lindgren S, Janzon L. Prevalence of swallowing complaints and clinical findings among 50-79-year-old men and women. *Dysphagia* 1991;6:187–192.

9. Siebens H, Trupe E, Siebens A. Correlates and consequences of eating dependency in institutionalized elderly. *Am J Geriat Soc* 1986;34:192–198.

10. Kapoor N, Bassi A, Sturgess R, Bodger K. Predictive value of alarm features in a rapid access upper gastrointestinal cancer service. *Gut* 2005;54:40–5.

11. Wallander M-A, Johansson S, Ruigomez A, Garcia Rodriguez LA. Unspecified abdominal pain in primary care: the role of gastrointestinal morbidity. *Int J Clin Pract* 2007;61:1663–1670.

12. Southampton Primary Care Trust. West Hampshire Out of Hours Service. Southampton; 2006.

13. Beach Program AGPS, Classification U. Presentations of abdominal pain in Australian general practice. *Aust Fam Physcn* 2004;33:968–9.

14. Hamilton W. Earlier diagnosis of colorectal, lung and prostate cancer. MD thesis, University of Bristol; 2005.

15. Cannings-John R, Butler C, Prout H, *et al*. A case–control study of presentations in general practice before diagnosis of coeliac disease. *Br J Gen Pract* 2007;57:636–642.

16. McGee S. *Evidence Based Physical Diagnosis*, 2nd edn. St Louis: Saunders/Elsevier; 2007.

17. Hamilton W, Round A, Sharp D, Peters T. Clinical features of colorectal cancer before diagnosis: a population-based case–control study. *Br J Cancer* 2005;93:399–405.

18. Curless R, French JM, Williams GV, James OF. Colorectal carcinoma: do elderly patients present differently? *Age Ageing* 1994;23:102–7.

19. Chaplin A, Curless R, Thomson R, Barton R. Prevalence of lower gastrointestinal symptoms and associated consultation behaviour in a British elderly population determined by face-to-face interview. *Br J Gen Pract* 2000;50:798–802.

20. Carlsson L, Hakansson A, Nordenskjold B. Common cancer-related symptoms among GP patients. *Opportunistic screening in primary health care. Scand J Primary Health Care Suppl* 2001;19:199–203.

21. MacArthur C, Smith A. Factors associated with speed of diagnosis, referral, and treatment in colorectal cancer. *J Epidemiol Community Health* 1984;38:122–6.

22. Stapley S, Peters TJ, Sharp D, Hamilton W. The mortality of colorectal cancer in relation to the initial symptom and to the duration of symptoms: a cohort study in primary care. *Br J Cancer* 2006;95:1321–5.

23. Selvachandran S, Hodder R, Ballal M, Jones P, Cade D. Prediction of colorectal cancer by a patient consultation questionnaire and scoring system: a prospective study. *Lancet* 2002;360:278–83.

24. Lawrenson R, Logie J, Marks C. Risk of colorectal cancer in general practice patients presenting with rectal bleeding, change in bowel habit or anaemia. *Eur J Cancer Care* 2006;15:267–71.

25. Hamilton W, Peters TJ. *Cancer Diagnosis in Primary Care*. Oxford: Churchill Livingstone; 2007.

26. Hernandez JL, Riancho JA, Matorras P, Gonzalez-Macias J. Clinical evaluation for cancer in patients with involuntary weight loss without specific symptoms. *Am J Med* 2003;114:631–7.

27. Guralnik JM, Eisenstaedt RS, Ferrucci L, Klein HG, Woodman RC. Prevalence of anemia in persons 65 years and older in the United States: evidence for a high rate of unexplained anemia. *Blood* 2004;104:2263–8.

28. Weller D, Coleman D, Robertson R, *et al*. The UK colorectal cancer screening pilot: results of the second round of screening in England. *Br J Cancer* 2007;97:1601–5.

29. Hamilton W, Lancashire R, Sharp D, Peters TJ, Cheng K, Marshall T. The importance of anaemia in diagnosing colorectal cancer: a case–control study using electronic primary care records. *Br J Cancer* 2008;98:323–7.

30. Krausse R, Muller G, Doniec M. Evaluation of a rapid new stool antigen test for diagnosis of *Helicobacter pylori* infection in adult patients. *J Clin Microbiol* 2008;46:2062–5.

31. Moayyedi P, Soo S, Deeks J, *et al*. Eradication of *Helicobacter pylori* for non-ulcer dyspepsia. *Cochrane Database Syst Rev* 2006;(19):CD002096.

32. Pilotto A, Malfertheiner P. Review article: an approach to *Helicobacter pylori* infection in the elderly. *Aliment Pharmacol Ther* 2002;16:683–91.

33. Leonard J, Marshall J, Moayyedi P. Systematic review of the risk of enteric infection in patients taking acid suppression. *Am J Gastroenterol* 2007;102:2047–56.

34. Gassbarrini G, Holmes G. Coeliac disease in the elderly. *Gerontology* 2001;47:306–10.

35. Barrett J, Jiwa M, Rose P, Hamilton W. Pathways to the diagnosis of colorectal cancer: an observational study in three UK cities. *Fam Pract* 2006;23:15–19.

36. Cleary J, Peters TJ, Sharp D, Hamilton W. Clinical features of colorectal cancer before emergency presentation: a population-based case–control study. *Fam Pract* 2007;24:3–6.

37. Jones R, Latinovic R, Charlton J, Gulliford MC. Alarm symptoms in early diagnosis of cancer in primary care: cohort study using General Practice Research Database. *Br Med J* 2007:334:1040.

38. Gibbs JF, Rajput A, Chadha KS, *et al*. The changing profile of esophageal cancer presentation and its implication for diagnosis. *J Natl Med Assoc* 2007;99:620–6.

39. Martin IG, Young S, Sue-Ling H, Johnston D. Delays in the diagnosis of oesophagogastric cancer: a consecutive case series. *Br Med J* 1997;314:467–70.

40. Bowrey D, Griffin S, Wayman J, Karat D, Hayes N, Raimes S. Use of alarm symptoms to select dyspeptics for endoscopy causes patients with curable esophagogastric cancer to be overlooked. *Surg Endosc* 2006;20:1725–8.

41. Brotze S, McElhinney S, Weston A. The frequency of Barrett's esophagus in high risk patients with chronic GERD. *Gastrointest Endosc* 2005;61:226–31.

42. Basu K, Pick B, de Caestecker J. Audit of a Barrett's epithelium surveillance database. *Eur J Gastroenterol Hepatol* 2004;16:171–5.

43. Panter SJ, O'Flanagan H, Bramble MG, Hungin APS. Empirical use of antisecretory drug therapy delays diagnosis of upper gastrointestinal adenocarcinoma but does not effect outcome. *Aliment Pharmacol Ther* 2004;19:981–8.

44. Takhar AS, Palaniappan P, Dhingsa R, Lobo DN. Recent developments in diagnosis of pancreatic cancer. *Br Med J* 2004;329(7467):668–73.

Chapter 10

Diabetes and endocrine problems

Simon Croxson and Roger Gadsby

Introduction

This chapter will focus on diabetes since this is common, has a significant morbidity and mortality and can be well managed in primary care. Thyroid disease and Addison disease are also covered. Diabetes in elderly people has special problems such as residential care and dementia, as well as the great variability of the subjects and the presence of multiple comorbidities which can influence diabetes treatments and priorities.

The difficulty is that there is a paucity of randomised controlled trials in the older person looking at real outcomes. Some hypoglycaemic agent trials do contain older people, but the numbers of those aged >80 years are minimal, and outcomes are generally glucose levels achieved and safety (both important) rather than outcomes of avoiding vascular events, and quality of life measures. Blood pressure trials generally give better evidence, but the problems of recruiting frail older people into a clinical trial are very significant. Many of the appropriate trials have been reviewed by Sinclair, and published under the aegis of the European Union of Geriatric Medicine Society.[1]

As in all areas of elderly care, close links between primary and secondary care are vital; good liaison can obtain appropriate treatment for frail older people in residential care without the need to be dragged up to a hospital clinic or ward. It is important that this process continues, despite the UK Government's attempts to fragment care and split professionals.

The Quality and Outcomes Framework (QOF) of the general practitioner (GP) contract introduced in 2004 has a number of clinical indicators for diabetes.[2] There are 93 points that can be achieved by fulfilling all the indicators. There has been an improvement in the process and outcome scores in diabetes achieved by practices year by year since its introduction, suggesting that the QOF is an important lever for improving diabetes care. There are QOF indicators for hypothyroidism, but for no other endocrine problems.

The GP contract QOF allows individuals to be excluded for varying reasons. If the clinician feels that achieving targets is not in the individual patient's best interests, then 'exception reporting' allows the practice to exclude individual patients from the disease indicators in particular circumstances.

Diabetes: epidemiology, and diagnosis

The prevalence of diabetes varies in different populations, varying by ethnicity, geographical area and date and method of study; much diabetes is undiagnosed, so screening by glucose tolerance test (GTT) is required to fully assess the prevalence.[3]

Among UK elderly, the prevalence is ~10% in white British elderly, 25% in Indo-Asian British elderly and 25% in residents of care homes; 30–50% of these subjects are undiagnosed. There is a delay of at least 4–7 years, but more probably 10 years, between onset of diabetes and diagnosis among subjects of all ages.

There are many reasons to diagnose diabetes; the most pertinent are that diagnosis allows management of vascular risk factors, and that deaths from diabetic hyperglycaemic comas characteristically occur in older subjects not known to have diabetes.

Although the fasting plasma glucose is preferred by many, it has a low sensitivity and the frail, slim, older person with undiagnosed diabetes will often have a fasting plasma glucose in the impaired fasting plasma glucose range, or even within the normal range, despite a clearly elevated post-challenge glucose level. In the Bristol population, 30% of subjects with impaired fasting plasma glucose (IFG) (6.0–6.9 mmol/l inclusive) have diabetes and in the Gujerati population of Leicester, 85% of IFG subjects had diabetes. Isolated post-challenge hyperglycaemia carries an increased mortality compared to subjects with normal glucose tolerance. A raised glycosylated haemoglobin or fructosamine is specific, but again has low sensitivity, and osmotic symptoms have low sensitivity and specificity.

So, what test? In free-range elderly people, a postprandial glucose of ≥7.8 mmol/l has the best sensitivity/specificity as a screening tool prior to further investigations; if this is clearly ≥11.1 mmol/l, then this suggests diabetes, and one would merely confirm the diagnosis; but if the postprandial glucose is in the 7.8–11.0 mmol/l range, further tests are required. One could do a fasting plasma glucose test, and if not a diabetic value, proceed to a test 2 h after 75 g anhydrous glucose conveniently given as 113 ml polycal, or one could go straight to a full 2 point (fasting and 2 h levels) GTT. A single abnormal plasma glucose is highly suggestive of diabetes, and technically one would want confirmatory evidence such as osmotic symptoms, another significantly raised plasma glucose value, or specific complications which means retinopathy. However, in the Melton survey based on a well, primary care population, if the 2 h value was ≥13 mmol/l, retesting was always positive for diabetes.[4] World Health Organization criteria[5] are summarized in Table 10.1.

After a diagnosis of diabetes, one has to decide which type. Ninety-five per cent of diabetes in elderly people is type 2 diabetes mellitus (T2DM), but the incidence of type 1 diabetes mellitus (T1DM) is the same from age 30 to 80 years,[6,7] and secondary diabetes (presumably from chronic

Table 10.1 World Health Organization[5] criteria for diabetes diagnosis (mmol/l)

	Venous plasma	Capillary whole blood
Diabetes		
Fasting or	≥7.0	≥6.1
2 h post load	≥11.1	≥11.1
IGT		
Fasting and	<7.0	<6.1
2 h post load	≥7.8 <11.1	≥7.8 <11.1
Normal		
Fasting and	<6.0	<5.6
2 h post load	<7.8	<7.8

IGT, impaired glucose tolerance.
Only venous plasma and capillary whole blood glucose values are given.

pancreatitis, and steroids) is a disease of older people.[6] Also, T1DM in elderly people can be a slow-onset, latent autoimmune diabetes of the adult (LADA), and T2DM can present as diabetes with ketoacidosis (DKA), or ketosis-prone T2DM,[8] which is particularly common in those of African-Carribean origin. From a pragmatic point of view, one would detect the apparently T1DM subjects on standard clinical criteria;[9] either spontaneous significant ketosis, or two of the following: personal history of autoimmune disease, T1DM in a first-degree relative, significant osmotic symptoms, or significant weight loss (even if overweight at onset and still overweight). The LADA subjects will be identified over the first year since, as fast as one increases the oral hypoglycaemic agents, the plasma glucose rises further rather than falls. The ketosis-prone T2DM subjects will look clinically like a type 2 person (overweight, non-white ethnicity, family history of T2DM) presenting as DKA and initial management will be as a hospital inpatient; but as a GP, it would be worth questioning whether African-Carribean subjects diagnosed as T1DM do in fact have T2DM. With secondary diabetes, there may also be evidence of T2DM, and we will discuss management later.

At presentation, the type 2 diabetic person is usually overweight; so the underweight 'type 2 diabetic person' should ring warning bells; the differential includes T1DM (including LADA), insulin-deficient type 2 diabetes,[10] thyrotoxicosis and malabsorption as causes of secondary diabetes, and coexistent malignancy since carcinoma pancreas, breast, uterus and colon are more common in diabetic people.

If there is doubt about the type of diabetes, specialist review measuring antibodies, and indices of beta-cell function and insulin resistance such as glucagon-stimulated C-peptide release could be invaluable.[11]

Impaired fasting glucose and impaired glucose tolerance

Impaired fasting glucose is a fasting glucose level between normal and abnormal; as discussed above, a glucose tolerance test is required to accurately define these subjects' glucose tolerance.

Impaired glucose tolerance (IGT) is a non-diabetic fasting glucose level with a 2 h GTT value between normal and diabetic. IGT carries an increased risk of future diabetes and vascular disease. Management is thus to avoid diabetes by diet and exercise, to avoid vascular events by aggressive management of vascular risk factors and to screen for diabetes every 1–3 years.

Drugs that worsen glucose tolerance

There is clear evidence from Anglo-Scandinavian Cardiac Outcomes Trial (ASCOT) that a beta-blocker/thiazide combination is particularly good at precipitating diabetes,[12] so one would not use this in people at risk of diabetes unless there were no other options. If one gives them to a diabetic person, the impact on their glycaemic control seems minimal, generally,[13] and the problem of hypoglycaemia unawareness with beta-blockers is generally not significant; however, sometimes there is a deterioration in glucose control or development of hypoglycaemia unawareness, so patients need to be monitored for worsening glycaemia and warned about possible hypoglycaemia unawareness. The effect of steroids is well known and can precipitate DKA in subjects not known to have diabetes.

Finally, the atypical antipsychotics quetiapine and olanzapine can precipitate diabetes.[14]

If prescribing a drug such as the above that might precipitate diabetes, it is advisable to warn the patient or their carers to report osmotic symptoms or drowsiness and to check random plasma glucose levels as above; the chance of developing diabetes is related to the standard risk factors of ethnicity, obesity and family history.

Hyperglycaemic emergencies

Elderly people may suffer three sorts of hyperglycaemic emergency; these often occur in those not known to have diabetes. Early diagnosis and referral is essential for optimum patient outcomes.

Diabetic ketoacidosis will manifest as decreased conscious level, 'gone off legs' with hyperglycaemia and ketosis.[15] However, it should be noted that in the setting of poor carbohydrate intake or profuse vomiting, the plasma glucose may not rise dramatically, or even at all, known as 'euglycaemic diabetic ketoacidosis'. Thus it is vital not only to test for glucose levels using a fingerprick meter but also to be able to test for ketones. If the person will produce no urine, one can measure the ketone β-hydroxybutyrate on the Optium Exceed® (Abbott Diabetes Care, Maidenhead, UK) home blood glucose meter; here ≥3.0 mmol/l (or ≥3 on urine testing) suggests significant ketosis and the need for hospital admission.

The older type 2 diabetic person also classically gets hyperomolar non-ketotic coma (HONK)[15] which has now been renamed the hyperosmolar hyperglycaemic state because there is some crossover between HONK and DKA. Again, the patient will be off legs, drowsy, etc., may well be in a residential care home with no known diabetes, and there may be a history suggestive of a urinary tract infection. Why some get HONK and some DKA is not totally clear, but it may well be more to do with counter-regulatory hormones than the theory that T2DM subjects produce a small amount of insulin which suppresses lipolysis; also hyperosmolarity decreases ketogenesis. Again, the fingerprick glucose level must be measured and taken with the clinical picture for diagnosis and hospital inpatient treatment.

Finally, some elderly patients with renal impairment can achieve quite high plasma glucose values without disturbance of consciousness, but with hyponatraemia (each 3 mmol/l glucose equates to ~1 mmol/l sodium);[16] they need to be treated and monitored, but do not need to be managed as per DKA which risks fluid overload. These subjects often need a few days in hospital to stabilize, and be supported and monitored.

Thus in the older person, the questions to be asked regarding management at home are:

- Is the patient confused, ill or vomiting?
- Is there supervision at home lest they deteriorate?
- Plasma glucose and ketone levels?

Hypoglycaemia

We will consider this initially in the setting of diabetes, and then consider spontaneous hypoglycaemia.

The problem of hypoglycaemia cannot be emphasized enough. It occurs with insulin and sulphonylureas, and over the first few years of the UK Prospective Diabetes Study (UKPDS), hypoglycaemia was as common on glibenclamide as on insulin.[17]

The first problem is poor patient recognition; in older people becoming hypoglycaemic, the sympathetic symptoms are poorly appreciated and are appreciated at a lower plasma glucose value, i.e. there is less time before neuroglycopenia occurs with confusion and decreased conscious level. Their hypoglycaemic symptoms also differ from younger people's so that they are more likely to have neurological symptoms of slurred speech, confusion and weakness than younger people. Patients and medical staff are poor at appreciating hypoglycaemia, which can present as 'gone off legs', acute confusion, transient ischaemic attack, stroke, and fits; in any diabetic person on hypoglycaemic treatment who has a 'funny turn' or neurological deficit, fingerprick glucose estimation is vital.

If the older person has had a hypo which is corrected by themselves, or their family giving oral glucose (15 g rapidly acting carbohydrate such as three dextrosol tablets or glass of Lucozade followed by 15 g long-acting carbohydrate, e.g. two biscuits or a large slice of bread), then they can stay at home. If they have needed external help, then there should be someone else at home lest hypo recurs; if they have needed parenteral glucose or glucagon, then they need admission to hospital for 24 h observation, at least. It is thought that glucagon is contraindicated in sulphonylurea hypoglycaemia since these subjects have some beta-cell function which is later stimulated by the pharmacological dose of glucagon. Finally, the cause of the hypoglycaemia must be elucidated and addressed.

Risk factors for hypoglycaemia in older people include:[18]

- choice of sulphonylurea or insulin
- male gender
- any co-morbid conditions such as cardiac, hepatic or renal impairment
- recent discharge from hospital or change in dose
- alcohol excess
- chronic confusion.

Hypoglycaemia does occur in older people not on insulin or sulphonylurea, but is rare.[15] Causes include:

- surreptitious administration of hypoglycaemic treatment by a 'carer'
- acute overwhelming illness, e.g. sepsis
- spuriously low fingerprick plasma glucose measurements in shocked, peripherally shut-down subjects.
- insulinoma or tumours producing insulin-like substance
- alcohol intoxication
- Addison disease.

They may need secondary care to fully investigate the causes, but in our experience, the subjects are admitted to hospital as 'gone off legs' or stroke, and hypoglycaemia is then found.

Management of hyperglycaemia

The main drivers to improve glycaemic control in older diabetic people are to improve quality of life and cognition[19] and to avoid metabolic decompensation and infection; it may be that improved glycaemic control protects against development of small vessel and large vessel disease, but the older diabetic person may not live long enough to derive this benefit.[20] But what glycaemic targets? There have been no large long-term trials of the value of glucose control in older people. It is clear that lower glycosylated haemoglobin (HbA1c) in large trials such as Diabetes Control and Complications Trial (DCCT) and UKPDS avoided microvascular and macrovascular complications; these studies are often cited as stating that one should aim for a DCCT-aligned HbA1c (upper limit normal range 6.2%) value of 7.0% since this was the best compromise between risk of complications and risk of hypoglycaemia; what the authors actually said was that one should aim for HbA1c levels as low as safely possible. Different organizations presently advocate different HbA1c levels, from 6.5% to 7.5%. The 2008 National Institute of Health and Clinical Excellence (NICE) guidelines recommend a usual HbA1c target of 6.5% for those controlled on lifestyle, metformin and/or sulphonylurea but an HbA1c target of 7.5% for those on more complex glucose lowering regimens. It is important to note that the HbA1c represents an average plasma glucose, i.e. it may disguise dramatic swings.

In older people, it is vital to have an individual assessment of the patient. If one is using agents that do not cause hypoglycaemia, then one could aim for a very low target, e.g. within the normal range; but if using agents which might cause hypoglycaemia, then <7.5% would be reasonable, and if hypoglycaemia was a problem despite adjusting the medication, then one would accept a higher HbA1c. In very frail older people, the consensus view is that an HbA1c <8.0% would be acceptable.[21] Guidelines do not emphasize enough the target to avoid hypoglycaemia.

Which agents to use?

There is a wide choice which creates difficulty. The choice of oral agents really depends on the comorbid conditions contraindicating various agents, the glucose reduction required and the risk of hypoglycaemia. The exception is that an underweight diabetic person mainly has poor beta-cell function and little insulin resistance, so insulin is generally required, although a carefully supervised trial of a sulphonylurea would be reasonable in the absence of ketones. Generally, when one adds the third agent, one does not get so much glucose lowering as when one added the second agent. Most oral agents drop the HbA1c by 1–1.5%.

The NICE glucose-lowering algorithm is readily accessible in downloadable form,[22] as is the American Diabetes Association/European Association for the Study of Diabetes (ADA/EASD) algorithm.[23] They are rather convergent and go 'lifestyle, metformin, another oral agent or insulin'.

Initial management: diet, exercise and consider metformin

Although diet and exercise are a cornerstone of managing hyperglycaemia, it may not provide long-term control; hence the joint EASD/ADA guidelines[24] recommend lifestyle plus metformin if a person with diabetes has a raised HbA1c at initial assessment. The NICE guideline in the UK recommends that lifestyle change alone should be the initial therapy, and only if this is unsuccessful should metformin be added as the drug of first choice.

The standard diet is low refined carbohydrate, high complex carbohydrate, low saturated fat and use of monosaturated fats.[25] This does permit 50 g of refined carbohydrate per day if taken with a meal containing fibre to retard its absorption. However, given the poor calorie intake in some older people, one may allow frail older people to have more fat in the diet. A dietician's assessment is invaluable, but one can get a rough idea of diet one's self; in particular, hyperglycaemic people with thirst can consume large quantities of sugary drinks such as lemonade. Patients value written information and the Nutrition Advisory Group for Elderly People of the British Dietetic Association produce excellent guides, straightforward and easy to read and understand.[26]

The biguanides are some of the oldest hypoglycaemic drugs, but we are still learning about them. Metformin is the biguanide of choice since it has the lowest, most predictable risk of lactic acidosis and has been validated in UKPDS.[27] It produces no weight gain, does not cause hypoglycaemia, may prevent vascular events and is extremely economical.[13,28]

The main concern is the risk of lactic acidosis; this is a disease of the elderly population and in the past was generally fatal; with metformin, lactic acidosis occurs predominantly in the setting of renal impairment and age is not an independent risk factor for lactic acidosis.[28] When used carefully, the population prevalence of lactic acidosis is similar to that of the background population, and hypoglycaemia from sulphonylureas is a greater problem.[28]

The present consensus is that with eGFR >50, standard dose metformin (2 g/day) can be used; with eGFR <30, do not use metformin; with eGFR 30–50, proceed with caution, i.e. 1 g/day metformin and monitoring of renal function to ensure that it remains stable.

Previously heart failure needing >80 mg furosemide per day contraindicated metformin; but it now appears that in these cases, the heart failure was responsible for the lactic acidosis,[29] rather than the metformin; so cautious use of metformin in heart failure might be reasonable, providing that the heart failure is stable, that renal function is stable and the patient is not hypoxic.

Similarly, liver disease is a contraindication to metformin, even though metformin is renally excreted and not hepatotoxic. Metformin was trialled in non alcoholic steato-hepatitis, and although not beneficial, did not harm the patients;[30] so again, if stable and discussed with the patient, use in hepatic impairment could be considered. For difficult decisions like these, consultation with secondary care may be appropriate.

Gastrointestinal (GI) side-effects are the patient's main concern; interestingly the diarrhoea can start after several years of metformin (although generally soon after starting). If one gives metformin after food, one minimizes the nausea and anorexia, so we generally forget to tell the overweight subjects this. With the diarrhoea, a lower dose sometimes avoids it, and the modified-release (MR) preparation avoids it in 50% of patients;[31] the MR metformin is designed to reduce GI side-effects, not to make it once per day, so one still needs to give two or three doses per day. Recently a 750 mg MR tablet has been introduced with same size and cost as the 500 mg MR tablet; although both are still large, both are extremely cost effective.

In tube-fed patients, a liquid metformin preparation is available, but it is expensive; a second cheaper suspension should appear in 2009.

In normal renal function individuals, one would aim for 1.5–2 g/day; larger doses give more side-effects, but minimal extra plasma glucose reduction.

Metformin doubles the risk of vitamin B_{12} deficiency, which might present as neuropathy or cognitive impairment. One could fully investigate B_{12} deficiency on and off the metformin, but if one removes the metformin, half will still have B_{12} deficiency, and one has removed a valuable agent, perhaps now needing insulin injections. It is simplest to merely replace the B_{12} with intramuscular hydroxycobalamin, although some patients are treated with oral cyanocobalamin to good effect.

Sulphonylureas

These agents stimulate beta-cell function, have been in use for almost 50 years, and have been validated in UKPDS.[17] They are economical and can be used with various comorbidities, although the presence of comorbidities increases the risk of hypoglycaemia; they also cause weight gain.

There are few studies in elderly populations apart from the observational studies in populations showing the risk of hypoglycaemia with the longer-acting agents. Based on the work of Harrower,[32] it seems that tolbutamide and gliclazide are the sulphonylureas to use since they had lowest (but not zero) rate of hypoglycaemia, and more subjects to achieve target HbA1c at 1 year. Glimepiride was not included in that trial, and is attractive because of the once daily dosing and availability of a broad range of tablet sizes, so that the dose is one tablet daily (1–4 mg); however, the hypo rate was significantly higher than with gliclazide MR.[33] Gliclazide MR and plain gliclazide have a similar rates of attained HbA1c and hypoglycaemia.

When using sulphonylureas, it is vital to ensure an adequate diet; in some parts of the UK, mobile meals deliver food Monday to Friday, leaving the patients to go hypoglycaemic at the weekend.

The NICE guidelines recommend that for most people with type 2 diabetes, a sulphonylurea should be the next drug to be added once lifestyle change plus metformin at maximally tolerated doses does not achieve the agreed HbA1c target.

Thiazolidinediones (TZDs) or glitazones

These agonists of the peroxisome proliferator-activated receptors (gamma) decrease insulin resistance.

There is evidence that rosiglitazone increases myocardial infarctions and that pioglitazone decreases the myocardial infarction rate. Pioglitazone is associated with slight decreases in blood pressure (BP) and significant decreases in triglyceride levels, which may explain this. We will consider just pioglitazone in this group.

The advantages of pioglitazone are that it does not cause hypoglycaemia (on its own), decreases adverse vascular events in those who have had one already,[34] delays insulin use[35] and significantly decreases the plasma glucose; it is also beneficial in non-alcoholic steato-hepatitis[36] and can be used in severe renal impairment (chronic kidney disease (CKD) stage 5).

The first disadvantage is peripheral oedema; pioglitazone increases the hospital admission rate with heart failure, but not the mortality rate.[37] Echocardiogram studies show no decline in left ventricular function on the TZDs. We feel that TZDs cause some fluid retention, but not heart failure. The significance is that one would not use a TZD in overt heart failure; one warns the patients of the risk and, if they get a small amount of oedema, 50 mg daily of spironolactone often resolves the issue;[38] significant oedema needs TZD withdrawal.

The second disadvantage is the slight increase in distal fractures (<1% incidence per year); the TZDs probably do cause a slight negative bone balance. At present, we are not sure how to manage this, but we ensure adequate calcium and vitamin D intake, and perform DEXA (dual-energy X-ray absorptiometry) scans.

The third disadvantage is weight gain which is similar to that of a sulphonylurea.[39]

Pioglitazone does take longer to work and to wear off (2–4 weeks) after stopping, compared with other oral agents.

When using pioglitazone, we are cognisant of the pricing structure; so, if adding to a sulphony-lurea, we would start at 15 mg per day and gently build up to avoid hypoglycaemia, but if adding to an agent with almost zero risk of hypo, we would start at 45 mg per day. The metformin/pioglitazone fixed-dose combination product is very competitively priced, for a TZD.

Acarbose

This agent inhibits intestinal alpha-glucosidase and hence retards the breakdown of complex carbohydrates. The dramatic flatulence and lack of hard endpoint data limit its use. However, it does not cause hypoglycaemia on its own, and does not cause weight gain and is relatively economical. Liver and renal impairment are cautions with acarbose. In practice, we give 25 mg at the start of each meal and, if tolerated, after 1 month increase the dose to 50 mg with each meal. Larger doses cause even more wind for little further hypoglycaemic effect. It can also be used with insulin to decrease postprandial hyperglycaemia, and it decreases laxative requirements.

Prandial glucose regulators, nateglinide and repaglinide

These two agents are classed together but show significant differences. Neither have hard outcome data.

Repaglinide is derived from the non-sulphonylurea end of the glibenclamide molecule; when taken, it transiently stimulates beta-cell function, so it is taken at the start of each meal at a dose of 1–4 mg. It has a lower (but not zero) rate of hypoglycaemia than glibenclamide, low risk of weight gain, can be used in significant renal impairment and is ideal in those with erratic dietary habits. It is as potent as other standard oral hypoglycaemic agents, and can be used as a prandial supplement to a basal insulin regimen.

Nateglinide is a heavily modified phenylalanine molecule which resensitizes the beta-cell to secrete insulin in the presence of food; the drug is taken regularly three times daily, and if food is eaten insulin release is augmented, but if no food is taken nothing happens. It is safe in significant hepatic impairment and can be used in significant CKD. The studies suggest that it does not cause hypoglycaemia on its own, but we have found some of our very frail elderly subjects experiencing mild symptomatic hypoglycaemia on nateglinide. One can titrate the dose from 60 mg three times daily up, and this is what we do in the frail elderly; in the fitter subjects, we start at 120 mg three times daily and do not generally escalate to 180 mg three times daily; lower doses do not make them hypo and larger doses do not have much more of a hypoglycaemic effect. The reason that this drug is not more widely used is that it is less potent than other standard oral hypoglycaemic agents with an HbA1c reduction generally of ~0.6%.

The prandial glucose inhibitors can be mixed with all other oral hypoglycaemic agents except sulphonylureas, since both stimulate insulin release by the same final pathway.

Dipeptidyl peptidase-4 inhibitors (DPP-4 inhibitors)

Most are familiar with the two problems of T2DM, insulin resistance and impaired beta-cell function. However, other abnormalities contribute significantly to the hyperglycaemia including inappropriate hyperglucagonaemia, and a decrease in the incretin effect whereby oral intake of food increases insulin secretion. Glucagon-like peptide 1 (GLP-1) suppresses the hyperglucago-naemia, mediates the incretin effect, increases beta-cell function, slows gastric emptying and induces satiety. One can increase GLP-1 levels by inhibiting its breakdown with a DPP-4 inhibitor tablet, or giving an injectable mimetic such as exenatide. The use of these drugs in elderly people has recently been reviewed.[40]

Insulin therapy

This is required for those with T1DM, and given time, most people with T2DM experience deterioration in glucose control rendering insulin necessary. The decision to start insulin in T1DM is straightforward, once the diagnosis has been made. In T2DM, one generally does not get an improvement in HbA1c with traditional insulins unless the HbA1c is >8.5%, although this might be because we tend to supplement with basal insulin, and because lower HbA1c levels are driven more by postprandial glucose excursions, rather than the background/fasting plasma glucose.

There is a wide range of short-acting, long-acting, ready-mixed insulins in both traditional and analogue formats as well as the GLP-1 mimetics, exenatide and related agents.

The T1DM person will probably be under secondary care; but the person with T2DM can initiate insulin in primary care. A full discussion is beyond the scope of this chapter, but there are several options regarding the insulin and regarding the tablets. Choice of insulin regimen depends on who will give it, when they can give it, patient dietary habits, and degree of glycaemic control required; it is also not set in tablets of stone, so that if one regimen does not work, then it is very reasonable to try another.

The NICE guideline recommends that once daily basal insulin therapy should be considered as an option to be added if lifestyle change plus maximally tolerated doses of metformin plus sulphonylurea do not achieve agreed HbA1c target levels.

Once daily glargine; this can be given at anytime, but obtains better control with paradoxically fewer hypos if given in the morning and has fewer hypos and better HbA1c than once daily isophane insulin;[41] the Optiset pen is prefilled; one can set and forget the dose adjustment collar so that the patient does not have to set the dose; however, the plunger is stiff, and it only goes up to 40 units. The prefilled Solostar pen has an easier plunger, can give 80 units and is easy to dial. The problem with this regimen is that the fasting plasma glucose is relatively easy to control, but the glucose levels may rise during the day; options at this stage are either to add in some rapid-acting insulin at breakfast and or lunchtime, or to revert to a shorter-acting insulin, possibly levemir, or a traditional isophane NPH insulin such as Insulatard, or a ready-mixed insulin, e.g. Novomix 30 at breakfast time, or to accept the poor control. We would not recommend the reloadable glargine cartridge pens for older people (Opticlick) because they are very difficult to use.

Patients on Levemir, once daily, tend not to gain weight, particularly if given at bedtime; it also has a lower rate (but not zero) of hypoglycaemia in older people compared with isophane insulin. The prefilled Innolet (eggtimer) device is superb for older people; the insulin is also available in a traditional disposable pen (Flexpen) which older folk find difficult to use at large dose because the plunger gets stiff, and a reloadable pen (Novopen 3) which is excellent if the patient can reload it. The problems with Levemir are that it sometimes needs to be given twice per day (which is not generally a problem if patients are giving it themselves) and sometimes it may need a larger dose than other insulins.

The Novomix 123 regimen[42] uses Novomix 30 which is given before the main meal of the day to control the glucose level before the next meal; once controlled, one assesses whether the glucose levels are controlled at other times, and if not, add some Novomix 30 before the next largest meal. This is a bit complicated for the physician and the patient has to do more monitoring, but it is useful in those who eat just one meal per day.

Exenatide is a different agent that mimics GLP-1, does not cause hypos on its own and leads to weight loss which is greater than one would expect from the nausea that it produces. It is only suitable for treating T2DM. It is given by a prefilled pen twice per day, initially 5 μg twice daily and then 10 μg twice daily after 1 month; the advantages are that no titration is required and weight is lost. However, it only drops the HbA1c by 1% and thus one would probably need to leave patients on any sulphonylurea that they were taking, increasing the risk of hypoglycaemia.[43] The NICE guideline recommends that Exenatide therapy should be considered as an option to be added if lifestyle change plus maximally tolerated doses of metformin plus sulphonylurea do not achieve agreed HbA1c target levels, only in people with a body mass index of ≥35 kg/m². NICE also recommends that Exenatide be continued only if beneficial response occurs and is maintained (at ≥1% HbA1c reduction in 6 months and weight loss of ≥5% at 1 year).

Traditional insulins, e.g. isophane NPH, can be used; they need resuspending by shaking 20 times, and even with this, there is more variability than with analogue insulins; however, they have been used for decades and validated in UKPDS.[17] For T2DM, an overnight regimen seems to be as good as others, but avoids so much weight gain. Often one finds that the glucose levels are acceptable before breakfast and then escalate during the day, requiring a second dose for breakfast. These insulins are recommended by NICE for initial use on the basis of their cost-effectiveness.

Traditional ready-mixed insulin twice per day, e.g. mixtard 30 twice daily or Novomix 30 twice daily. One can try this, and one could split the dose ⅔ a.m., ⅓ p.m. if main meal lunchtime or ½ a.m., ½ p.m. if main meal evening. Studies show that generally once daily long-acting analogue achieves better control in T2DM.

An intensive basal bolus insulin regimen entails one (or sometimes two) injections of long-acting basal insulin and a shot of rapid-acting insulin before each meal. It is straightforward to adjust, generally, but it needs many injections and blood glucose tests to obtain the full benefit. We often get here in stages with a background insulin initially and then, given time, adding in the prandial doses as needed; it is very valuable for ill diabetic inpatients and then we can revert back to their usual less complicated regimen on discharge.

It is vital to teach the patients/carers about the insulin device, and review diet, and management of hypoglycaemia; this can be done by a diabetes specialist nurse based in hospital or primary care.

Starting dose depends on the patient; if starting someone who is otherwise well on insulin at home on their own, we are always cautious: 6 units per day in a frail woman with renal impairment, or 10 units per day in the fitter subjects. The dose is almost guaranteed to be too little; thus it is necessary to titrate the dose which requires the patient (or carer) to measure the blood glucose. Adjustment of the dose can be made by patient or carer (add 2–4 units each week until the fasting glucose tests are <7.0 mmol/l, unless going hypo works well with once daily glargine and Levemir) or by nurse or by doctor; it does not matter who does it, as long as it is done.

Home blood glucose meters

There are many on the market and they continue to improve each year; for the older person, one is looking for a straightforward meter with a large display, a memory and no need to insert a coding chip, calibration strip or cartidges of test strips. Several are on the market, and it is easy to teach most patients how to use them. There is always debate about the indication for home blood glucose monitoring (HBGM), but Diabetes UK have an invaluable consensus view,[44] which is:

◆ Only test if the management will be altered.

◆ Increase testing during intercurrent illness or if considering escalating treatment.

◆ Self blood glucose monitoring is expensive.

◆ For patients on diet plus agents unlikely to cause hypoglycaemia: monitor via HbA1c, and only use HBGM if unable to use HbA1c.

◆ For patients on sulphonylurea: monitor during titration (once to twice per day).

◆ For T2DM patients on basal insulin supplementation: test fasting daily whilst titrating; when stable, test once per day at various times.

◆ For subjects on multiple insulin doses per day: test twice per day whilst titrating if on regimen of two doses per day, and four times per day if on regimen of four doses per day; test at different times.

The NICE guideline recommends that self-monitoring of blood glucose should be only offered as part of self-management education.

One would also note that the amount of testing may vary; for routine assessment of glucose control, a full profile once per week may be more than adequate, but patients should test more frequently if unwell, and before driving a car if on insulin with its risk of hypoglycaemia.

Hypertension

The great value of antihypertensive treatment in elderly diabetic subjects has been assessed in many studies. For instance, in Syst-Eur, treatment with a dihydropyridine calcium channel blocker avoided strokes in non-diabetic subjects, but in diabetic subjects, this treatment avoided stroke, cardiac events and death.[45] On the other hand, in HOT,[46] the aggressively treated diabetic person did worse than the poorly treated non-diabetic person on some hard outcome measures.

The current BP targets from the NICE guidelines[47] are <140 systolic and <80 diastolic BP, whereas JBS 2 and BHS 4 guidelines suggest a target of <130 systolic.[48,49] HOT[46] demonstrated benefit with a 140/81 achieved BP, and ADVANCE[50] showed benefit with a 135/75 mm achieved BP. However, these studies are biased towards elderly patients in their sixties rather than those in their eighties; HYVET shows the benefit of a <150 systolic target in octogenarians.[51] So in the younger, fitter subjects, we aim for a 130 systolic target, but would accept a 150 systolic target in the frail older person. Given the large BP reductions needed by some patients to reach the target, and the difficulty tolerating multiple agents, missing the target is quite common despite trying.

Choice of first-line agent is often an irrelevant question since multiple agents are required. Given the benefit of a calcium channel blocker/angiotensin-converting enzyme inhibitor (ACEI) combination in ASCOT,[26] one could argue in favour of these, or in favour of an ACE/indapamide combination given in the ADVANCE study,[50] or in favour of an angiotensin receptor blockers (ARBs) given the benefit in the LIFE diabetes subgroup,[52] or the equivalence to ACE in ONTARGET.[53] Indeed, the simplest thing to state would be to avoid use of beta-blocker for hypertension; although beta-blockers decrease BP, their effect on avoiding stroke and heart failure is not as great as other agents.[12,13,52] One would consider beta-blocker if one were treating another problem such as tachycardia, angina, post-myocardial infarction prophylaxis or heart failure, but there might be another agent that would also treat several problems.

The BP control algorithm from NICE[54] is basically the ABCD algorithm without the B, as in BHS 4.[55]

It is often easier to control BP than blood sugar; given the dramatic benefit of BP intervention in UKPDS[56] and Syst-Eur,[45] can one focus on the BP and forget the blood sugar? UKPDS 75[57] shows that the benefits of BP and blood sugar control are additive, so one has to try one's best to control both.

Dyslipidaemia

The Heart Protection Study had three important messages:[44] (i) a random, not fasting, total cholesterol was used; (ii) that treating diabetic subjects with a random total cholesterol ≥3.5 mmol/l is beneficial, even in the lowest tertile of raised cholesterol; (iii) this applied to subjects aged 75–80 years at start of study.

The benefit of cholesterol reduction in individuals aged 70–82 years was also shown in PROSPER.[58]

When looking at older subjects, we would look at the person's biological age and treat accordingly; side-effects of the statin are generally independently related to age and renal impairment; in significant CKD (stage 4–5), one would use atorvastatin.

Antiplatelet and anticoagulant agents

Antiplatelet agents have been advised for use in older people with diabetes, bearing in mind peptic ulcer disease,[46,48] but recent work suggests that they may not be beneficial except for those with established cardiovascular disease.[59] Atrial fibrillation is more common in diabetic people and carries worse outcomes which are improved by warfarin; in all ages, warfarin decreases the thromboembolic rate from 8.6 to 2.8 events per 100 patient-years.[60]

Feet and neuropathy

There are several excellent books on this topic.[61,62]

An annual assessment of feet is required regarding neuropathy (using monofilament), peripheral vascular disease, deformity, skin condition and state of footwear and insole.

If the patient has had a previous ulcer, or has several risk factors for foot ulcers, he/she should be referred to an orthotist for consideration of surgical shoes (if they are walking), to avoid ulceration and infection.

An infected foot is a limb-threatening condition and is a major cause of hospitalization; it must be treated aggressively and empirically.[62] Superficial infections are often aerobic Gram-positive cocci, but deeper infections are characteristically due to multiple different organisms; the infected diabetic foot may not show marked signs of severe infection, so one needs a high degree of clinical suspicion. If patients develop an infected foot ulcer, we would use a 3 week oral course of broad spectrum antibiotics such as augmentin or clindamycin, and any necrotic tissue needs urgent debridement, e.g. by state-registered podiatrist. A short course of a low dose of a narrow spectrum antibiotic may allow the foot to worsen dramatically. For worsening or persisting foot problems, referral to a multidisciplinary diabetic foot clinic is proven to save lower extremities from amputation. The elderly amputee has a small chance of becoming independently mobile again.

Neuropathy may be due to the diabetes, but given the multiple co-morbidities in elderly people and in particular the high prevalence of vitamin B_{12} deficiency, one must consider other causes, ask about alcohol intake, and measure B_{12}, thyroid function and serum electrophoresis.

Eyes

Patients should have an annual assessment of their eyes unless already under ophthalmologist care, or blind, or cannot cooperate with laser or cataract extraction. Digital retinal photography is the optimum tool with best sensitivity/specificity compared with careful exam by consultant ophthalmologist (which is clearly not feasible for the large population needing screening). It is then just necessary to ensure that local patients are being screened. If they cannot get to the screening centre, opticians will visit at home or in residential care, but their payment is minimal for the time concerned unless they sell spectacles at the same time; alternatively, one could have physicians visit nursing homes for an annual review, although this too would need consideration of funding (see Chapter 16).

Kidneys

One must check renal function and for microalbuminuria.

The use of eGFR is invaluable; since older people may have little muscle mass, their serum creatinine value can be unremarkable in the setting of quite advanced renal impairment (see Chapter 14).[63]

Microalbuminuria

If microalbuminuria is present the QOF clinical indicator says that the person should be treated with an ACE or an ARB (if ACE is not tolerated); these agents have been shown to reduce microalbuminuria and decrease the rise in creatinine in T2DM.[13] However, the main problem for older diabetic patients with microalbuminuria is vascular death rather than end-stage renal disease,[64] and one would be doing the utmost to prevent vascular disease anyway. Vascular risk was dramatically reduced by giving ramipril 10 mg at night in the HOPE study;[65,66] initially, this was thought to be due to a special property of ramipril (although it had been seen in meta-analyses of ACEIs in post-myocardial infarction studies) since the BP the next morning was only minimally decreased, but it may be explained by the 16 mm systolic fall in BP overnight.[67] Indapamide has been shown to reduce microalbuminuria in diabetes in the NESTOR study,[68] but only the HOPE study showed hard outcomes of avoiding vascular events and reduction in mortality.

Diabetes and mental health

Diabetes is associated with a 2–3-fold increase in dementia; this is generally considered to be vascular in origin, but Alzheimer's type dementia might be more prevalent than in the non-diabetic population. Dementia may progress more rapidly in the diabetic population.

The first step is avoidance; there is evidence that good BP control is associated with less risk of developing dementia; there is no evidence that aspirin use, control of lipids or control of blood glucose is beneficial; indeed, there is limited case report evidence that profound hypoglycaemia can cause permanent cognitive loss.

Although guidelines do recommend annual testing for cognitive impairment using a Folstein Mini-Mental State Examination score, this rarely happens in practice. Cognitive impairment may present in several ways, but loss of glycaemic control may be the first obvious sign in the older diabetic person. Plasma glucose may arise from poor drug or dietary compliance, but the patient may present with hypoglycaemia either due to lack of diet, or due to taking insulin twice, having forgotten that the first dose has been taken.

There is also an increased risk of depression with diabetes—hardly a surprise—but depression is a risk factor for future diabetes. Treatment of depression can improve self-care and the presence of depression should be considered and sought, e.g. with a Geriatric Depression Score or similar tool (see Chapter 22).

Residential care

Diabetes is an independent risk factor for admission to residential care, with a prevalence of 25% in UK care homes. If a patient is well controlled on oral agents, then residential care homes (private rest homes, local authority social care homes) may be appropriate. However, we have grave concerns about insulin-treated diabetic subjects going into these homes; the residents may need nursing home care for administration of insulin, blood glucose monitoring and care during inter-current illness; residential care home staff generally cannot give insulin and it is difficult for district nurses to manage all the insulin injections in their area that the patients cannot give themselves.

Special attention must be given to the risk of hypoglycaemia. Upon admission to care homes, blood glucose levels may drop due to enforced medication compliance, inability to be indiscreet with diet, and poor dietary intake. It is known that 50% of care home residents do not receive their required calorie intake.[69] With time, the resident may eat less, lose weight and be at further risk of hypoglycaemia. The management is to be aware of the problem, monitor glucose levels, be more relaxed about diet, e.g. avoid sugary drinks, sweets etc., and use agents that do not produce hypoglycaemia if possible.

Similarly, the residents' BP may drop as their weight decreases, with a consequent reduction in need for medication. With the poor renal function in care home residents and poor oral intake, we tend to remove ACEIs, ARBs and diuretics first, although of course each patient needs individual assessment.

Residents of nursing homes generally have short survival due to their severe frailty and comorbid conditions, which is why they went into the home in the first instance. Age and poor renal function are independent risk factors for adverse reactions to statins, which are unlikely to benefit the resident long term; we generally stop statins when patients go into nursing home care, but maintain them in subjects going into residential care homes. Again, each patient needs individual consideration.

If the subjects can comply with laser therapy or a cataract extraction under local anaesthetic, then they need an eye examination each year. This can be very difficult to organize and options include doctors or opticians visiting the home to review the eyes or taking the patient to the routine eye examinations that should be present in each district.

Nursing home residents have at-risk feet; they need regular simple podiatry from whomever can administer it, and attention to pressure areas by an appropriate registered general nurse (see Chapter 26).

Falls

People with T2DM have a 70% increased risk of osteoporotic fractures due to their increased risk of falls;[70] this is probably related to their risk factors for falls which include visual impairment, peripheral neuropathy, hypotension, hypoglycaemia and cognitive impairment. A referral to a falls service may help (see Chapter 13).

Care during intercurrent illness

This has no evidence base behind it, apart from case reports. There are many guidelines available on the internet, but we particularly like the West Suffolk[71] and the DARTS Tayside[72] guidelines.

Patients should ensure adequate fluid intake and test more frequently, if they are performing HBGM, and should test for ketones if plasma glucose is high, e.g. ≥13 mmol/l, although patients' clinical state is just as important.

The patient should know when to call for help, e.g. if unable to eat or drink, if repeated vomiting or diarrhoea, if hyperglycaemia (e.g. ≥25 mmol/l) or hypoglycaemia, if significant ketosis, and in the older person in particular if they become drowsy or confused. The patients should know whom to call for help.

One would continue hypoglycaemic agents generally, and ensure adequate carbohydrate intake.

If the patient is taking insulin, and becoming hyperglycaemic, then they can increase the insulin, quick-acting if one has a choice, by 2–4 units per dose until better.

If they are having difficulty eating, then they could take a small carbohydrate-containing drink each hour such as 100 ml milk, 100 ml pure fruit juice, 50 ml of Lucozade, 150 ml of normal lemonade or a scoop of ice cream.

There are concerns regarding the patient with vomiting in particular, but also diarrhoea; if this persists, and the blood glucose level becomes abnormal and patients generally need inpatient care, especially if insulin-treated. There is also a concern about renal function deteriorating in this scenario; to try to avoid this, we would consider stopping ACEIs, ARBs, and diuretics temporarily in this setting; with the risk of lactic acidosis in renal impairment with metformin, one might consider omitting the metformin for 24 h, and monitoring with HBGM. If someone is this ill for >24 h, they probably need inpatient care.

One should also check that the heels are not at risk from pressure sores.

Thyroid disease

Thyroid disease is common in elderly people, but studies show that they have fewer symptoms of hyper- or hypothyroidism than younger people. Thyroid disease is common in elderly people with prevalences of hyperthyroidism of 0.5–2.3% and of diagnosed overt hypothyroidism of 2–7.4%.

One would test in specific indications such as cognitive impairment, atrial fibrillation, weight loss, peripheral neuropathy or entrapment neuropathies, or proximal myopathy. It is not worth screening the whole population routinely, but people with previous hyperthyroidism, those on amiodarone, and hypothyroid patients should be tested each year. It may be worth screening women aged >50 years since 1 in 70 may have unknown thyroid disease, and screening diabetic people every 5 years; it is not worth routinely screening men or younger women, and there are many recommendations on whom to screen routinely.[73]

The assessment of thyroid disease has been made much simpler by the introduction of the supersensitive thyroid-stimulating hormone (TSH) assay 15 years ago; but now one finds subjects with normal free T4, and abnormal TSH levels; their management is outlined in Table 10.2.

Mild subclinical hypothyroidism with TSH 6–10 and normal T4 may progress to overt hypothyroidism; some reviewers feel that it has no associated morbidity or mortality, whereas the suggestion of increased mortality seems to be most likely in younger people. For mild subclinical hypothyroidism, observation with annual thyroid function test (TFTs) is advised rather than treatment.[74]

In subclinical hypothyroidism when the TSH is >10, the progression to overt hypothyroidism in the next year is so high that thyroxine treatment is warranted.[74]

Treatment of hypothyroidism is with thyroxine 25 μg daily, increasing by 25 μg each month until TSH is normalized with annual review of TFT once stable.[75] In the setting of cognitive impairment, one often finds that the occurrence of hypothyroidism is present by chance, not causally, so that the subjects continue to decline cognitively despite treating the hypothyroidism.

In subclinical hyperthyroidism, at present the recommendation is merely to observe, since it will often revert to normal.[73,74]

There is a choice of treatment for thyrotoxicosis; one can improve patients' symptoms rapidly with an oral antithyroid drug such as carbimazole 40 mg daily, possibly with propranolol. Thence options are to titrate the carbimazole to normalize TFTs (and the free thyroxine often becomes normal before the TSH), to continue the carbimazole but add in thyroxine building up to 100–150 μg daily (block and replace therapy), or radioactive iodine. The carbimazole may cause agranulocytosis, hepatitis, skin rashes, etc., and are an extra tablet burden. A review of whether to titrate the oral antithyroid drug or to block and replace concluded that trial data were poor, that titration seemed to have fewer side-effects, and that perhaps radioactive iodine should be considered. The radioactive iodine may need a second dose, has a high chance of late hypothyroidism and the patient must be continent; however, it is our preferred choice to avoid tablets and their risks. Toxic goitre is more common than Graves disease in the older person and requires a larger dose of radioactive iodine.

During severe illness, any abnormality of thyroid function can occur, but it is generally suppressed TSH and low thyroxine levels; if the patient survives (and this is a marker that they may not) then the thyroid function will generally normalize.[15,76] Thus in the very sick person, the TFTs should be interpreted with the clinical picture (as all tests should be).

Amiodarone is a major problem; it is an effective antiarhythmic with a small, negatively inotropic effect; however, it is 39% iodine by weight and has a half-life in older people of ~60 days. Amiodarone often induces transient changes in thyroid function, so abnormal values always need repeating (as they do anyway); mild abnormalities of thyroid function are common and it is important not to overinterpret small abnormalities but to monitor them. But amiodarone-associated hypothyroidism occurs in 6–14% of the population and is more common in elderly females. The most straightforward approach is to continue the amiodarone, and add in thyroxine

Table 10.2 Thyroid function test interpretation

TSH (mIU/l)	Free thyroxine	Interpretation	Management
Elevated	Subnormal	Overt hypothyroidism	Confirm and treat
4.5–10	Normal	Mild subclinical hypothyroidism	Monitor annually
>10	Normal	Subclinical hypothyroidism	Confirm and treat
Suppressed	Elevated	Overt hyperthyroidism	Confirm and treat
<0.45	Normal	Subclinical hyperthyroidism	Monitor annually

TSH, thyroid-stimulating hormone.

72. DARTS Tayside Diabetes Network. *Sick Day Rules for Patients onTablets*. Dundee: DARTS Tayside Diabetes Network; 2008. Available at: http//taysidedn.dundee.ac.uk/Documetns/Uploaded/SickDayRulespatientsonTablets%20.pdf.

73. Mohandas R, Gupta KL. Managing thyroid dysfunction in the elderly. Answers to seven common questions. *Postgrad Med* 2003;113:54–6.

74. Surks MI, Ortiz E, Daniels GH, *et al.* Subclinical thyroid disease: scientific review and guidelines for diagnosis and management. *J Am Med Assoc* 2004;291:228–38.

75. Premawardhana LDKE, Lazarus JH. Management of thyroid disorders. *Postgrad Med* 2006;82(971):552–8.

76. Umpierrez GE. Euthyroid sick syndrome. *South Med J* 2002;95:506–13.

77. Pavord SR, Girach A, Price DE, Absalom SR, Falconer-Smith J, Howlett TA. A retrospective audit of the combined pituitary function test, using the insulin stress test, TRH and GnRH in a district laboratory. *Clin Endocrinol (Oxf)* 1992;36:135–9.

Chapter 11

Haematological conditions

David Allsup and Michael Small

Introduction

Haematological abnormalities in elderly patients represent a frequent challenge to the primary care physician. Whereas acute, symptomatic conditions such as acute leukaemia are easily managed with prompt referral to a haematology unit, the interpretation of incidentally identified abnormalities in a full blood count or a coagulation screen may be more challenging, especially in the asymptomatic patient. Additionally, the use of more sophisticated diagnostic methods has resulted in an increased detection of lymphoproliferative disorders such as chronic lymphocytic leukaemia (CLL) and monoclonal gammopathy of uncertain significance (MGUS), conditions often with a prolonged asymptomatic phase but which may in some cases progress to overt disease states. Such early identification of haematological abnormalities may be perceived as advantageous but considerable anxiety may be caused in the minds of patients, and of the physician, as regular follow-up is often advised even though it may only be a minority who eventually undergo disease progression and require therapy.

Many studies have identified a fall in the mean haemoglobin concentration with increasing age;[1] however, these findings are inconsistent and often derived from studies with small sample sizes. There is therefore no case for a distinct normal range for red cell parameters in the elderly population and similarly leukocyte and platelet counts remain stable throughout adult life. This stability of the blood counts occurs in spite of a decrease in marrow cellularity at sites such as the sternum and iliac crest where normal haematopoiesis is gradually replaced by fatty tissue.[2] However, pathologies manifesting with a haematological abnormality do increase in prevalence with advancing years, indicating that elderly patients with an abnormality in the blood count should be investigated for underlying disease rather than attributing such an abnormality to the ageing process.

Anaemia

The World Health Organization defines anaemia as a haemoglobin level of <13 g/dl for adult males and of <12 g/dl for females. With increasing age the incidence of anaemia rises, with 11% of men and 10.2% of women aged >65 years being anaemic rising to >20% in both sexes aged >85 years.[3] In many cases the anaemia will be mild and asymptomatic, and in 83% of cases a thorough assessment will reveal an underlying cause.[4] Anaemia in elderly people is associated with an increase in all-cause mortality and possibly also with impairment in quality of life, though the possibility that the underlying pathology responsible for the anaemia is the actual cause of these outcomes cannot be discounted.[5]

The initial approach to investigation of anaemia in an elderly patient is identical to that in a younger individual, with a thorough history and examination required prior to an interpretation of laboratory results. Anaemias are usefully subclassified by the size of the red cells into microcytic,

normocytic and macrocytic. The presence of concurrent abnormalities in the leukocyte or platelet count in the anaemic patient can also give diagnostic clues to the astute physician.

Microcytic anaemia

A microcytic anaemia in an elderly patient almost always indicates underlying iron deficiency.
The diagnosis is confirmed by an assessment of the serum ferritin, which may be low; serum iron
and the percentage saturation of the iron-binding protein transferrin, also low, or by an increased
concentration of serum transferrin receptor, though this latter investigation is infrequently performed. Examination of a blood film will reveal characteristic hypochromic microcytes with
'pencil cells' in the presence of iron deficiency. Interpretation of these results can be confounded
by the fact that ferritin is an acute phase protein whose plasma concentration can be spuriously
elevated in the presence of concurrent inflammation or malignancy. Confirmation of iron deficiency should prompt a search for a source of gastrointestinal (GI) bleeding such as a gastric or
colonic malignancy, oesophago-gastritis or ulceration, which are present in 62% of patients
investigated.[6] Effort should not be expended on faecal occult blood analysis in the presence of
confirmed iron deficiency due to the relatively high incidence of occult GI malignancy in this
population. Dietary causes of iron deficiency are rare and a source of blood loss from the GI tract
should always be sought before ascribing the iron deficiency anaemia to dietary insufficiency.[6]
Other causes of a microcytic anaemia include anaemias of chronic disease, haemoglobinopathies
and rarely sideroblastic anaemia.

Case History 1: iron deficiency anaemia

A widow aged 82 years presents to her practioner feeling tired all the time. She is an infrequent attendee at
the surgery. On further questioning she reports being more breathless when going upstairs and has had some
epigastric pain after eating. She has been taking citalopram 20 mg once daily since her husband died last year
as well as aspirin 75 mg once daily. On examination she is pale, has a mild tachycardia and some tenderness
in the epigastrium. The patient doesn't want to make much fuss and asks if you can prescribe a tonic to pick
her up. You arrange some initial blood tests and advise her to attend again in a week. Her results show a
microcytic hypochromic anaemia prompting you to arrange for a ferritin level before seeing her again. The
ferritin is low, confirming iron-deficient anaemia. The patient declines an endoscopic examination of the
stomach and is commenced on a proton pump inhibitor for a possible gastritis and ferrous sulphate 200 mg
three times a day. After several months her anaemia improves and she feels better.

Six months later she re-presents with dysphagia and recurrent iron deficiency anaemia. She is now willing
to undergo an endoscopic examination which reveals a large carcinoma at the gastro-oesophageal junction.

Macrocytic anaemia

Macrocytic anaemias are commonly due to megaloblastosis secondary to deficiencies of vitamin
B_{12} or folic acid, haemolysis, hypothyroidism, liver disease and alcohol abuse. Haematological
pathologies such as myelodysplasia, myeloma and other malignant infiltrations of the bone marrow can also present with a macrocytosis. Appropriate investigations include estimations of
vitamin B_{12} and folate, a reticulocyte count and direct antiglobulin test (formerly known as the
Coombs test) as well as liver and thyroid function tests. Folate levels can be assessed using either
a serum folate or red-cell folate assay; however, both methods have their limitations and a normal
result should not automatically deter the physician from diagnosing folate deficiency if other
features favour the diagnosis, particularly if there are megaloblastic features in the blood film and
the serum B_{12} is normal. Likewise megaloblastic anaemia due to B_{12} deficiency can, in certain
circumstances, occur in the presence of a normal assay result for serum B_{12}.

B_{12} deficiency is most commonly due to pernicious anaemia and is readily diagnosed by the detection of anti-intrinsic factor antibodies or following a gastric biopsy. Other possible causes of low serum B_{12} levels include previous gastric or ileal resections, terminal ileal disease and intestinal bacterial overgrowth. Folate deficiency may also be secondary to malabsorptive states and because of limited body stores may also be due to poor oral intake. This is particularly relevant in the elderly population where up to 35% have evidence of folate deficiency.[7]

An elderly patient with an undiagnosed macrocytic anaemia, after exclusion of other causes and in the absence of other cytopenias or features to suggest haematological malignancy, should therefore be given a trial of folate and B_{12} supplementation, even if assays for these vitamins are normal before referral to haematologist for consideration of an examination of the bone marrow.

Normocytic anaemia

Normocytic anaemias therefore describe the anaemias when the MCV lies within the normal range. These anaemias may also be secondary to deficiencies of iron, B_{12} or folic acid occurring either in isolation or combination. The anaemia of chronic disease (ACD) is characterized by normocytic normochromic anaemia with a haemoglobin concentration of typically between 7 and 10 g/dl and is found in 19.7% of anaemic patients aged >65 years.[3] ACD is associated with malignancy, inflammatory conditions such as rheumatoid arthritis and Crohn's disease as well as with chronic infections. To reflect this aetiological relationship, ACD has also been described as the anaemia of chronic inflammation.[8] The pathological defect in ACD is one of a failure of incorporation of iron into haemoglobin resulting in chronic anaemia. Investigation classically reveals a low serum iron concentration and a normal or low serum transferrin with a reduced saturation of transferrin-iron-binding sites. The serum ferritin is usually within the normal range and if examination of bone marrow iron stores is undertaken these will be normal with increased storage of iron in macrophages. The diagnosis of ACD is made in the presence of a stable anaemia occuring against a background of chronic inflammation and when other possible causes for the anaemia have been excluded.

Therapy for ACD is directed at the underlying cause, but often this can be difficult to achieve particularly in the presence of malignancy. Erythropoietin injections are effective in iron-replete patients but care needs to be taken to avoid overcorrection of the haemoglobin to >11–12 g/dl as this has been associated with adverse outcomes.[9] Iron supplementation has no role in patients with ACD with normal iron stores but may be effective in patients refractory to erythropoietin, particularly when given parenterally.[10] Other anaemias should have the underlying cause treated as appropriate, with, for example, supplementation of iron, folic acid or B_{12} depending on the deficiency identified.

Despite extensive investigation, 34% of patients aged >65 years will have unexplained anaemia[3] and it is this group who should be considered for referral to a haematology department. A proportion of these patients will have a myelodysplastic syndrome as a cause of their anaemia. Indicators of an underlying myelodysplasia are a progressive anaemia with no identifiable cause, the presence of concurrent neutropenia and thrombocytopenia, dysplastic features in the blood film and palpable splenomegaly or hepatomegaly. A bone marrow examination to assess the morphology of the marrow and to search for any chromosomal rearrangements can help in the confirmation of this diagnosis.

Neutrophil abnormalities

The neutrophil count remains remarkably static throughout adult life ($1.7–7.5 \times 10^9/l$) with no evidence of a decline in those aged >60 years. The neutrophilic response to infection may be blunted in an elderly population and there is a progressive age-related defect in neutrophil-mediated phagocytosis that may contribute to an increase in the incidence of infections.[11] Neutropenia and neutrophilia are relatively common incidental findings in this population and are usually of little relevance but can, on occasion, be indicative of a primary haematological abnormality.

Neutropenia

Isolated neutropenia in older people is commonly secondary to bacterial or viral infections, medication, immune-mediated peripheral consumption and connective tissue diseases such as rheumatoid arthritis. Mild neutropenia (neutrophils $>1 \times 10^9/l$) is associated with a low risk of infection with the risk increasing with neutrophil counts of $0.5–1 \times 10^9/l$ and being of greatest risk in the presence of severe neutropenia as defined by a neutrophil count of $<0.5 \times 10^9/l$.[12] Severe neutropenia requires urgent assessment due to the significant morbidity and mortality associated with neutropenic sepsis in these patients.

Often an underlying cause can be identified in mild-to-moderate neutropenia and no further action is required. However, patients with unexplained, progressive or severe neutropenia should be referred to a haematologist for assessment. Myelodysplastic syndromes may present in elderly people with an isolated neutropenia, as can large granular lymphocytic proliferations, a heterogeneous group of lymphoproliferative disorders (LPDs) characterized by a mild lymphocytosis and neutropenia. The use of prophylactic antibiotics in asymptomatic patients with severe neutropenia is controversial due to the associated risk of antibiotic resistance. Granulocyte-colony-stimulating factor injections may normalise the neutrophil count in neutropenic patients but should only be used in the presence of sepsis, or a high risk of sepsis, and a neutrophil count of $<1 \times 10^9/l$.

Neutrophilia

An elevated neutrophil count is not primarily associated with adverse health outcomes and usually occurs in response to significant disease states. Sepsis, chronic inflammation, malignancy, corticosteroids and cigarette smoking are commonly associated with an elevation of the neutrophil count. A persistent neutrophilia in the absence of an obvious cause should prompt a search for an occult malignancy or chronic sepsis. Occasionally an elevated neutrophil count may indicate an underlying myeloproliferative disorder, a diagnosis made more likely by the presence of coexistent polycythaemia, thrombocytosis or hepatosplenomegaly. Chronic myeloid leukaemia and chronic neutrophilic leukaemias are rare conditions that can present with a mild neutrophilia and which are characterized by rearrangements of chromosomes 9 and 22 identified by cytogenetic or molecular analysis of peripheral blood or bone marrow.

Lymphocytoses

The immune system has two main mechanisms with which to counter infectious agents, the innate immune response and the humoral, or adaptive, response. Innate immunity provides an immediate response to possible infections and is mediated by neutrophils, macrophages, eosinophils, natural killer cells, complement proteins and pre-formed IgM antibodies. The innate response is rapid in onset but generic and non-specific. By contrast, the adaptive immune response is based upon the generation of specific memory B- and T-lymphocytes that can rapidly promote the formation of immunoglobulin molecules that display specificity towards proteins associated with an infectious agent.

Immunosenescence describes a complex process characterized by a progressive impairment in innate and humoral immunity that occurs throughout adult life and ultimately results in an increased risk of infection or death. In addition to a decline in neutrophil function, numerous age-related changes in T- and B-lymphocytes have been described that are also thought to contribute to immunosenescence. Whereas the absolute lymphocyte count remains unchanged throughout adult life there is a progressive age-related decrease in the ratio of naive to memory T-cells, in addition to the development of complex functional and cell signalling abnormalities within T-cell subsets. This T-lymphocyte dysregulation may cause secondary B-cell abnormalities with consequential impairment of the antibody response in the elderly patient.[13]

An elevated lymphocyte count ($>3.5 \times 10^9$/l) is a common pathological abnormality which, if transient and associated with an obvious infection, can be confidently labelled as being reactive in nature. More troublesome is the persistent lymphocytosis often identified incidentally. Such a lymphocytosis can be a reactive phenomenon caused by a concurrent disease state or can represent a primary lymphocyte disorder. Common causes of a sustained reactive lymphocytosis in older people include autoimmune disorders, occult non-haematological malignancy, splenectomy, hyposplenism, chronic inflammation and cigarette smoking. By contrast, disorders such as CLL, monoclonal B-lymphocytosis (MBL), marginal zone lymphoma, follicular lymphoma, mantle cell lymphoma, hairy cell leukaemia and large granular lymphocytic leukaemia are all potential causes of a primary lymphocytosis with CLL and MBL being by far the most prevalent.

In children and young adults, viral infections predominate as a cause of lymphocytoses, LPDs being extremely rare. However, in older individuals a sustained lymphocytosis, in the absence of an underlying autoimmune or inflammatory disorder, is more likely to be secondary to LPD, most commonly MBL.

Monoclonal B-lymphocytosis

MBL describes a heterogeneous group of subclinical LPDs characterized by a population of clonal B-lymphocytes detectable in the peripheral blood at a level of $<5 \times 10^9$ cells/l. Usually the clonal cells detected in MBL are phenotypically identical to those present in CLL, but the latter condition is diagnosed when the clonal cell level is $>5 \times 10^9$/l. MBL is a common incidental diagnosis present in up to 5.5% of the population aged >65 years, but in many of these cases the proportion of clonal B-cells is exceedingly low and can often be associated with a normal total lymphocyte count.[14] The clinical relevance of the detection of small populations of clonal B cells in otherwise asymptomatic individuals can be debated, especially as the rate of progression to an overt LPD such as CLL is low at 1–2% per year.[15]

Chronic lymphocytic leukaemia

CLL is diagnosed following the identification of clonal B cells, with a characteristic immunophenotype, $>5 \times 10^9$ cells/l or in association with tissue involvement as evidenced by lymphadenopathy or hepatosplenomegaly. It is the commonest leukaemia in the West with an estimated annual incidence in the USA of 2–6 cases per 100 000,[16] predominantly affecting men aged >50 years.[17] Some CLL patients survive for many years with no adverse symptoms whereas others have a rapidly progressive disease that is often refractory to treatment. The majority of patients present with early stage disease (stage A) that is associated with a median survival of >10 years and usually do not need therapy at presentation. By contrast, those CLL patients presenting with anaemia or thrombocytopenia due to extensive bone marrow involvement (stage C) have a poor prognosis and need treatment.[18] At least half of all CLL patients have a favourable genetic phenotype (somatically hypermutated V_H genes) and may have a survival similar to age-matched controls.[19]

Treatment for CLL is only indicated in the presence of symptoms and is non-curative; this is also true for most other LPDs such as follicular and marginal zone lymphomas.

Elderly patients with a persistent unexplained lymphocytosis should be referred for investigation if there are coexistent features to suggest LPD such as lymphadenopathy or hepatomegaly, if there are associated cytopenias or in the presence of systemic symptoms (weight loss, night sweats or fevers). In the absence of these features the asymptomatic patient with an incidentally identified lymphocytosis can be safely monitored in the community assuming that it is non-progressive and the patient remains well.

Paraproteins

Paraproteins, or M proteins, are monoclonal immunoglobulin molecules detectable in the serum and are common incidental findings. The presence of a paraprotein denotes the existence of a population of clonal B-lymphocytes producing immunoglobulin molecules all of which are of the same isotype (IgG, IgA, IgM or rarely IgD) and of the same specificity and affinity for a single antigenic domain. Immunoglobulin molecules are composed of heavy and light chains, with the lower molecular weight light chains undergoing glomerular filtration and reabsorption in the proximal renal tubule. In conditions of a marked excess of light chain production the ability to reabsorb the filtered light chain is overwhelmed and the protein becomes detectable in the urine, where it is described as Bence Jones protein.[20]

The prevalence of paraproteins is high in the elderly population and increases with age.[21] Often a paraprotein is found following the unexpected detection of a raised total protein performed as part of a routine biochemical profile. Further investigations in the form of serum protein electrophoresis subsequently demonstrate an increase in immunoglobulin, which is then characterized by immunofixation. However, serum protein electrophoresis, assessment of immunoglobulins and immunofixation are often specifically requested by physicians seeking to diagnose myeloma in elderly patients with symptoms such as anaemia, renal impairment or bone pains.

The common causes of a paraprotein include monoclonal gammopathy of uncertain significance (MGUS), multiple myeloma, solitary plasmacytomas, amyloidosis and LPDs such as CLL and Waldenström's macroglobulinaemia. In addition paraproteins may be found in association with acute or chronic infections, autoimmune conditions, inflammatory disorders and non-haematological malignancies.

Multiple myeloma

The initial approach to a patient with a paraprotein should be directed at the exclusion of multiple myeloma or an LPD as a possible cause of the paraprotein. Myeloma is commonly associated with either an IgG, IgA or light-chain-only paraprotein. Occasionally myeloma may be associated with an IgD paraprotein,[22] while IgM myeloma is an extremely rare and distinct entity.[23] The common clinical features associated with myeloma include bone pain possibly associated with lytic lesions or osteoporosis, renal impairment, anaemia, hypercalcaemia, symptomatic hyperviscosity, amyloidosis and recurrent bacterial infections. These symptoms have been described as myeloma-related organ or tissue impairment (ROTI). The diagnosis of myeloma rests on demonstrating a paraprotein in the presence of one or more ROTI features and the identification of clonal plasma cells in the bone marrow or in a plasmacytoma.[24] Myeloma therapy is indicated in the presence of symptoms and can include radiotherapy to painful bone lesions, corticosteroids and oral alkylating agents. Novel agents such as thalidomide, the thalidomide analogue lenalidomide and the proteasome inhibitor bortezimib can also be effective in elderly patients. Autologous stem cell transplantation is an effective therapy that can prolong overall survival but is restricted to patients without significant comorbidities and with a good performance status. All patients with symptomatic myeloma should be considered for therapy with a bisphosphonate such as sodium clodronate, pamidronate or zolendronate as these are proven to reduce bone pain and fractures.[25]

Case History 2: back pain and a raised erythrocyte sedimentation rate (ESR)

A woman aged 89 years presents to the nurse practitioner with a 3 month history of feeling tired all the time. She has aches and pains all over and thinks she has lost weight. The nurse practitioner is concerned and so arranges some blood tests and a follow-up appointment with the doctor at the end of the week. One week later the lady reattends and the doctor notes that most of the pain is in the patient's lower back, which is sufficiently severe to keep her awake at night. The results of the investigations are as follows, with normal ranges in parentheses:

Haemoglobin 11.0 g/dl (12.5–16 g/dl).

Platelets 400×10^9/dl (150–400).

White cell counts 4.0×10^9/dl (4–11), with a normal differential count.

ESR 90 mm/h (<35).

Renal function is normal with a glomerular filtration rate of 70 ml/min. Liver function tests and serum calcium are also normal.

Albumin 30 g/l (36–48).

Total protein 91 g/l (62–78).

Plain X-rays of the lumbar spine are arranged and show generalized osteopenia with some degenerative changes.

One week later, serum electrophoresis and subsequent immunofixation reveals the presence of a 32 g/l IgG kappa paraprotein with low IgA and IgM. The lady is referred to the local haematology department where a bone marrow examination demonstrates the presence of 25% plasma cells within the aspirate sample, confirming a diagnosis of multiple myeloma. In view of her symptoms (back pain and mild anaemia) she is commenced on therapy with the oral alkylator melphalan. She is poorly tolerant of this therapy and later opts for supportive therapy with analgesia and transfusion of red cells as required.

Monoclonal gammopathy of uncertain significance

MGUS is diagnosed in the presence of a paraprotein but where there are no clinical features to suggest myeloma. A diagnosis of MGUS is made in the presence of a paraprotein with a concentration of <30 g/l and where there are <10% plasma cells in the bone marrow and no evidence of myeloma-related tissue damage.[24] The prevalence of MGUS is 3.2% at age >50 years and 5.3% at age >70 years,[21] with a risk of progression to myeloma or a similar malignancy of 1% per annum.[26]

IgM paraproteins constitute ~20% of all paraproteins and are associated with an underlying LPD in 30% of cases at presentation.[27] After a median of 60 months the probability of a patient with an isolated IgM paraprotein (IgM MGUS) developing an overt B-cell malignancy is 11.7%.[28]

Patients with a paraprotein should be referred for investigation if they have any myeloma ROTI features or other abnormalities such as lymphadenopathy to suggest a haematological malignancy. However, the asymptomatic patient with a paraprotein can be safely monitored in the community on an infrequent but regular basis. Such community-monitored paraprotein patients should have a full blood count, biochemical profile with serum calcium estimation and estimation of immunoglobulins performed every 4–6 months to monitor for signs of progression to myeloma.

Raised plasma viscosity and ESR

Estimation of the plasma viscosity (PV) and the ESR are methods for the indirect assessment of total plasma protein. With an increase in plasma protein there is an associated rise in viscosity, which can then be assessed in the haematology laboratory via the PV and ESR.

The normal PV range is 1.5–1.6 mPa/s and rises with age but shows no variation between genders.[29] An elevated PV can indicate an acute phase increase in fibrinogen or immunoglobulins and can be of use in monitoring a known inflammatory process such as rheumatoid arthritis. In a patient known to have a paraprotein the PV should be assessed to detect the hyperviscosity syndrome that may need urgent therapeutic plasmapheresis and treatment of the underlying condition.

Assessment of the PV is often undertaken in the elderly patient presenting with non-specific symptoms. In this context an elevated PV could indicate an underlying inflammatory or neoplastic process and should prompt the physician to assess the patient for myeloma, but the patient's clinical features should dictate what, if any, further investigations are required.

The bruising patient

Disorders of haemostasis in elderly people are common abnormalities, which may present a challenge to the physician. Thrombocytopenia along with haemostatic abnormalities manifesting with prolongation of *in vitro* clotting times such as the prothrombin, activated partial thromboplastin and thrombin times (PT, APTT, TT) may manifest with bruising, bleeding from mucosal surfaces, life-threatening haemorrhage or be completely asymptomatic.

The normal range for the platelet count in elderly adults is the same as that for younger adults,[30] but there may be an increase in platelet activation and aggregation which has been postulated to be related to the increased incidence of thrombosis in this patient group. There are general age-related increases in the concentration of clotting factors such as factors V, VII, VIII, IX and von Willebrand factor which, although possibly also being associated with an increased thrombotic risk, do not translate into different normal ranges for the PT, APTT and TT in the elderly.[31]

When elderly patients present with bruising or bleeding, the history should be directed at defining the nature of the symptoms and whether they are of recent onset or whether there is a lifelong bleeding tendency. Patients should be questioned about bleeding associated with surgery, dental extractions and in females about haemorrhage associated with childbirth and menstruation. A lifelong bleeding tendency may suggest a constitutional disorder such as von Willebrand disease, mild haemophilia A or B (severe disease presents in childhood) or a platelet function defect. Symptoms of more recent onset suggest an acquired disorder such as idiopathic thrombocytopenic purpura (ITP), thrombocytopenia due to marrow failure, medication or liver disease or a disorder of haemostasis such as disseminated intravascular coagulation (DIC), the coagulopathy of liver disease or acquired haemophilia. A review of the patient's medication will highlight drugs such as non-steroidal anti-inflammatory drugs or anticoagulants that may have haemorrhagic complications as side-effects.

Thromobocytopenia

Thrombocytopenia is a common cause of bleeding and investigation is directed at the exclusion of possible causes such as those producing bone marrow failure (leukaemia, lymphoma, myelodysplasia and aplastic anaemia), connective tissue diseases, liver disease, chronic DIC, medications and infectious agents. Because of the increased incidence of haematological malignancies in the elderly population compared with younger patients, practice guidelines suggest that patients aged

>60 years with unexplained thrombocytopenia should be considered for a bone marrow examination,[32] though in practice this is often only performed when therapy is being considered to elevate the platelet count. Once all possible causes of a low platelet count have been excluded, then a diagnosis of ITP can be made. ITP typically has a relatively benign course in young adults and children but in elderly individuals is associated with an increased risk of bleeding.[33] First-line therapy for ITP consists of corticosteroids and is indicated in the presence of symptoms or if the platelet count is $<30 \times 10^9/l$. Intravenous immunoglobulin is an alternative therapy in those where high-dose corticosteroids might be associated with unacceptable side-effects.[32] An elderly patient with thrombocytopenia should be referred to a haematologist if there are features to suggest a coexistent haematological malignancy, if the thrombocytopenia is progressive or is below a level where intervention may be required should the patient require an invasive surgical procedure ($<80 \times 10^9/l$). The stable thrombocytopenic patient with a platelet count of $>80 \times 10^9/l$ can be safely monitored in the community.

Prolongation of the APTT

A prolonged APTT in the presence of a bleeding tendency should prompt a referral to a haematologist for investigation for a possible constitutional disorder of haemostasis such as mild haemophilia A and B, factor XI deficiency or von Willebrand disease. Acquired haemophilia is a rare but serious disorder where anti-factor VIII autoantibodies induce a severe bleeding tendency with an associated mortality of ~20% in those patients requiring treatment.[34]

The commonest cause of bruising in older people is senile purpura, where an age-associated increase in skin fragility results in spontaneous cutaneous bleeds in the presence of normal haemostasis. Senile purpura affects up to 10% of the population aged between 70 and 90 years and often results in unsightly pseudoscars.[35] Tragically, abuse of elderly individuals is more common than appreciated, affecting up to one in four vulnerable individuals,[36] and may present with bruising or injuries possibly of unusual appearance or distribution. Unexplained bruising in a vulnerable elder should lead to the consideration of physical abuse (see Chapter 24).

References

1. Nilsson-Ehle, H., Jagenburg, R., Landahl, S., Svanborg, A, Westin, J. (1989) Decline of blood haemoglobin in the aged: a longitudinal study of an urban Swedish population from age 70 to 81. *Br J Haematol* 71, 437–42.
2. Hartsock, R. J., Smith, E. B, Petty, C. S. (1965) Normal variations with aging of the amount of hematopoietic tissue in bone marrow from the anterior iliac crest. A study made from 177 cases of sudden death examined by necropsy. *Am J Clin Pathol* 43, 326–31.
3. Guralnik, J. M., Eisenstaedt, R. S., Ferrucci, L., Klein, H. G, Woodman, R. C. (2004) Prevalence of anemia in persons 65 years and older in the United States: evidence for a high rate of unexplained anemia. *Blood*, 104, 2263–8.
4. Joosten, E., Pelemans, W., Hiele, M., Noyen, J., Verhaeghe, R, Boogaerts, M. A. (1992) Prevalence and causes of anaemia in a geriatric hospitalized population. *Gerontology* 38, 111–7.
5. Caro, J. J., Salas, M., Ward, A, Goss, G. (2001) Anemia as an independent prognostic factor for survival in patients with cancer: a systemic, quantitative review. *Cancer* 91, 2214–21.
6. Rockey, D. C, Cello, J. P. (1993) Evaluation of the gastrointestinal tract in patients with iron-deficiency anemia. *N Engl J Med* 329, 1691–5.
7. Ortega, R. M., Manas, L. R., Andres, P., *et al.* (1996) Functional and psychic deterioration in elderly people may be aggravated by folate deficiency. *J Nutr* 126, 1992–9.
8. Weiss, G, Goodnough, L. T. (2005) Anemia of chronic disease. *N Engl J Med* 352, 1011–23.

9. Henke, M., Laszig, R., Rube, C., *et al.* (2003) Erythropoietin to treat head and neck cancer patients with anaemia undergoing radiotherapy: randomised, double-blind, placebo-controlled trial. *Lancet* 362, 1255–60.

10. Auerbach, M., Ballard, H., Trout, J. R., *et al.* (2004) Intravenous iron optimizes the response to recombinant human erythropoietin in cancer patients with chemotherapy-related anemia: a multicenter, open-label, randomized trial. *J Clin Oncol* 22, 1301–7.

11. Butcher, S. K., Killampalli, V., Chahal, H., Kaya Alpar, E, Lord, J. M. (2003) Effect of age on susceptibility to post-traumatic infection in the elderly. *Biochem Soc Trans* 31, 449–51.

12. Bodey, G. P., Buckley, M., Sathe, Y. S, Freireich, E. J. (1966) Quantitative relationships between circulating leukocytes and infection in patients with acute leukemia. *Ann Intern Med* 64, 328–40.

13. Mcglauchlen, K. S, Vogel, L. A. (2003) Ineffective humoral immunity in the elderly. *Microbes Infect* 5, 1279–84.

14. Vogt, R. F, Marti, G. E. (2007) Overview of monoclonal gammopathies of undetermined significance. *Br J Haematol* 139, 687–9.

15. Rawstron, A. C. (2007) Monoclonal B-cell lymphocytosis: good news for patients and CLL investigators. *Leuk Lymphoma* 48, 1057–8.

16. Call, T. G., Phyliky, R. L., Noel, P., *et al.* (1994) Incidence of chronic lymphocytic leukemia in Olmsted County, Minnesota, 1935 through 1989, with emphasis on changes in initial stage at diagnosis. *Mayo Clin Proc* 69, 323–8.

17. Diehl, L. F., Karnell, L. H, Menck, H. R. (1999) The American College of Surgeons Commission on Cancer and the American Cancer Society. The National Cancer Data Base report on age, gender, treatment, and outcomes of patients with chronic lymphocytic leukemia. *Cancer* 86, 2684–92.

18. Binet, J. L., Auquier, A., Dighiero, G., *et al.* (1981) A new prognostic classification of chronic lymphocytic leukemia derived from a multivariate survival analysis. *Cancer* 48, 198–206.

19. Hamblin, T. J., Davis, Z., Gardiner, A., Oscier, D. G, Stevenson, F. K. (1999) Unmutated Ig V(H) genes are associated with a more aggressive form of chronic lymphocytic leukemia. *Blood* 94, 1848–54.

20. Pratt, G. (2008) The evolving use of serum free light chain assays in haematology. *Br J Haematol* 141, 413–22.

21. Kyle, R. A., Therneau, T. M., Rajkumar, S. V., *et al.* (2006) Prevalence of monoclonal gammopathy of undetermined significance. *N Engl J Med* 354, 1362–9.

22. Wechalekar, A., Amato, D., Chen, C., Keith Stewart, A, Reece, D. (2005) IgD multiple myeloma—a clinical profile and outcome with chemotherapy and autologous stem cell transplantation. *Ann Hematol* 84, 115–7.

23. Feyler, S., O'Connor, S. J., Rawstron, A. C., *et al.* (2008) IgM myeloma: a rare entity characterized by a CD20-CD56-CD117- immunophenotype and the t(11;14). *Br J Haematol* 140, 547–51.

24. B.C.S.H. (2006) Guidelines on the diagnosis and management of multiple myeloma 2005. *Br J Haematol* 132, 410–51.

25. Djulbegovic, B., Wheatley, K., Ross, J., *et al.* (2002) Bisphosphonates in multiple myeloma. *Cochrane Database Syst Rev*, CD003188.

26. Kyle, R. A., Therneau, T. M., Rajkumar, S. V., *et al.* (2002) A long-term study of prognosis in monoclonal gammopathy of undetermined significance. *N Engl J Med* 346, 564–9.

27. Roberts-Thomson, P. J., Nikoloutsopoulos, T, Smith, A. J. (2002) IgM paraproteinaemia: disease associations and laboratory features. *Pathology* 34, 356–61.

28. Morra, E., Cesana, C., Klersy, C., *et al.* (2004) Clinical characteristics and factors predicting evolution of asymptomatic IgM monoclonal gammopathies and IgM-related disorders. *Leukemia* 18, 1512–7.

29. I.C.S.H. (1984) Recommendation for a selected method for the measurement of plasma viscosity. International Committee for Standardization in Haematology. *J Clin Pathol* 37, 1147–52.

30. Tsang, C. W., Lazarus, R., Smith, W., Mitchell, P., Koutts, J, Burnett, L. (1998) Hematological indices in an older population sample: derivation of healthy reference values. *Clin Chem* 44, 96–101.

31. Franchini, M. (2006) Hemostasis and aging. *Crit Rev Oncol Hematol* 60, 144–51.

32. B.C.S.H. (2003) Guidelines for the investigation and management of idiopathic thrombocytopenic purpura in adults, children and in pregnancy. *Br J Haematol*, 120, 574–96.

33. Cortelazzo, S., Finazzi, G., Buelli, M., Molteni, A., Viero, P, Barbui, T. (1991) High risk of severe bleeding in aged patients with chronic idiopathic thrombocytopenic purpura. *Blood* 77, 31–3.

34. Collins, P. W., Hirsch, S., Baglin, T. P., I.C.S.H. (2007) Acquired hemophilia A in the United Kingdom: a 2-year national surveillance study by the United Kingdom Haemophilia Centre Doctors' Organisation. *Blood*, 109, 1870–7.

35. Kaya, G, Saurat, J. H. (2007) Dermatoporosis: a chronic cutaneous insufficiency/fragility syndrome. Clinicopathological features, mechanisms, prevention and potential treatments. *Dermatology* 215, 284–94.

36. Cooper, C., Selwood, A, Livingston, G. (2008) The prevalence of elder abuse and neglect: a systematic review. *Age Ageing* 37, 151–60.

Chapter 12

Locomotor problems in older people

Nada Hassan and David Scott

Introduction

Approximately 30% of the general population have musculoskeletal symptoms either of arthritis or back pain. In England and Wales, between 1.3 and 1.75 million people have symptomatic osteoarthritis and a further 0.25–0.5 million have rheumatoid arthritis. About one in seven visits to the general practitioner (GP) involves a musculoskeletal disorder, the commonest being osteoarthritis (OA), back pain, gout, fibromyalgia and bursitis/tendonitis, with back pain being the most frequent cause of chronic disability. The prevalence of physical disability in the community increases with age.[1] The economic burden of such musculoskeletal diseases is also high, accounting for up to 1–2.5% of the gross national product of Western nations.[2]

The aim of this chapter is to highlight the management of some of the commonest musculoskeletal disorders encountered in general practice among older people.

Osteoarthritis

Osteoarthritis is the most common degenerative musculoskeletal disorder that affects weight-bearing joints. It is more common in women than men aged >50 years with an estimated prevalence of 2–3% (10% knee OA for those aged >55 years).

Predisposing factors include old age, obesity, smoking and certain occupations requiring bending and heavy lifting. It is estimated that 80% of the population will have radiographic evidence of OA by the age of 65 years, and 60% of those will be symptomatic.

Clinical picture

The main presentation is that of a deep, achy, joint pain exacerbated by extensive use with occasional stiffness, especially after immobility. The commonest sites involved are the cervical and lumbar spine, first carpometacarpal and metatarsal joint, proximal interphalangeal joint, distal interphalangeal joint, hips and knee joints.

Clinical examination reveals reduced range of movement of the affected joint with crepitus and tenderness on palpation. Joint mal-alignment may also be visible.

Heberden and Bouchard nodes (which represent palpable osteophytes in the distal and proximal interphalangeal joints respectively) are characteristic findings especially in women. Erosive OA is quite rare but is typically bilateral and symmetrical, particularly affecting the distal interphalangeal joints of the hands (F:M ratio of 12:1).

Laboratory and radiographic features

Most laboratory investigations in OA are normal, including inflammatory markers (erythrocyte sedimentation rate (ESR) and C-reactive protein (CRP)). Synovial fluid analysis shows mild inflammatory characteristics (synovial white blood cell count (WBC) <2000/mm³). X-Ray changes include joint space narrowing (loss of the articular cartilage), sclerosis and osteophyte formation (due to the attempted repair and bone regeneration inside the joint), subchondral bone cysts (due to synovial fluid being forced by the pressure of weight into the exposed bone), and occasionally fractured osteophytes result in the formation of loose bodies.

In erosive OA, there can be a more inflammatory component to the history (increased stiffening, soft tissue swelling) with the formation of erosions but affecting distal and proximal interphalangeal joints as in classical OA and in contrast to rhematoid arthritis (RA) (Figure 12.1).

A magnetic resonance imaging (MRI) scan may show partial or full-thickness cartilage defects as well as bone marrow oedema (indicated by decreased T1 and increased T2 signal from the subchondral bone).

Treatment of osteoarthritis

In 2008 treatment was reviewed by the National Institute for Health and Clinical Excellence (NICE) which stressed the following:

- ◆ Healthcare professionals should offer accurate verbal and written information to all people with osteoarthritis to enhance understanding of the condition and its management.
- ◆ Holistic assessment of the effect of OA on the patient, including effects on activities of daily living, mood, sleep etc.
- ◆ Exercise should be a core treatment for patients with osteoarthritis, irrespective of age, co-morbidity, pain severity or disability. This includes local muscle strengthening and general aerobic fitness.
- ◆ Supervised fitness programmes, advice on weight loss especially for obese or overweight patients, ambulatory aids, splints, hydrotherapy are all effective.
- ◆ The use of local heat or cold should be considered as an adjunct to core treatment.
- ◆ Consider the use of transcutaneous electrical nerve stimulation as an adjunct to core treatment for pain relief.
- ◆ Advice on appropriate footwear (including shock-absorbing properties) as part of core treatment for people with lower limb osteoarthritis. Bracing, joint supports and insoles may also

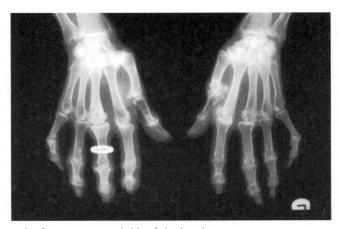

Fig. 12.1 Radiograph of severe osteoarthritis of the hands.

be helpful, as may assistive devices such as walking sticks and tap turners. Seek advice from physiotherapists and occupational therapists (see Chapter 27).

♦ Electro-acupuncture should not be used to treat people with osteoarthritis.

Drug treatment

Analgesics and NSAIDs

1) Paracetamol can be used for pain relief (regular dosing may be required). It can be used with topical non-steroidal anti-inflammatory drugs (NSAIDs) ahead of oral NSAIDs, cyclo-oxygenase 2 (COX-2) inhibitors or opioids.

2) When offering treatment with an oral NSAID/COX-2 inhibitor, the first choice should be either a standard NSAID or a COX-2 inhibitor. In either case, these should be co-prescribed with a proton pump inhibitor (PPI), choosing the one with the lowest cost.

3) There is no evidence that any of the available NSAIDs is more effective than any other for osteoarthritis of the knee or hip. It usually takes 2–4 weeks to evaluate the efficacy of NSAIDs. So if one is ineffective for that period, try another.

4) Opiates can be used when other treatments have failed or are not appropriate.

COX-2 inhibitors

These are used for patients with a low cardiovascular risk who have a history of peptic ulcer, gastrointestinal bleeding, or gastrointestinal intolerance to NSAIDs (including salicylates) and whose joint pains are inadequately controlled using paracetamol.

Dietary supplements

Glucosamine and chondroitin sulphate are dietary supplements which have been reported to retard further cartilage loss in some, but not all studies. There is contradictory evidence for their use, hence the NICE guidelines did not recommend them.

Local intra-articular injections

Both glucocorticoid and hyaluronan have been used intra-articularly to help alleviate symptoms in mild–moderate cases and in patients with monoarticular or pauciarticular osteoarthritis. However, hyaluronan injections were not recommended by NICE for the treatment of osteoarthritis.

Topical capsaicin

Capsaicin, the active principle of hot chilli pepper, exerts its therapeutic effect by enhancing the release of substance P from unmyelinated C nerve fibres. Substance P is then rapidly depleted and signal transmission of pain from C fibres to higher neurocentres is reduced in the area of administration. When used in patients with OA, studies showed help in pain reduction by 4 weeks compared with placebo.[3]

Arthroscopic lavage and debridement

This should not be offered as part of treatment for osteoarthritis, unless there is knee osteoarthritis with a clear history of mechanical locking (not gelling, 'giving way' or X-ray evidence of loose bodies).

Joint replacement surgery

This should be considered for patients with osteoarthritis who experience joint symptoms (pain, stiffness and reduced function) that have a substantial impact on their quality of life and are refractory to non-surgical treatment. Referral should be made before there is prolonged and established functional limitation and severe pain.

Gout

This is a disease characterized by tissue deposition of monosodium urate crystals as a result of hyperuricaemia (>417 μmol/l (7 mg/dl) in males and >357 μmol/l (6.0 mg/dl) in females), but only 15% of patients with hyperuricaemia develop gout.

The disease has a common presentation in primary care with a prevalence that increases with age and rise of serum uric acid. Data from the UK General Practice Research Database from 1990 to 1999 showed an incidence of gout of 12–18 new cases per 10 000, with a prevalence of nearly 7% in men aged >65 years.[4] Males are generally more affected with a ratio of M:F of 2–7:1. Ninety per cent of patients with gout are under-excreters of uric acid (<800 mg/day).

Gout can present as:

1) Acute gouty arthritis.

2) Chronic tophaceous gout (infrequently seen with current effective therapies).

3) Uric acid nephrolithiasis.

4) Gouty nephropathy.

Gout is increasingly recognized in elderly patients, particularly women on diuretics (especially thiazides), and in these patients associated tophi are seen.

In acute gouty arthritis, the attack is characterized by severe pain, redness, swelling, and disability reaching maximum intensity over several hours with complete resolution almost inevitably occurring within a few days to several weeks, even in untreated cases. The signs of inflammation associated with acute gout often extend beyond the joint involved, giving the impression of arthritis in several contiguous joints, tenosynovitis, dactylitis (sausage digit), or even cellulitis.

At least 80% of initial attacks involve a single joint, typically the first metatarsophalangeal joint (known as podagra). Involvement of the ankles, wrists, knees, or the olecranon bursa occurs more commonly with recurrent episodes of gouty arthritis. Shoulders, hips, sterno-clavicular joints, and even the spine and sacroiliac joints may become affected, causing diagnostic confusion.

Monoarticular gouty arthritis can give a clinical picture indistinguishable from acute septic arthritis, including fever, leukocytosis, and elevated ESR. On rare occasions, acute gout and septic arthritis may even coexist. It is therefore important to perform a synovial fluid analysis to look for crystals in these circumstances.

Polyarticular gouty arthritis rarely occurs as an initial manifestation (<20%) but is more common late in the course of untreated gout. The classical sites for tophi (extra articular deposits of uric acid) are the pinna of the ears, the bursa of the elbow and knees, the Achilles tendon and the dorsal surface of the MCP joints.

Investigations

Serum uric acid level may be normal in an acute attack (levels actually fall at the onset of the attack) and so the gold standard test is the isolation of uric acid crystals in the synovial fluid. X-Rays may be normal in the acute stage but subsequently joint erosions, deformities and perio-steal new bone formation may be seen.

Treatment of acute gout

According to the latest guidelines from the British Society for Rheumatology and British Health Professionals in Rheumatology (2007):

1) Rest and elevate the affected joint (expose it to a cool environment).

2) Avoid dehydration.

3) Advise on weight reduction to achieve ideal body weight.

4) Avoid intake of purine-rich food e.g. liver, kidneys, shellfish and yeast extracts as well as red meat.

5) Inclusion of skimmed milk and/or low fat yoghurt, soy beans and vegetable sources of protein and cherries, in the diet should be encouraged.

6) Restrict alcohol consumption to <21 units/week in men and <14 units/week in women. Beer, stout, port and similar fortified wines are best avoided.

7) Start analgesics and anti-inflammatory drug therapy (maximum doses) immediately and continue for 1–2 weeks, if there are no contraindications. The majority of attacks subside in 3–5 days.

8) In patients with increased risk of peptic ulcers, bleeds or perforations, co-prescription of gastro-protective agents should follow standard guidelines for the use of NSAIDs and COX-2 inhibitors.

9) Colchicine can be used as an alternative but is slower to act (500 µg 2–4 times per day).

10) Allopurinol should not be commenced during an acute attack, but in patients already established on allopurinol, it *should be continued* and the acute attack should be treated conventionally.

11) Steroids can be used, intra-articularly in monoarthritis, orally or parentrally in refractory cases or if patients are unable to tolerate NSAIDs or colchicine (e.g. 120 mg of i.m. Depo-Medrone® or 60 mg of i.m. triamcinolone). Oral regimens include prednisolone 20 mg for 10 days or adrenocorticotrophic hormone 40–80 IU for 3 days.

12) If diuretics are being used to treat hypertension, an alternative antihypertensive agent should be considered, e.g. angiotensin II receptor blockers (ARBs), but in patients with heart failure, diuretic therapy should not be discontinued.

13) Avoid use of high doses of aspirin (600–2400 mg/day). Low doses (75–150 mg/day) have insignificant effects on the plasma urate, and should be used as required for cardiovascular prophylaxis.

14) Patients with gout and a history of urolithiasis should be encouraged to drink >2 l of water daily and avoid dehydration. Alkalinization of the urine with potassium citrate (60 mEq/day) should be considered in recurrent stone-formers.

When to treat with uric-acid-lowering drug therapy

The British Society for Rheumatology has also reviewed the use of uric-acid-lowering drugs. The basic advice for patients with acute attacks is the same as those having more than two acute attacks per year. Tradition has it that we should wait 1–2 weeks after the inflammation has settled but there is actually no evidence base for this. In patients in whom there is a risk of not starting allopurinol, it is better to get on with it so long as cover is given for the risk of flares as outlined below.

Other indications include tophaceous gout, chronic gouty arthritis with bony erosions, uric acid stones, patients who need to continue treatment with diuretics and patients with renal insufficiency. Asymptomatic hyperuricaemia (uric acid >714 μmol/l (>12 mg/dl)) carries a risk of urate nephrolithiasis, hence uric-acid-lowering drugs can also be used.

Start with allopurinol (xanthine oxidase inhibitor) at a dose of 50–100 mg/day and increasing by 50–100 mg increments every few weeks (maximum dose 900 mg), aiming for a plasma urate level of <300 μmol/l.

Uricosuric agents can be used as second-line drugs in patients who are under-excretors of uric acid and in those resistant to, or intolerant of, allopurinol. The preferred drugs are sulfinpyrazone (200–800 mg/day) in patients with normal renal function or benzbromarone (50–200 mg/day) in patients with mild/moderate renal insufficiency.

It is important to recognize that acute attacks of gout are more frequent after initiating uric-acid-lowering drugs and that this risk can last for as long as 6 months. It is therefore advisable to consider low dose maintenance analgesia such as with colchicine (0.5 mg twice per day) or even anti-inflammatory agents for this length of time.

Polymyalgia rheumatica

Polymyalgia rheumatica (PMR) is the commonest inflammatory rheumatic disease of older people and represents one of the commonest indications for long-term steroid therapy in the community.[5]

Several criteria have been adopted to diagnose the condition, the latest from Jones and Hazleman[6] which include:

1) Bilaterally painful shoulders, neck ± pelvic girdle without muscle weakness.

2) Morning stiffness >30 min.

3) Symptom duration of >2 months.

4) ESR >30 mm/h or CRP >6 mg/ml.

5) Rapid response to steroids.

6) To exclude any other diagnosis including inflammatory arthritis or malignancy.

It is almost only described in patients above the age of 50 years, with a slight predilection to women.

The ESR is usually elevated >30 mm/h, and the response to corticosteroid therapy is generally dramatic with 70% improvement in patient global response within 1 week and normalization of inflammatory markers within 3–4 weeks.

Autoimmune responses are believed to play a prominent role in polymyalgia rheumatica, with bursitis, synovitis and tenosynovitis of the proximal shoulder and hip girdles being characteristic features.

PMR mimics include rheumatoid arthritis (particularly late onset), remitting symmetrical seronegative synovitis with pitting oedema (RS3PE), systemic lupus erythematosus, polymyositis, spondyloarthropathy, fibromyalgia, bacterial endocarditis, thyroid dysfunction and cancer.

There are no diagnostic tests for PMR and it is important to exclude these diagnoses by careful history, examination and by appropriate investigations. Baseline bloods should include ones to exclude mimics, including full blood count, urea and electrolytes (U&Es), liver function tests (LFTs), bone profile, myeloma screen, thyroid-stimulating hormone, creatine kinase, rheumatoid factor (RF) and antinuclear antibodies (ANAs) plus baseline urinalysis and a chest X-ray.

Some 20% of PMR patients have histological or clinical evidence of giant cell arteritis, so it is important to ask for relevant questions to exclude it such as temporal headaches, scalp tenderness, jaw or tongue claudication and visual symptoms.

PMR tends to run a self-limited course lasting between 9 months and sometimes as long as 5 years. Relapses are most likely to occur in the first 18 months and may be as high as 25%, with no way of predicting which patients will relapse.

Treatment

◆ Start with oral prednisolone 15–20 mg once daily, for 3 weeks.[7] Reduce oral prednisolone to 12.5 mg/day for 3 weeks, 10 mg/day for 4–6 weeks and then reduce by 1 mg every 4–6 weeks.[8]

◆ An alternative is to use intermittent intramuscular methylprednisolone at a dose of 120 mg every 3 weeks for 4 doses, then reduce dose by 20 mg/month every 12 weeks up to 48 weeks.[9]

◆ It is the rate of reduction that determines the relapse more than the actual starting steroid dosage. A gradual reduction over 2 years is often required.[10]

◆ Steroid-sparing medications including methotrexate[11] and azathioprine[12] have been studied in patients in whom corticosteroid reduction has proved difficult. Insufficient supporting evidence is available to consider any of these drugs for primary therapy.

◆ Trials have shown loss of bone mineral density in PMR patients treated with steroids,[13] hence patients should be commenced on calcium and vitamin D and bisphosphonates.

Evaluation of a single swollen joint

It is very important to take a careful history and to perform a detailed examination of an acutely swollen joint. The most important cause to rule out is sepsis with symptoms usually present for <2 weeks. This can be associated with constitutional symptoms of high grade fever, weight loss and malaise. Early recognition is vital as it has a case fatality of up to 11% and can result in severe joint destruction within days. The British Society for Rheumatology algorithm for investigation and management is shown in Figure 12.2.

Differential diagnoses of monoarthritis include:

1) Infection (bacterial, viral, mycobacterial, fungal, spirochete).

2) Crystal arthritis (monosodium urate, calcium pyrophosphate dihydrate (pseudogout), calcium oxalate and hydroxyapatite crystals).

3) Haemoarthrosis which occurs in the setting of trauma or anticoagulation or clotting disorders.

4) Systemic rheumatic disease (RA, systemic lupus erythematosus), seropositive spondyloarthropathies and sarcoidosis).

5) Tumours (chondrosarcoma, osteoid osteoma, pigmented villonodular synovitis or metastatic disease). Myelodysplastic and leukaemic disorders may cause arthralgia or an acute arthritis.

6) Local osteonecrosis or meniscal tear.

Infection

Septic arthritis can be caused by several organisms depending on the host immune response. Predisposing factors include:

1) Trauma.

2) Local infection or septicaemia.

3) Intravenous drug abuse.

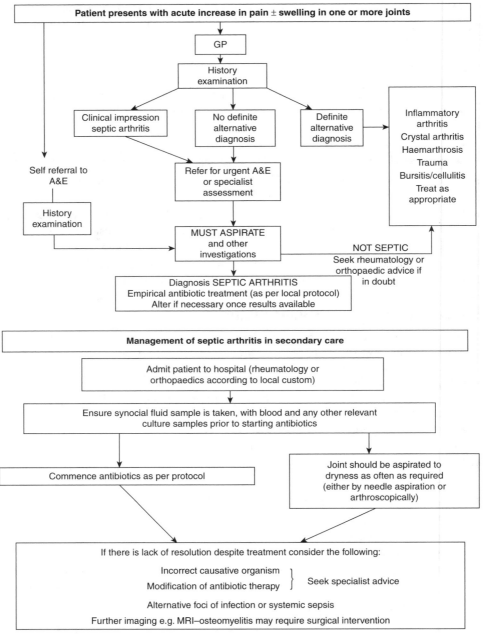

Fig. 12.2 British Society of Rheumatology algorithm for the investigation and management of suspected septic arthritis.
A&E, accident and emergency; MRI, magnetic resonance imaging.

4) Recent invasive procedure.

5) Pre-existing joint disease including prosthetic joints.

6) Steroids and immunosuppressant drugs (including previous intra-articular joint injections).

The commonest organism to cause septic arthritis is *Staphylococcus aureus* followed by streptococci and Gram-negative organisms. It typically affects large joints such as the hips and knees, although the wrists and ankles are also sometimes involved.

Gastrointestinal or genitourinary complaints and recent sexual exposures suggest possible infectious portals of entry, or may be associated with a seronegative spondylo-arthropathy or reactive arthritis. Recent travel to endemic regions and the immune status of the host may predispose to unusual infectious agents.

Trauma

For trauma to cause genuine joint pain and swelling, it is usually mentioned in the history. Intra-articular fractures, dislocations, ligamentous sprains and complete tears (e.g. of the anterior or posterior cruciate ligaments of the knee), and meniscal damage are often associated with haemarthrosis. If that is suspected, an urgent referral to the orthopaedic team is advised.

Crystalline disease

Gout usually presents with an acute response with severe pain, redness, swelling, and disability (see above). Pyrophosphate arthropathy (pseudogout) commonly affects the knee joints but can also be seen to involve the shoulders, wrists and ankles, especially in older people where bilateral wrist involvement can occur.

In all cases, the affected joint usually shows evidence of synovitis with soft tissue swelling, warmth and usually a joint effusion. Patients with septic arthritis, crystal-induced arthritis, or fracture are usually unable to bear weight, with reduced active and passive range of movement.

Patients with suspected septic arthritis will need urgent hospital referral, where the following investigations and management can be undertaken.

Investigations

Basic blood tests include full blood count, inflammatory markers (ESR/CRP), U&Es, LFTs, plus other tests including ANAs, RF (or anti-cyclic-citrullinated peptide (CCP)) and HLA-B27 are performed if other systemic rheumatic diseases are suspected.

Other important investigations include blood cultures ×2 (essential), swabs (e.g. throat, skin for culture and sensitivity), MSU and in cases of suspected tuberculosis, sputum ×3 plus an early morning urine specimen.

Imaging

It is important to undertake baseline X-rays in the acute stage, but this is more to exclude other problems such as trauma, fractures, tumours, joint effusions, or even chondrocalcinosis. If more information is required because of difficulty in making a diagnosis, MRI can be helpful in detecting osteomyelitis that may not be obvious on a plain X-ray.

Synovial fluid analysis

This is the gold standard investigation. It *should be performed as soon as possible* and the urgent sample sent for Gram stain, crystals, white cells and cultures (preferably before starting antibiotics). It ideally should be examined microscopically for evidence of bacterial infection within 4 h. Hip aspiration may be guided by ultrasonography (seek specialist advice).

Synovial biopsy

This is rarely required. The main indication is in patients with refractory monoarthritis where there is a possibility of atypical infections (e.g. tuberculosis, fungi and viruses) or evaluation for other rarities such as sarcoidosis or a malignancy.

Treatment

Management depends on the underlying cause. In suspected cases of septic arthritis even in the absence of fever, intravenous antibiotics should be instigated as soon as possible, according to local protocols, and a potentially infected prosthetic joint should always be referred to an orthopaedic surgeon.

In cases of crystalline arthropathy, once infection is ruled out NSAIDs can be prescribed or local steroid injections performed. Other causes of acute painful monoarthritis are treated depending on the underlying cause (see Figure 12.2).

Rheumatoid arthritis

Rheumatoid arthritis (RA) is a chronic, systemic, inflammatory disorder of unknown aetiology. It has been postulated that genetic factors (high risk of disease concordance in twins), sex hormones and possibly infectious agents (e.g. Epstein–Barr virus, parvovirus and cytomegaovirus) may contribute to the autoimmune mechanism. Genetic factors were also studied and an association with HLA-DR4 and HLA-DR1 noted.

The prevalence of RA is ~0.5–1% of the population worldwide. According to the Norfolk Arthritis Register (NOAR), the annual incidence is ~36/100 000 for women and ~14/100 000 for men (F:M ratio of 3:1). It is rare in men aged <45 years of age, but the incidence rises in women aged ≤45 years.[14]

The arthritis is usually symmetrical, affecting the small joints of the hands and feet. If untreated the disease may lead to joint destruction due to erosion of cartilage and bone.

RA has a wide clinical spectrum ranging from mild disease to a severe form with extra-articular manifestations.

To diagnose RA, the American College of Rheumatology criteria (1987) are adopted (requiring four to diagnose) which include:

1) Morning stiffness for ≥1 h and present for ≥6 weeks.

2) Swelling of three or more joints for ≥6 weeks.

3) Swelling of wrist, metacarpophalangeal, or proximal interphalangeal joints for ≥6 weeks.

4) Symmetric joint swelling for 6 weeks.

5) Hand X-ray changes typical of RA that must include erosions or unequivocal bony decalcification.

6) Rheumatoid subcutaneous nodules.

7) Positive rheumatoid factor.

The disease onset is usually insidious, with the predominant symptoms being pain, stiffness, and swelling of joints. It can, however, present acutely in 10–25% of cases. Typically, the metacarpophalangeal (MCP) and proximal interphalangeal joints of the fingers, the wrists, and metatarsophalangeal (MTP) joints of the toes are sites of arthritis early in the disease. Involvement of axial and central joints is less common, occurring in 20–50% of patients.

Morning stiffness is a common feature in those with active RA, usually lasting more than an hour. Up to one-third of patients have the acute onset of polyarthritis associated with myalgia, fatigue, low grade fever, weight loss and depression.

It has been noted especially in the elderly groups that RA can present with 'polymyalgia rheumatica' type features with a good response to steroids and the synovitis becoming more apparent on steroid withdrawal.

Examination in the active stage reveals evidence of synovitis with swollen and tender joints typically elicited by tangential squeezing at the MCP and MTP joints. As the disease progresses, deformities occur including ulnar deviation, volar subluxation of the MCP joints, swan neck and *boutonnière* deformities of the fingers. And with further progression muscle wasting and tendon ruptures may occur.

Clinical evidence of active disease can be measured by performing a disease activity score (DAS 28) which involves counting the numbers of tender and swollen joints as well as laboratory tests of disease activity and patient's global assessment on the disease activity.

Extra-articular manifestations are more frequently noted in males with positive pheumatoid factor and ANAs; these commonly include sicca symptoms and the presence of rheumatoid nodules, which reflect a more severe disease.

Other general features include fever, weight loss and lymphadenopathy. Organ-specific involvements include:

◆ Lung/heart involvement causing exudative pleural effusions, lung nodules, related interstitial lung disease and pleuro-pericarditis.

◆ Eye involvement causing scleritis, episcleritis, keratoconjuctivitis and corneal melt syndrome.

◆ Skin: leg ulcers and vasculitis.

◆ Blood involvement causing anaemia, thrombocytosis and rarely Felty's syndrome (low neutrophil count and splenomegaly, occurring in <1% of cases).

◆ Cental nervous system involvement causing entrapment neuropathies and mononeuritis multiplex. Cervical myelopathy can result from atlanto-axial subluxation.

◆ Amyloidosis can affect any organ, especially the kidneys and heart.

RA patients were shown to have higher risks of infections,[15] cardiovascular disease[16] and lymphomas related to both duration and severity of the disease. Life expectancy of RA patients was noted to be less than age- and sex-matched control populations, especially in patients with severe, polyarticular disease due to the presence of other co-morbidities.[16] It is important to assess patients clinically as well as functionally. The Stanford Health Assessment Questionnaire (HAQ) is one of the best-known methods to self-report on functional capabilities.

Investigations

Blood tests

1) Anaemia: the commonest types are the normochromic normocytic anaemia of chronic disease and iron deficiency anaemia related to NSAID use. Anti-folate drugs such as methotrexate can cause a macrocytic anaemia.

2) Low WBC count can be observed as a result of drug related bone marrow toxicity, particularly with disease modifying drugs, or as part of Felty's syndrome.

3) High inflammatory markers, including ESR, CRP. Serum alkaline phosphatase, platelet count, globulin and ferritin levels can also be raised in the active stage.

4) RF is positive (titres >1:80) in 75–80% of cases. It is usually associated with nodulosis and extra-articular features and, according to the NOAR database, a high titre RF is an important

variable in predicting continuing severity of radiographic damage during the first 5 years after presentation with inflammatory polyarthritis.[18]

5) Anti-cyclic-citrullinated peptide (CCP) is highly specific for RA (96–98%) and shows a positive predictive value for erosive disease in early RA.[19] The anti-CCP antibody status is most informative in RF-negative patients.[20] This test is not routinely available in primary care.

Imaging

♦ X-ray findings in RA include: peri-articular osteopenia, joint space narrowing, erosions and subluxation. Early erosions predict aggressive disease and predict outcome.[21] X-Rays of the cervical spine are important to evaluate vertical or horizontal C1–C2 subluxation, especially in the flexed lateral view.

♦ Ultrasound is important in detecting synovitis,[22] erosions and effusions. It is also used to examine tendons for tendonitis and tears.

♦ MRI allows accurate visualization of the bone, joints and soft tissue and can detect early disease (bone marrow oedema) before plain X-rays.

♦ Bone scans can reveal areas of high intake but are not widely used for this purpose.

Management of RA

♦ The latest recommendations from NICE [23] require early referral to a specialist for any person with suspected persistent synovitis of undetermined cause. It is particularly important if RA is suspected as it has been noted that 70% of joint erosions detected on X-rays of hands and feet occur in the first 2 years of disease.

♦ Non-pharmacological and preventive treatments include rest, especially of an acutely painful joint. Physical, occupational and dietary therapy such as omega-3 fatty acid supplementation[24] are important as well as general measures to protect bone structure and function.

♦ Range-of-motion exercises help to preserve or to restore joint motion. Patients with RA should have access to specialist physiotherapy, with periodic review to improve general fitness and encourage regular exercise, and learn exercises for enhancing joint flexibility, muscle strength, and managing other functional impairments. They should also have access to a multidisciplinary team (MDT) that can provide the opportunity for periodic assessment of the effect of the disease on their lives and access to a named member of the MDT (for example, the specialist nurse) who is responsible for coordinating their care.

♦ Drug therapy is the mainstay of treatment for all patients except for those in clinical remission. These include:

1) *Analgesics* such as topical agents (e.g. capsaicin) and oral agents like acetaminophen, propoxyphene, tramadol, and more potent opioid agents (e.g. oxycodone).

2) *Non-steroidal anti-inflammatory drugs* have both analgesic and anti-inflammatory properties but do not alter disease outcomes. Selective COX-2 inhibitors may be substituted for non-selective NSAIDs in some patients who are at higher risk for adverse gastroduodenal effects.

3) *Glucocorticoids* can be used acutely orally, intravenously, or by intra-articular injection. Oral doses equivalent to ≤15 mg/day of prednisolone are effective in relieving joint pain.

4) *Disease-modifying anti-rheumatic drugs (DMARDs)* have the potential to reduce or prevent joint damage, preserve joint integrity and function, reduce health costs, and maintain economic productivity.[25] In patients with newly diagnosed active RA, offer a combination

of DMARDs (including methotrexate and at least one other DMARD, plus short-term glucocorticoids) as first-line treatment as soon as possible, ideally within 3 months of the onset of persistent symptoms. Other examples of DMARDs include hydroxychloroquine, sulfasalazine, methotrexate, and leflunomide. Used less often are gold salts, D-penicillamine, azathioprine, and cyclosporine. Tetracycline derivatives (e.g. doxycycline, minocycline) can inhibit activity of metalloproteinases involved in joint destruction by rheumatoid synovium but are rarely used. Many localities have shared care protocols for the prescribing and monitoring of DMARDs, often as part of a DES (directly enhanced service).

5) *Anticytokine therapies (biologics)* are based upon an increased understanding of the biology of RA. Examples include the anti-tumour necrosis factor (TNF)-alpha agents such as etanercept, infliximab and adalimumab, and the interleukin-1 receptor antagonist, anakinra. Other biological therapy includes abatacept (CTLA4-Ig) and the B-cell depleting monoclonal antibody, rituximab.

◆ Several studies indicate that early use of glucocorticoids followed by rapid reduction of dose and discontinuation, in combination with concomitant, sustained use of a regimen of traditional DMARDs that includes methotrexate, is superior to monotherapy or step therapy with traditional DMARDs.[26]

◆ A combination of methotrexate or another DMARD with anti-TNF agents is effective in reducing disease activity and reducing the rate of radiographic progression of joint disease.[27]

Other parameters that need addressing are:

1) Bone protection, since RA alone appears to cause a gradual loss of bone mineral density.

2) Modifying risk factors for atherosclerosis.

3) Avoidance of live vaccines in patients receiving immunosuppressive drugs.

4) Careful monitoring of drug toxicities.

5) Effects of RA on mood and sleep: actively look for depression and treat if present.

6) Effect of RA on activities of daily living, and possible need for advice from physiotherapy or occupational therapy colleagues about assistive devices (see Chapter 27).

Conclusion

Rheumatological conditions are common in older people. Many can be investigated and managed in primary care, but others need prompt referral to secondary care for further investigation and management. Shared care protocols for some conditions (e.g. DMARD monitoring) underline the importance of close primary and secondary care working. Many rheumatological conditions benefit from consideration about rehabilitation (see Chapter 27) and the potential role of other health professionals, such as physiotherapists and occupational therapists. Chronic pain is strongly associated with depression in older people and this should be actively looked for and managed if detected (see Chapter 22).

References

1. Urwin M, Symmons D. Estimating the burden of musculoskeletal disorders in the community: the comparative prevalence of symptoms at different anatomical sites, and the relation to social deprivation. *Ann Rheum Dis* 1998;57:649–55.

2. Reginster J-Y. The prevalence and burden of arthritis. *Rheumatol J* 2002;41(Suppl 1):3–6.

3. Deal CL, Schnitzer TJ, Lipstein E, *et al*. Treatment of arthritis with topical capsaicin: a double-blind trial. *Clin Ther* 1991;13:383.

4. Mikuls TR, Farrar JT, Bilker WB, Fernandes S, Schumacher HR, Jr, Saag KG. Gout epidemiology: results from the UK General Practice Research Database, 1990–1999. *Ann Rheum Dis* 2005;64:267–72.

5. Smeeth L, Cook C, Hall AJ. Incidence of diagnosed polymyalgia rheumatica and temporal arteritis in the United Kingdom, 1990 to 2001. *Ann Rheum Dis* 2006;65:1093–8.

6. Jones JG, Hazleman BL. Polymyalgia rheumatica and giant cell arteritis – a difficult diagnosis. *J R Coll Gen Pract* 1981;31(226):283–9.

7. Scharf J, Nahir M. Low-dose steroid treatment in polymyalgia rheumatica. *NY State J Med* 1977;77:368–9.

8. Behn AR, Perera T, Myles AB. Polymyalgia rheumatica and corticosteroids: how much for how long? *Ann Rheum Dis* 1983;42:374–8.

9. Dasgupta B, Dolan AL, Panayi GS, Fernandes L. An initially double-blind controlled 96 week trial of depot methylprednisolone against oral prednisolone in the treatment of polymyalgia rheumatica. *Br J Rheumatol* 1998;37:189–95.

10. Delecoeuillerie G, Joly P, Cohen de Lara A, Paolaggi JB. Polymyalgia rheumatica and temporal arteritis: a retrospective analysis of prognostic features and different corticosteroid regimens (11 year survey of 210 patients). *Ann Rheum Dis* 1988;47:733–9.

11. Van der Veen MJ, Dinant HJ, van Booma-Frankfort C, van Albada-Kuipers GA, Bijlsma JW. Can methotrexate be used as a steroid sparing agent in the treatment of polymyalgia rheumatica and giant cell arteritis? *Ann Rheum Dis* 1996;5:218–23 *(erratum appears in Ann Rheum Dis 1996;55:563)*.

12. De Silva M, Hazleman BL. Azathioprine in giant cell arteritis/polymyalgia rheumatica: a double-blind study. *Ann Rheum Dis* 1986;45:136–8.

13. The deleterious effects of low-dose corticosteroids on bone density in patients with polymyalgia rheumatica. *Br J Rheumatol* 1998;37:292–9.

14. Symmons DPM, Barrett EM, Bankhead CR, Scott DGI, Silman AJ. The incidence of rheumatoid arthritis in the United Kingdom: results from the Norfolk Arthritis Register. *Br J Rheumatol* 1994;33:735–739.

15. Doran MF, Crowson CS, Pond GR, O'Fallon WM, Gabriel SE. Frequency of infection in patients with rheumatoid arthritis compared with controls: a population-based study. *Arthritis Rheum* 2002;46:2287–2293.

16. Wållberg-Jonsson S, Johansson H, Ohman ML, Rantapää-Dahlqvist S. Extent of inflammation predicts cardiovascular disease and overall mortality in seropositive rheumatoid arthritis. A retrospective cohort study from disease onset. *J Rheumatol* 1999;26:2562–71.

17. Symmons DPM, Silman AJ. The Norfolk Arthritis Register (NOAR). *Clin Exp Rheumatol* 2003;21(Suppl 30):S94–S99.

18. Bukhari M, Lunt M, Harrison BJ, Scott DG, Symmons DP, Silman AJ. Rheumatoid factor is the major predictor of increasing severity of radiographic erosions in rheumatoid arthritis: results from the Norfolk Arthritis Register Study, a large inception cohort. *Arthritis Rheum* 2002;46:906–12.

19. Kroot E-JJA. The prognostic value of anti-cyclic citrullinated peptide antibody in patients with recent-onset rheumatoid arthritis. *Arthritis Rheum* 2000;43:1831–1835.

20. Bukhari M, Thomson W, Naseem H, Bunn D, Silman A, Symmons D, Barton A. The performance of anti-cyclic citrullinated peptide antibodies in predicting the severity of radiologic damage in inflammatory polyarthritis: results from the Norfolk Arthritis Register. *Arthritis Rheum* 2007; 56:2929–2935.

21. Welsing RB *et al.* The relationship between disease activity and radiologic progression in patients with rheumatoid arthritis: a longitudinal analysis. *Arthritis Rheum* 2004;50:2082–20934.

22. Grassi W, Filippucci E, Farina A, Salaffi F, Cervini C. Ultrasonography in the evaluation of bone erosions. *Ann Rheum Dis* 2001;60:98–104.

23. NICE Clinical Guideline 79. Rheumatoid arthritis: the management of rheumatoid arthritis in adults. National Institute for Health and Clinical Excellence. 2009. www.nice.org.uk.

24. Geusens P, Wouters C, Nijs J, Jiang Y, Dequeker J. Long-term effect of omega-3 fatty acid supplementation in active rheumatoid arthritis. A 12-month, double-blind, controlled study. *Arthritis Rheum* 1994;37:824–9.

25. American College of Rheumatology Ad Hoc Committee on Clinical Guidelines. Guidelines for the management of rheumatoid arthritis: 2002 update. *Arthritis Rheum* 2002;46:328.

26. Boers M, Verhoeven AC, Markusse HM, *et al.* Randomised comparison of combined step-down prednisolone, methotrexate and sulphasalazine with sulphasalazine alone in early rheumatoid arthritis. *Lancet* 1997;350:309.

27. Hyrich KL, Symmons DP, Watson KD, Silman AJ. Comparison of the response to infliximab or etanercept monotherapy with the response to cotherapy with methotrexate or another disease-modifying antirheumatic drug in patients with rheumatoid arthritis: results from the British Society for Rheumatology Biologics Register. *Arthritis Rheum* 2006;54:1786–94.

Chapter 13

Falls and osteoporosis

Finbarr Martin and Denise Kendrick

Introduction

A fall is 'an event whereby an individual comes to rest on the ground or another lower level with or without a loss of consciousness'. There are other definitions but this simple one adopted by the National Institute of Health and Clinical Excellence (NICE)[1] makes sense in clinical practice. It includes a spectrum of events with syncope at one end and loss of balance due to postural instability at the other. A fall is a symptom, not a diagnosis, and although assessment can be a clinical challenge, it is worthwhile as the frequency of falls can be reduced and the devastating consequences can be minimized.

Impact of falls and fractures on individuals and services

Falls are a major cause of disability and the leading cause of injury-related death in people aged >75 years in the UK.[2] In UK primary care populations about a third of people aged >50 years have at least one fall each year, the rate rising with age to >60% in nonagenarians, and being generally higher in women.[3,4] Many falls go unreported, but in 1999, there were 647 721 fall-related emergency department attendances in the UK, with attendance rates rising to one in ten of those aged >75 years.[5] Nearly a third of all attendances resulted in hospital admission, making a total of >200 000 per year. The risk of admission is ten-fold higher for the older age group. In addition, many people are helped off the floor by ambulance crews but not conveyed to hospital, and these do not appear in the statistics.

Falls have psychological as well as physical consequences. There is a strong relationship between falls and anxiety and depression.[6] Post-fall anxiety significantly impacts upon rehabilitation and return of functional independence. Fear of falling may both precede and follow falls. It is an independent risk factor for future falls.

More than 300 000 people each year receive hospital treatment in the UK for fragility fractures. The commonest is hip fracture, >70 000,[7] of whom 10% die within a month and the excess mortality is 20% at 1 year. The average age of hip fracture patients is increasing and the associated frailty may explain why the 1 year case fatality rate appears to be increasing.[8]

Health and social care costs of fragility fractures amount to around £2 billion, most of which relates to the hip fractures. Current projections suggest that by 2020, this sum will rise by 50%.[9] About 60% of the cost of falls is National Health Service costs, half for acute inpatient care and much of the rest on long-term care. Identifying all falls-related service activity is challenging but recent estimates suggest that it may account for between 10% and 25% of local health and social care spending on older people, taking the total costs to about £3 billion per year.[10]

Box 13.1 Important 'intrinsic' risk factors for falls[a]

Lower limb weakness (includes proximal and distal muscle groups).
Balance deficit (particularly dynamic balance).
Gait abnormalities.
Visual impairment (includes acuity and contrast sensitivity).
Mobility limitation (includes self-perceived difficulty).
Cognitive impairment.
Impaired functional status.
Postural (orthostatic) hypotension.
Fear of falling (particularly with self-imposed activity limitation).

[a] In order of magnitude of association and adapted from a review of 16 studies by Rubenstein.[11]

Assessing and managing falls risk in the community

There is a spectrum of risk among older people. Risk factors have been identified by case–control comparative studies or by prospective cohort studies investigating baseline characteristics for their ability to predict subsequent falls (Box 13.1).[11] Approaches to the classification of risk factors have varied. Some studies have focused on muscle strength or cognition, others on specific medical conditions. Generally there is distinction of intrinsic patient factors from external factors such as domestic hazards, though in practice the risk is a product of the two. For example, the famous 'loose rug' may become hazardous only to the person with poor vision or muscle weakness combined with poor judgement. Likewise most patients survive 'culprit medications' successfully until compromised by other factors including acute illness.

The management approach depends upon the degree of risk. For many the risk is low and the preventive approach is not falls-specific. Taking regular physical exercise, maintaining social contacts, eating healthily, having regular eye checks and medication reviews are all likely to contribute. Older people who begin to experience mobility difficulties and may therefore modify or reduce their usual activities are at greater risk, particularly if fear of falling results in significant activity limitation.[12] For patients with specific conditions such as Parkinson's disease (postural instability and orthostatic hypotension), stroke (asymmetrical weakness, visual neglect, etc.), or lower limb osteoarthritis (pain, proximal weakness, reduced ankle flexibility) all of which result in additional falls risk, the reduction of this risk can be incorporated into their clinical management, but unrelated risk factors must also be addressed. Then there are those who have already fallen and perhaps sustained significant injury or fragility fracture. Secondary falls and fracture prevention must follow management of the injury and any immediate precipitating conditions.

Thus general practitioners (GPs), practice and community nurses, therapists and social care providers all have important roles to play. But research with older people across this spectrum of risk has shown that prevention of falls is not their prominent perspective, whereas maintaining mobility and independence is.[13] So opportunities to identify those who have fallen or are at increased risk will arise in the context of other requests for help. In such contacts, older people should be routinely asked about falls in the previous year, mobility difficulties or fear of falling.[1] There is no risk assessment tool shown to have very high overall predictiveness in primary care, but using the five-question Falls Risk Assessment Tool (Box 13.2) may help, as 57% of those scoring ≥3 on this tool will fall within 6 months.[14]

Those reporting a fall, or at increased risk of falls, should be seen by their GP for an assessment of balance and gait deficits and considered for their ability to benefit from interventions to

Box 13.2 The falls risk assessment tool

- Fall in the previous year.
- Taking four or more medications per day.
- History of stroke or Parkinson's disease.
- Patient reporting problems with balance.
- Unable to get out of chair at knee height, without using arms.

improve strength and balance.[1] Medical contraindications are few but would include unstable angina. For those able to participate and without significant visual or cognitive impairment, this is the most effective preventive approach.[15] Realistically it may take several consultations to comprehensively assess and manage falls risk, as illustrated in the four-part Case Study on Mrs J.

Case Study   Mrs J's first consultation

Mrs J is aged 76 years. She has a history of hypothyroidism, hypertension, a total abdominal hysterectomy and bilateral salpingo-oophorectomy at age 40 years for fibroids, knee osteoarthritis, and bilateral cataracts. She takes atenolol 50 mg once per day, bendroflumethazide 2.5 mg once per day, levothyroxine 75 μg once per day and co-codamol 2 tablets four times per day. She is a non-smoker, lives alone but attends with her daughter. She complains of fatigue and difficulty getting about recently, and she fears becoming housebound. Her daughter adds that mum tripped when going shopping last year and is worried that she will fall again as she now seems unsteady on her legs.

History

She was used to walking 20 min to the shops each day till she had a chest infection four months ago, lost 4 kg in weight and stayed at home for 6 weeks. Walking is now limited to 250 m before having to rest because of fatigue and weakness. It is also difficult to get in and out of the bath and out of the chair. Last year's falls were due, she perceives, to a broken paving stone which she hadn't seen but she is worried about another fall. Her mother fractured her hip aged 78 years. Since her husband died 2 years ago, she is very lonely, cries most days, and memory, concentration and appetite are not as good as they used to be. She feels tired all the time, sleeps 6 h at night, plus 2 h every afternoon in her chair. She denies depression and considers her feelings to be normal in the circumstances. She has nocturia two or three times per night, but no incontinence. Her ankles are slightly swollen and she sometimes feels light-headed when she stands up from sitting down. Her cataracts make it difficult to read the instructions on her medicines, but she takes them as recommended. She drinks two glasses of wine per night to help her sleep.

Examination

Pallor, no shortness of breath when she walked into your room. Pulse 76 bpm regular, blood pressure 120/70 mmHg sitting, minimal ankle oedema, quadriceps wasting and weakness, otherwise examination is normal. OA changes in both hands and knees. She uses her arms to help her get up from a chair and the Timed Up and Go test takes 16 s, but gait appears normal. Body mass index (BMI) is 18.6 kg/m^2.

Investigations: full blood count, urea and electrolytes and estimated glomerular filtration rate, liver function tests, thyroid function tests, C-reactive protein and RBS (random blood sugar). Refer to practice nurse for lying and standing blood pressure (see Box 13.3).

Assessment

Risk factors for a fall: previous fall, impaired vision, impaired mobility and balance, and four or more medications per day. Risk factors for osteoporosis: age, gender, early menopause, low BMI, maternal hip fracture at age >75 years.

Box 13.3 Measurement of orthostatic (postural) hypotension

- ◆ Measure supine blood pressure (BP) after minimum 10 min lying down, relaxed.
- ◆ Stand and measure BP (support patient if necessary) 1 and 3 min after standing.
- ◆ Orthostatic hypotension is defined as ≥20 mmHg systolic and/or ≥10 mmHg diastolic drop of BP or if the systolic BP falls to <100 mmHg.
- ◆ It is most likely to be present on rising initially in the morning, so may be missed at surgery.
- ◆ A similar drop in BP may occur postprandially, especially after a full carbohydrate meal.

Her 10 year prospective fracture risk was estimated using the WHO Fracture Risk Assessment Tool (http://www.shef.ac.uk/FRAX/). Ten-year probability of a major osteoporotic fracture is 33% and of hip fracture is 27%.

Management
- ◆ Explain that several consultations will be needed to deal with her problems.
- ◆ Explain increased risk of falling and of fracture and that reviewing medication, home hazard assessment, strength and balance training and correction of vision have all been shown to be effective in reducing falls.
- ◆ Discuss referral to community occupational therapy for assessment of home hazards and advice on maintaining safe independent activity.
- ◆ Discuss referral to community physiotherapy for gait assessment and retraining and consideration for a strength and balance training programme.
- ◆ Review in 2 weeks.

There is no reliable adequately validated clinical tool for assessing gait and balance performance to predict future falls among community-dwelling older people.[16] NICE recommends selecting a suitable approach locally. We recommend the Timed Up and Go (TUG) test as a feasible and quick test of functional mobility (see Box 13.4). The cut-off score suitable for identifying risk will depend on the sample population and the balance to be struck between high sensitivity (not missing a potential faller) and high specificity (not subjecting many future non-fallers to more rigorous assessments unnecessarily). Performance of TUG is significantly different between fallers and non-fallers among older adults living in the community;[17] those taking ≥14 s are at an increased

Box 13.4 Timed up and go test

- ◆ People should be observed and timed rising from a chair of standard height, without pushing up with their arms, walking 3 m, turning and returning to sit in the chair.
- ◆ If people can rise only by pushing up with their arms, or are unsteady or require assistance to complete this task, they require a fuller falls assessment.
- ◆ If people cannot initiate this task at all, further assessment is necessary but they may be at low risk for falling
- ◆ If people demonstrate no difficulty or unsteadiness, they may be at low risk and need no further assessment of gait and balance.

Box 13.5 What is a multifactorial falls risk assessment, and who needs it?[1]

A multifactorial assessment should be underaken by a health care professional with appropriate skills and experience and usually within a specialist falls service. Such an assessment should include:

- ◆ Falls history.
- ◆ Assessment of gait, balance, mobility and muscle weakness.
- ◆ Assessment of osteoporosis risk.
- ◆ Assessment of older persons' perceived functional ability and fear of falling.
- ◆ Assessment of visual impairment.
- ◆ Assessment of cognitive impairment and neurological examination.
- ◆ Assessment of urinary incontinence.
- ◆ Assessment of home hazards.
- ◆ Cardiovascular examination and medication review.

NICE guidance recommends that a multifactorial falls risk assessment should be performed for older people who:

- ◆ have had recurrent falls.
- ◆ present to medical attention because of a fall.
- ◆ demonstrate abnormalities of gait and balance.

risk of falls,[18] but cognitive impairment reduces its utility.[19] Asking patients to get up from a chair without using their arms assesses balance. Patients who are unable to do this are at an increased risk of hip fracture (odds ratio: 3.58; 95% confidence interval (CI): 1.17, 10.93).[20]

So far, Mrs J has had a fairly full assessment. Box 13.5 lists the domains of a full multifactorial falls risk assessment as described by NICE guidance.

Case Study Mrs J's second consultation

Mrs J returns 2 weeks later.

Assessment
Blood tests reveal chronic kidney disease stage 3. She has orthostatic hypotension (BP 124/75 mmHg lying and 110/65 mmHg standing).

Investigations
Serum calcium and phosphate, DEXA scan (see Box 13.6) and food diary for 1 week to assess calcium and vitamin D intake.

Management
- ◆ Expedite cataract operation.[21]
- ◆ Review medication and explain that antihypertensives are causing orthostatic hypotension, and discuss stopping one of the antihypertensives and monitoring BP.
- ◆ Suggest paracetamol instead of co-codamol.
- ◆ Explain that swollen ankles result from reduced mobility and sleeping in the chair and suggest elevation. Explain reduced need for sleep with increasing age; suggest trying not to sleep during the day, as this may be contributing to poor night-time sleep, and may increase the risk of falls.

◆ Explain that two glasses of wine at night might appear to help sleep, but may increase risk of falling at night, and suggest reducing to one glass per night.

◆ Give Help the Aged leaflets *Staying Steady*[22] (this includes advice about reduction of falls risk and information about strength and balance exercises) and *Healthy Bones*.[23] If she cannot read them, ask her daughter to phone for large-print leaflets.

Referral to a community- or hospital-based specialist falls service should be considered for completion of the multifactorial risk assessment if the skills or facilities for this are not available in primary care.

Correcting vision as part of multifactorial falls management which includes an assessment of home hazards and strength and balance training reduces the risk of falls by 33% (rate ratio: 0.67; 95% CI: 0.51, 0.88).[24] There is, however, some evidence that improving vision without attending to other risk factors could increase falls.

Sleeping during the day is also a risk factor for falls (odds ratio: 1.32; 95% CI: 1.03, 1.69) and hip fracture (hazard ratio: 1.33; 95% CI: 0.99, 1.78).[25]

Home hazard assessments as part of multifactorial interventions reduce the risk of falls in community-dwelling older people by between 14% and 27%.[1] The assessment should be carried out by a health care professional and should include mitigation of identified hazards in the home, evaluation of the older person's ability to safely use mobility aids, if appropriate, and evaluation of ability to perform activities of daily living. The evidence suggests that this is most effective in those with multiple falls or at very high risk,[26] and whereas the hazard removal may be important for some, at least half the falls reduction is of outdoor falls, suggesting that the advice/education aspect is also important. There is no good evidence, however, that this approach is sufficient as a *single* intervention in fallers or those at risk.

Strength and balance training provided by a trained health professional and individually tailored to the patient reduces falls by 20%.[27]

At this stage it should be clear if there are indications for referral to a consultant-led specialist falls service, for:

◆ investigation of syncope;

◆ investigation of recurrent falls unexplained by the multifactorial falls risk assessment, as these patients have a significant prevalence of syncope, even if this is not recalled by the patient or witnessed by others;[28]

◆ diagnostic assessment of unexplained gait and balance abnormalities, as these may represent early neurodegenerative or cerebrovascular disease.

Case Study   Mrs J's third consultation

Assessment

Mrs J's food diary shows that her only regular calcium intake is half a pint of milk and one yoghurt per day. She always covers up in the sun. Calcium and phosphate levels are normal. Latest BP is 132/80 mmHg lying and 125/75 mmHg standing. You explain that fatigue can sometimes be due to feeling a bit low or down, and she completes the Geriatric Depression Scale and scores 4/15 (borderline for depression) (see Chapter 22).

Management

◆ Explain that intake of calcium and vitamin D is too low, even though serum calcium level is normal. Discuss changing diet and, if it is unlikely that she can get 1000 mg calcium and 10 μg vitamin D per day, suggest calcium and vitamin D supplement. She is less dizzy on standing and agrees to referral for occupational therapy assessment visit and an exercise programme.

◆ Explain that she may have depression and ask her to consider this possibility and review in 2 weeks.

The recommended daily intake of calcium is 1000 mg/day for postmenopausal women and vitamin D intake is 10 μg once daily. The Scottish Intercollegiate Guideline Network (SIGN) guidelines on osteoporosis give details of the calcium content of a range of foods.[29] The place of calcium and vitamin D supplementation in reducing falls and fractures has been unclear due to inconsistent trial results, perhaps associated with difference in the vitamin D status of the trial participants and the trial preparations used. A recent meta-analysis concluded that supplementation for people aged ≥50 years conferred a reduced risk of any fracture of 12% (risk ratio: 0.88; 95% CI: 0.83, 0.95), the greatest effect being with a daily dose of 1200 mg of calcium and 800 IU of vitamin D.[30]

Case Study   Mrs J's fourth consultation

Assessment

Mrs J has now had her first cataract operation which has gone well. The DEXA scan showed osteoporosis and she has started a bisphosphonate, which she is tolerating well. The occupational therapist has provided a range of aids, organised an alarm in case she falls and taught her how to get up after a fall. She has started the strength and balance exercises, and has started walking a bit further each day. She thinks that her mood is now improved due to reducing alcohol intake, increasing activity and cutting out sleep during the day.

Management

Encourage continuation with the exercises and suggest review in 1 month to assess depression.

Antidepressants of all types increase the risk of falls and fractures.[32] Both depression[33] and treatment with selective serotonin reuptake inhibitors may also reduce bone density.[34]

Assessing and managing fracture risk in older people in the community

Osteoporosis is the most common bone disease in both men and women, and its major impact on patients and services is through osteoporotic fractures. The epidemiology shows a transition from Colles fractures, peaking in the first decade or so after the menopause, through to (often asymptomatic) vertebral collapse to hip fractures, the average age for which is now >80 years in England.[35] Pubic rami and subcapital fractures of the humerus are also common from age 70 years onwards. Whilst osteoporosis is generally considered to be more prevalent in women, more than half the men aged ≥50 years with a hip fracture have osteoporosis. The incidence of any limb fracture (per 1000 person-years) in European women aged ≥50 years is 19 and 7.3 for men, with distal forearm fracture rates of 7.3 and 1.7, hip fracture rates of 1.3 and 0.8 and vertebral fracture rates of 10.7 and 5.7 for women and men respectively.[36] Lifetime fracture prevalence exceeds 50% in middle-aged men and 40% in women aged >75 years. White people are affected more than other ethnic groups across all ages and both genders.[37]

Osteoporosis is defined according to bone mineral density (Box 13.6).[38]

Bone mineral density is a better predictor of fractures than blood pressure is of stroke, with a relative risk of hip fracture of 2.6 for each 1 SD decrease in bone mineral density at the hip.[39] Bisphosponates significantly reduce the risk of hip, wrist and vertebral fractures in postmenopausal women with osteoporosis or those with a previous vertebral compression fracture.[40,41] Although osteopenia defines an intermediate risk group, since its prevalence is greater than osteoporosis, it represents a substantial portion of the population at risk for fracture. In fact, ~80% of fragility fractures occur in people without osteoporosis by the World Health Organization definition,[42] leading to the suggestion that the focus of fracture prevention must rest with identifying those at risk of falls rather than those with osteoporosis.[43]

Box 13.6 DEXA (dual-energy X-ray absorptiometry) scans for diagnosing osteoporosis

WHO definitions are based on comparisons of bone mineral density (BMD) with reference to the number of standard deviations (SDs) from the BMD in an average 25-year-old woman (T-score):

Normal	T-score of ≥–1 SD
Osteopenia	T-score of –1 to –2.5 SD
Osteoporosis	T-score <–2.5 SD
Established osteoporosis	T-score <–2.5 SD, with ≥1 fragility fractures

Reference standards have been published for the different measurement sites.

The prediction of fracture risk is usually based on BMD measurements at the femoral neck.

At present there are no comprehensive guidelines on who should be offered a DEXA scan, but local guidelines are likely to include factors such as:

◆ Untreated early menopause (aged <45 years).

◆ Prolonged amenorrhoea (>6 months).

◆ Primary hypogonadism.

◆ Fragility fracture aged <75 years.

◆ Secondary osteoporosis, e.g. endocrine, anorexia, malabsorption, chronic renal failure, chronic liver disease.

◆ X-Ray evidence of osteopenia or vertebral abnormalities found on investigation for loss of height or thoracic kyphosis.

◆ Maternal hip fracture aged <75 years.

◆ Low BMI (<19 kg/m^2).

◆ Corticosteroids 7.5 mg per day for ≥3 months.

◆ New fractures while taking bisphosphonates for ≥1 year.

Osteoporosis is usually primary, related to a range of factors affecting bone metabolism. These may not be modifiable, such as gender, age, a family history of fragility fractures (including loss of height of ≥2 inches suggesting vertebral fractures), years since becoming postmenopausal and Caucasian ethnicity. Modifiable factors include physical activity levels, body weight, smoking, alcohol intake, and low calcium or vitamin D intake.[44]

Secondary osteoporosis is associated with chronic inflammatory conditions, notably inflammatory bowel disease, rheumatoid arthritis and chronic liver disease, poor nutrition, notably coeliac disease and anorexia nervosa, and metabolic disturbances which directly affect bone metabolism such as male hypogonadism, hyperparathyroidism, renal disease and glucocorticoid excess.

The NICE clinical guideline on the assessment of fracture risk and the prevention of osteoporotic fractures is likely to be finalized in 2009, following completion of the NICE technology appraisals (TAs) on treatment of osteoporosis for the primary and secondary prevention of fragility fractures. Thus at present the only published NICE guidance is the TA on secondary

Box 13.7 Secondary prevention of osteoporotic fragility fractures (postmenopausal women only)[45]

Bisphosphonates (alendronate, etidronate and risedronate) are recommended for:

Aged ≥75 years | *without* need of DEXA scan
Aged 65–74 years | if DEXA confirms osteoporosis
Aged <65 years | if DEXA shows BMD T score <–3
| or if DEXA shows BMD T score <–2.5
| *plus 1 or more* additional risk factor

In all cases adequate intakes of vitamin D (10–20 μg, 400–800 IU) and calcium (1 g daily) are assumed, or supplementation should be prescribed.

Additional risk factors

- BMI <19 kg/m^2.
- Maternal hip fracture aged <75 years.
- Untreated premature menopause.
- Co-morbidities associated with bone loss: inflammatory bowel disease, rheumatoid arthritis, hyperthyroidism, coeliac disease, prolonged immobility.

An alternative for patients who cannot tolerate bisphosphonates is raloxifene. The main indicators of intolerance are usually oesophageal inflammation or bleeding.

Teriparatide (parathyroid hormone) is recommended for patients intolerant of, or unresponsive to, other treatments (based on another fragility fracture *plus* decline of BMD on a repeat DEXA) but only if the patient also has very severe osteoporosis (T score <–4) or T-score <–3 *plus* more than two fractures *plus* additional risk factors.

prevention (see Box 13.7) but this is limited to postmenopausal women, both steroid and male osteoporosis being excluded.[45]

A consequence of the guidance is that women aged >75 years with a fragility fracture do not need a DEXA scan prior to initiation of therapy. Guidance is currently lacking on more recent treatments such as strontium, for which there is a TA in preparation. SIGN has provided more extensive guidance including men in 2003.[46] In addition to advice on pharmacological agents, SIGN has recommended consumption (diet or supplements) of adequate calcium and vitamin D intake as in Box 13.7 and high intensity strength training and/or low impact weightbearing exercise. Although hormone replacement therapy is efficacious in prevention of fragility fractures, it is no longer considered suitable first-line therapy because of the associated excess cardiovascular and breast cancer deaths.

Male osteoporosis requires additional investigations, as illustrated in the following Case Study.

Case Study   Male osteoporosis

At the next consultation, Mrs J mentions her brother aged 78 years, who lives nearby her but is housebound. She mentions that he fell rising from a chair at home 8 months previously and sustained a fracture of the shoulder. The practice records indicate that this was a subcapital humerus fracture. He is on no regular medication, and other than several exacerbations of chronic obstructive pulmonary disease, he has no record of long-term conditions.

Subsequent assessment by the district nurse suggests that he has the following risk factors for falls: previous fall, inability to get up from chair without using arms, associated with reduced lower limb strength and orthostatic hypotension. He has the following risk factors for fractures: alcohol intake of average 4 units per day, BMI of 18.5 kg/m^2 and maternal hip fracture aged <75 years. He has lost nearly 10% body weight in the last 9 months, and describes poorly localized musculoskeletal discomfort.

What investigations does he need?

- Full blood count, renal function, electrolytes, liver function tests, calcium and phosphate.
- Serum testosterone: this may be low due to age and because of excess alcohol consumption. Subsequent hypogonadism is a potentially modifiable risk factor but for which there are no established treatment guidelines. Thyroid function: hyperthyoidism is associated with reduced bone mineral density and could explain some of his other symptoms.
- Vitamin D: this is likely to be low as a result of being housebound. Although no direct evidence exists for housebound frail men, it is reasonable to assume that supplementation is wise where levels are low.
- Plasma protein electrophoresis and urine sample for Bence Jones proteins: as myeloma is an important cause of secondary and male osteoporosis, often associated with diffuse bone pain and frequently not associated with abnormal bone biochemistry in early stages.
- Serum folate, since he is at risk for dietary reasons.
- DEXA scan? Since no guidance exists for men with fragility fractures, this could be performed if overall assessment leaves uncertainty about the probability of osteoporosis.

All the above investigations were normal except for Hb 10.2 g/l, with normal red cell indices and estimated glomerular filtration rate of 28 ml/min/1.73 m^2. These results indicate the need for further assessment as he may have chronic kidney disease stage IV (see Chapter 14). In addition, the usual doses of 800 IU of vitamin D in proprietary preparations may be ineffective, and activated vitamin D therapy (alphacalcidol or calcitriol) is likely to be needed as long as serum calcium is normal, in addition to a bisphosphonate for probable osteoporosis.

Managing falls and fracture risk in care homes

Up to 40% of care home admissions are related to recurrent falls. The risk of falling for residents is several-fold higher than for community dwelling people; variation reflecting the differences in care home populations but mobile individuals with cognitive impairment are at particularly high risk. A recent systematic review and meta-analysis suggested that there is insufficient evidence that multifactorial interventions (such as exercise training, staff education and medication reviews) in care homes reduce the risk of falls or fractures.[47] Where effectiveness was shown in a minority of individual studies, this did not benefit those with severe cognitive impairment. A Cochrane review 'Interventions for preventing falls in older people in residential care facilities and hospitals' is in progress.

What about injury prevention? Despite positive findings for efficacy in early studies, the latest evidence suggests that there is uncertainty around the effectiveness of hip protectors in institutional settings and there is no evidence to support their use in older people living at home.[48] Poor compliance is a problem due to discomfort, difficulty in putting them on, and in quick removal for toileting.

Auditing assessment and management of falls and fracture risk

A recent Healthcare Commission-funded national audit of the care of patients following fragility fractures indicated that most patients returning home from the emergency department following a fragility fracture were not offered a falls risk assessment, only one-third were on appropriate treatment for osteoporosis 3 months later and even after hip fracture <50% of patients were on appropriate osteoporosis treatment.[49] An evaluation of standards of care for osteoporosis and falls in primary care found that almost three-quarters of older women with a diagnosis of osteoporosis and a previous fragility fracture were prescribed appropriate treatment for osteoporosis, but that only 1 in 10 older women and 1 in 50 older men with a previous fragility fracture had a referral for a DEXA scan in their electronic medical record, and <1 in 50 older people recorded as being at high risk of falls had a recorded referral to a falls service or an exercise programme.[50] Although this may be partly explained by failure to enter data onto electronic records, it may also reflect care that does not meet current guidelines.

Conclusion

Falls reduction will occur with good multidisciplinary assessment and actions where appropriate. However, osteoporosis will increase with an ageing population and needs to be actively managed prior to patient frailty. The role of exercise is dealt with in Chapter 27.

References

1. National Institute for Health and Clinical Excellence. *Falls: The Assessment and Prevention of Falls in Older People*. Clinical Practice Guideline 21. London: Royal College of Nursing;NICE 2004.

2. Scuffham P, Chaplin P. The incidence and costs of accidental falls in the UK. Final Report. York Health Economic Form Consortium. York: University of York; 2002.

3. O'Neill TW, Varlow J, Reeve J, *et al*. Fall frequency and incidence of distal forearm fracture in the UK. *J Epidemiol Community Health* 1995;49:597–8.

4. Fleming J, Matthews FE, Brayne C; Cambridge City over-75s Cohort (CC75C) study collaboration. Falls in advanced old age: recalled falls and prospective follow-up of over-90-year-olds in the Cambridge City over-75s Cohort study. *BMC Geriatr* 2008;17:6.

5. Scuffham P, Chaplin S, Legood R. Incidence and costs of unintentional falls in older people in the United Kingdom. *J Epidemiol Community Health* 2003;57:740–4.

6. Vetter N, Ford D. Anxiety and depression scores in elderly fallers. *Int J Geriatr Psych* 1989;4:168–73.

7. Torgerson DJ, Iglesias CP, Reid DM. The economics of fracture prevention. In: Barlow DH, Francis RM, Miles A (eds), *The Effective Management of Osteoporosis*. London: Aesculapius Medical Press; 2001. p. 111–121.

8. Vestergaard P, Rejnmark L, Mosekilde L. Has mortality after a hip fracture increased? *J Am Geriatr Soc* 2007;55:1720–6.

9. Department of Health. *Hospital Episode Statistics (England) 2006*. Available from: http://www.hesonline.org.uk.

10. Personal communication from the Information Centre for Health and Social Care, March 2008.

11. Rubenstein LZ. Falls in older people: epidemiology, risk factors and strategies for prevention. *Age Ageing* 2006;35(Suppl 2):ii37–ii41.

12. Friedman SM, Munoz B, West SK, Rubin GS, Fried LP. Falls and fear of falling: which comes first? A longitudinal prediction model suggests strategies for primary and secondary prevention. *J Am Geriatr Soc* 2002;50:1329–35.

13. Yardley L, Todd C. *Encouraging Positive Attitudes to Falls Prevention in Later Life*. London: Help the Aged; 2005.

14. Nandy S, Parsons S, Cryer C, *et al*. Development and preliminary examination of the predictive validity of the Falls Risk Assessment Tool (FRAT) for use in primary care. *J Public Health* 2004;26:138–43.

15. Campbell AJ, Robertson MC. Rethinking individual and community fall prevention strategies: a meta-regression comparing single and multifactorial interventions. *Age Ageing* 2007;36:656–62.

16. Scott V, Votova K, Scanlan A, Close J. Multifactorial and functional mobility assessment tools for fall risk among older adults in community, home-support, long-term and acute care settings. *Age Ageing* 2007;36:130–9.

17. Gunter KB, White KN, Hayes WC, Snow CM. Functional mobility discriminates nonfallers from one-time and frequent fallers. *J Gerontol A Biol Sci Med Sci* 2000;55:M672–6.

18. Shumway-Cook A, Brauer S, Woollacott M. Predicting the probability for falls in community-dwelling older adults using the timed up & go test. *Phys Ther* 2000;80:896–903.

19. Rockwood K, Awalt E, Carver D, Macknight C. Feasibility and measurement properties of the functional reach and the timed up and go tests in the Canadian Study of Health and Aging. *J Gerontol A Biol Sci Med Sci* 2000;5:M70–3.

20. Benson R, Adachi JD, Papaioannou A, *et al.* Evaluation of easily measured risk factors in the prediction of osteoporotic fractures. *BMC Musculoskelet Disord* 2005;6:47.

21. Harwood RH, Foss AJ, Osborn F, Gregson RM, Zaman A, Masud T. Falls and health status in elderly women following first eye cataract surgery: a randomised controlled trial. *Br J Ophthalmol* 2005;89:53–9.

22. Help the Aged. *Staying Steady. Improving your strength and balance. Advice for older people.* London: Help the Aged; 2007. http://www.helptheaged.org.uk/NR/rdonlyres/F6D4F2BB-5DAD-42B4-8141-9354FE24AF6F/0/staying_steady_adv.pdf

23. Help the Aged. *Healthy bones. Caring for your bones. Advice for older people.* London: Help the Aged; 2007. Available from: http://www.helptheaged.org.uk/NR/rdonlyres/6F81A580-2867-4DE0-A25D-A15833F09669/0/HB07.pdf

24. Day L, Fildes B, Gordon I, Fitzharris M, Flamer H, Lord S. Randomised factorial trial of falls prevention among older people living in their own homes. *Br Med J* 2002;325(7356):128.

25. Stone KL, Ewing SK, Lui L-Y, *et al.* Self-reported sleep and nap habits and risk of falls and fractures in older women: The Study of Osteoporotic Fractures. *J Am Geriatr Soc* 2006;54:1177–83.

26. Nikolaus T, Bach M. Preventing falls in community-dwelling frail older people using a home intervention team (HIT): results from the randomized Falls–HIT trial. *J Am Geriatr Soc* 2003;51:300–5.

27. Gardner MM, Robertson MC, Campbell AJ. Exercise in preventing falls and fall related injuries in older people: a review of randomised controlled trials. *Br J Sports Med* 2000;34:7–17.

28. Parry SW, Steen IN, Baptist M, Kenny RA. Amnesia for loss of consciousness in carotid sinus syndrome: implications for presentation with falls. *J Am Coll Cardiol* 2005;45:1840–3.

29. Scottish Intercollegiate Guidelines Network. *Management of Osteoporosis. Guideline No. 71.* Annex 4. Calculate your calcium. Edinburgh: SIGN; 2003. Available at: http://www.sign.ac.uk/guidelines/fulltext/71/index.html.

30. Tang BM, Eslick GD, Nowson C, Smith C, Bensoussan A. Use of calcium or calcium in combination with vitamin D supplementation to prevent fractures and bone loss in people aged 50 years and older: a meta-analysis. *Lancet* 2007;370(9588):657–66.

31. Hartikainen S, Lönnroos E, Louhivuori K. Medication as a risk factor for falls: critical systematic review. *J Gerontol A Biol Sci Med Sci* 2007;62:1172–81.

32. Takkouche B, Montes-Martínez A, Gill SS, Etminan M. Psychotropic medications and the risk of fracture: a meta-analysis. *Drug Saf* 2007;30:171–84.

33. Haney EM, Chan BKS, Diem SJ, *et al.* Association of low bone mineral density with selective serotonin reuptake inhibitor use by older men. *Arch Intern Med* 2007;167:1246–51.

34. Diem SJ, Blackwell TL, Stone KL, *et al.* Depressive symptoms and rates of bone loss at the hip in older women. *J Am Geriatr Soc* 2007;55:824–31.

35. Clinical Effectiveness and Evaluation Unit. *National Clinical Audit of Falls and Bone Health in Older People-National Report.* Royal College of Physicians of London, 2007. Available at: http://www.

rcplondon.ac.uk/clinical-standards/ceeu/Current-work/Pages/Falls-and-Bone-Health-in-Older-People.aspx#national.

36. Ismail AA, Pye SR, Cockerill WC, *et al.* Incidence of limb fracture across Europe: results from the European Prospective Osteoporosis Study (EPOS). *Osteoporos Int* 2002;13:565–71.

37. Donaldson LJ, Reckless IP, Scholes S, Mindell JS, Shelton NJ. The epidemiology of fractures in England. *J Epidemiol Community Health* 2008;62:174–80.

38. World Health Organization. *Assessment of Fracture Risk and its Application to Screening for Postmenopausal Osteoporosis.* Geneva: WHO; 1994.

39. Marshall D, Johnell O, Wedel H. Meta-analysis of how well measures of bone mineral predict fractures. *Br Med J* 1996;312(7041):1254–9.

40. Wells G, Cranney A, Peterson J, *et al.* Alendronate for the primary and secondary prevention of osteoporotic fractures in postmenopausal women. *Cochrane Database Syst Rev* 2008;23(1):CD001155.

41. Wells G, Cranney A, Peterson J, *et al.* Risedronate for the primary and secondary prevention of osteoporotic fractures in postmenopausal women. *Cochrane Database Syst Rev* 2008;23(1):CD004523.

42. Stone KL, Seeley DG, Lui LY, *et al.* BMD at multiple sites and risk of fracture of multiple types: long-term results from the Study of Osteoporotic Fractures. *J Bone Miner Res* 2003;18:1947–54.

43. Järvinen TL, Sievänen H, Khan KM, Heinonen A, Kannus P. Shifting the focus in fracture prevention from osteoporosis to falls. *Br Med J* 2008;336(7636):124–6.

44. Melin AL, Wilske J, Ringertz H, Sääf M. Vitamin D status, parathyroid function and femoral bone density in an elderly Swedish population living at home. *Aging (Milano)* 1999;11:200–7.

45. National Institute of Health and Clinical Excellence. *TA87. Osteoporosis—Secondary Prevention: Quick Reference Guide.* London: NICE; 2005. Available at: http://www.nice.org.uk.

46. Scottish Intercollegiate Guideline Network. *Management of Osteoporosis—A National Clinical Guideline 71.* Edinburgh: SIGN; 2003. Available at: http://www.sign.ac.uk.

47. Oliver D, Connelly JB, Victor CR, *et al.* The prevention of falls and fractures in hospitals and care homes and effect of cognitive impairment systematic review and meta-analysis. *Br Med J* 2007;334(7584):82.

48. Parker MJ, Gillespie WJ, Gillespie LD. Hip protectors for preventing hip fractures in older people. *Cochrane Database Syst Rev* 2005;20(3):CD001255.

49. Royal College of Physicians Clinical Effectiveness and Evaluation Unit. *National Clinical Audit of Falls and Bone Health in Older People, 2007.* Available from: http://www.rcplondon.ac.uk/clinical-standards/ceeu/Current-work/Pages/Falls-and-Bone-Health-in-Older-People.aspx

50. Hippisley-Cox J, Bayly J, Potter J, Fenty J, Parker C. *Evaluation of Standards of Care for Osteoporosis and Falls in Primary Care.* Final Report to The Information Centre for Health and Social Care. Nottingham: Q Research; 2007.

Chapter 14

Kidney problems

Simon de Lusignan and John Feehally

Introduction

Kidney disease is usually asymptomatic and often only discovered on finding raised blood pressure (BP), abnormal urinalysis, or from routine surveillance of kidney function. Only when kidney disease becomes more severe do symptoms develop—including fluid overload and anaemia. Historically, kidney disease was thought of as a rare condition looked after by specialists. However, the routine reporting of estimated glomerular filtration rate (eGFR) alongside serum creatinine has led to the identification of large numbers of people with chronic kidney disease (CKD).

CKD is very common, affecting between 5% and 10% of the population. Approximately half of females aged >75 years and males aged >85 years have CKD. CKD is more prevalent in females and in people with cardiovascular disease, hypertension and diabetes.[1]

Many older people with CKD can be managed in the community. Indications for early referral include rapid deterioration in renal function, nephrotic syndrome, and features suggesting a multisystem disease with renal involvement.

Approximately 120–150 per million of population (pmp) develop end-stage renal disease (ESRD) and need to start renal replacement therapy (RRT: transplantation or dialysis) each year. There are ~750 pmp currently receiving RRT; 45% of these have a functioning renal transplant, the remainder receive various forms of dialysis. A practice of 10 000 would expect one or two people to start RRT each year; and have seven or eight who are receiving dialysis or have had a transplant. ESRD is more common with increasing age, and among older people the proportion who receive a transplant is much lower.

Late referral for RRT (defined as <90 days between referral and starting RRT) is associated with a poor outcome.[2,3] In the UK, a significant proportion of people with renal failure are referred late;[4] increasing age is one of the factors associated with late referral.

National guidelines are available to support the management of kidney disease, from the Renal Association[5] and National Institute for Health and Clinical Excellence (NICE).[6] Information about people who have received RRT is available from the UK Renal Registry. Equivalent guidelines and information sources exist in most other countries—and can be accessed via the European Renal Association.[7] Additionally, local renal specialist services also offer online guidelines for services in their locality.

In summary this chapter addresses key challenges for the non-specialist:

1) How to recognize kidney disease.

2) The management of CKD.

3) Rarer causes of kidney disease.

4) When to refer to specialist care.

Clinical markers of kidney disease

Many patients with kidney disease have no symptoms or physical signs, especially in the early stages. The commonest physical signs are oedema, hypertension, and abnormal urine testing. These clinical features taken with a small number of blood tests and urine tests, often combined with renal imaging, can be highly informative about the nature and severity of kidney disease.

Oedema

Fluid retention occurs in advanced kidney disease of all causes when the failing kidneys can no longer balance sodium and water intake. Oedema in kidney disease when renal function is preserved usually only occurs when there is nephrotic syndrome. Oedema in kidney patients is commonly an adverse affect of calcium channel blockers.

Blood pressure

Hypertension can be both the cause and consequence of kidney disease. Hypertension occurs in the great majority of people with advanced kidney disease. Hypertension becomes more common as GFR declines. Fluid retention is an important contributor to hypertension in advanced kidney disease.

Urine testing: dipstick, quantification of proteinuria

Urinalysis is highly informative and should be regarded as part of the initial examination in any patient in whom kidney disease is suspected, including all patients presenting with hypertension and diabetes.

Proteinuria

Proteinuria can occur in any kidney disease. It is characteristic of glomerular diseases (e.g. glomerulonephritis (GN) and diabetic nephropathy) but may be absent until the later stages of tubulointerstitial diseases (e.g. polycystic kidney disease). Most of the protein in the urine is usually albumin.

Proteinuria develops very slowly in diabetic nephropathy. Small amounts of albumin in the urine (microalbuminuria) are not detectable by conventional dipstick. However, detecting microalbuminuria is important in identifying patients at high risk of complications and needing intensive therapy. It is not certain whether a similar phase of microalbuminuria could be detected in other chronic kidney diseases but this seems probable. Microalbuminuria is measured by a urine albumin:creatinine ratio (ACR) on a 'spot' urine sample.

When there is overt proteinuria (i.e. dipstick 1+ or more) ACR is also useful in quantifying proteinuria; however, many laboratories measure urine protein:creatinine ratio (PCR) rather than ACR. An advantage of PCR is the identification of occasional patients with proteinuria, but no albumin in the urine, especially patients with free light chains in the urine with myeloma. NICE guidelines on chronic kidney disease [6] recommend that ACR rather than PCR should become the standard quantification in patients who are dipstick positive.

Haematuria

Dipsticks are used to identify patients with non-visible (microscopic) haematuria. The dipstick detects the presence of haemoglobin and therefore does not distinguish between patients with invisible haematuria, and occasional patients with haemoglobinuria; in practice this usually does not matter. There is no indication for urine microscopy for haematuria which is an unreliable test since red blood cells will often lyse in hypotonic urine before they get to the laboratory. Hence, negative microscopy does not prove the absence of haematuria.

In general, the combination of proteinuria and haematuria (in the absence of urinary tract infection (UTI)) suggests more severe kidney disease than haematuria or proteinuria alone.

Visible (macroscopic) haematuria

In the absence of urine infection, visible haematuria requires urological referral and evaluation. The two most important causes are renal tract malignancy and stones. Visible haematuria may be due to parenchymal renal disease in younger people when the urine will be brown rather than red, but this does not occur in older people.

Blood tests

Serum creatinine and eGFR

Exact measurement of glomerular filtration rate is not possible in clinical practice. Therefore simpler methods based on blood and urine tests have always been used to estimate GFR.

Since 2006 it has been routine for all clinical biochemistry laboratories in the UK to report estimated GFR (eGFR) as well as serum creatinine. eGFR is calculated using a formula which only requires age, gender, and serum creatinine. An additional factor is required for African-Caribbean ethnicity which otherwise underestimates eGFR. eGFR is not a precise measurement of GFR, but is significantly more accurate than serum creatinine. The formula for eGFR has been criticized, and its limitations are well known.[8]

It is especially reliable in patients with eGFR <60 (some laboratories do not give a value for eGFR when it is >60). Measurement of eGFR is a major element in a classification of CKD which has been widely adopted in recent years (see Table 14.2).

Renal imaging

Ultrasound scan is the first imaging modality for most patients with suspected kidney disease. Its advantages are that it is rapid and non-invasive.

Table 14.1 Renal ultrasound scan investigation of older people

Features on the scan	Additional comments
Renal size	
Shrunken kidneys (<9 cm length)	Indicates longstanding kidney disease but gives no information about cause.
Normal size	Does not exclude significant kidney disease, especially glomerular disease which may require renal biopsy for precise diagnosis.
Asymmetrical kidneys (>2 cm disparity)	Consider unilateral renal artery stenosis.
Renal outline	
Irregular outline	Implies patchy renal scarring, does not distinguish between vascular, infective, or congenital causes.
Hydronephrosis	Indicates obstruction to the renal tract. Does not always define level of obstruction, lower ureters poorly visualised.
Mass lesions	Reliably detects tumours >1 cm (benign or malignant).
Renal cysts	Detects simple cysts (common with increasing age) or conditions associated with multiple renal cysts, most commonly polycystic kidney disease.

Other tests which are less commonly useful

Serum sodium and potassium

See below ('Fluid and electrolyte problems').

Urine sodium and potassium

These should very rarely be measured in primary care. Urinary sodium in patients with hypertension is occasionally useful to establish concordance with recommendations for dietary salt restriction.

Serum calcium, phosphate, magnesium, parathyroid hormone, alkaline phosphatase

Disordered bone metabolism is an increasing problem as CKD progresses. Factors include vitamin D deficiency, and hyperparathyroidism. As CKD progresses, raised serum phosphate is usually the first abnormality followed by falling serum calcium. Alkaline phosphatase increases late as bone metabolism deteriorates. Paget's disease is an important differential diagnosis for rising alkaline phosphatase.

Chronic kidney disease

Introduction and definitions

Chronic kidney disease (CKD) describes people with impaired kidney function of ≥3 months duration whatever the cause. A classification of CKD developed in the USA by the Kidney Disease Outcome Quality Initiative (KDOQI) depends on eGFR has been widely adopted (Table 14.2).[9] It has been proposed that CKD stage 3 is further subdivided into stages 3a and 3b, and that all stages of CKD should have a 'p' added if there is significant proteinuria.[10] UK general practitioners have been set quality targets for management of CKD, but these only apply to people with eGFR <60 ml/min/1.73 m^2; i.e. with CKD stages 3–5.

Causes and consequences of CKD

Diabetes, hypertension, and atheromatous renovascular disease (ARVD) are the major causes of CKD in older people. In people with diabetes the prevalence of CKD is ~31%, compared to 6.9% in people without diabetes.[11] Hypertension is a frequent cause and consequence of CKD, and age-related decline in renal function is associated with high BP.[12] Cardiovascular co-morbidities are

Table 14.2 Stages of chronic kidney disease (CKD)

CKD stage	eGFR value (ml/min/1.73 m^2)	Name	Subdivision	Structural damage	Functional damage	QOF CKD
1	≥90	Kidney damage + normal or raised GFR		Yes	No	No
2	60–89	Kidney damage + mildly impaired GFR		Yes	Yes	No
3	30–59	Moderately impaired GFR	3a 45–59 3b 30–44	Possible	Yes	Yes
4	15–29	Severely impaired GFR		Possible	Yes	Yes
5	<15 or dialysis	Kidney failure		Possible	Yes	Yes

eGFR, estimated glomerular filtration rate; QOF, Quality and Outcomes Framework.

extremely common in CKD; three-quarters of people with CKD have one or more co-morbid circulatory diseases.[13] CKD is also independently associated with central obesity.[14] Medication can also contribute to impaired renal function (see 'Prescribing in kidney disease').

Other rarer causes of CKD in older people include: hereditary conditions (e.g. adult polycystic kidney disease); and inflammatory conditions (e.g. glomerulonephritis and vasculitis).

An increased prevalence of CKD in Black, South Asian and Hispanic populations may be related to the higher prevalence of hypertension, diabetes and obesity in these ethnic groups.

People with CKD are at increased risk of cardiovascular disease, and have a much greater risk of major adverse cardiovascular events than of progressing to ESRD. The degree of risk increases with the severity of CKD,[15] although the relative risks associated with reduced renal function are greater in younger people.

People with proteinuria are at greater risk of both progressive CKD and cardiovascular disease. Population-level data indicate than even minor increases in urine albumin excretion are associated with increased cardiovascular risk.[16] Although the general practice diabetic population are screened for microalbuminuria, proteinuria testing is equally important in risk stratification for people with hypertension and CKD without diabetes, although it is conducted less frequently. An ACR ≥70 mg/mmol (equivalent to proteinuria ~1 g/24 h) should prompt referral to a specialist unless explained by diabetes or other known cause.[2]

Identification of CKD

More than 80% of older people with CKD will be identified by routine urine testing or measurement of eGFR among those known to have diabetes, hypertension, or cardiovascular disease. CKD typically remains asymptomatic until CKD stage 4 when anaemia usually develops, or stage 5 when frank uraemic symptoms begin.

Management of BP and cardiovascular risk

Essential hypertension can cause progressive CKD but this is unusual if BP is well controlled from a time when GFR is preserved. Secondary hypertension occurs in most forms of renal disease and is a powerful amplifier of the risk of progression of CKD. By the time the patient presents with falling GFR, it is not always easy to work out, even with detailed investigation, whether the raised BP is the cause or consequence of CKD.

BP control is the main aim of CKD management, and evidence for benefit is strongest in those with proteinuria. Angiotensin-converting enzyme inhibitors (ACEIs) and angiotensin II receptor blockers (ARBs) are first-line treatment for hypertension. Current Renal Association guidance sets threshold levels for treatment and the targets for optimum BP management are shown in Table 14.3. The more recent NICE guidance simply sets a range: systolic between 120 and 140 mmHg,

Table 14.3 Blood pressure (BP, mmHg) thresholds for treatment and BP target

| | Renal Association | | | | QOF | | NICE | |
| | Proteinuria | | No proteinuria | | Proteinuria | | | |
	Systolic	Diastolic	Systolic	Diastolic	Systolic	Diastolic	Systolic	Diastolic
Threshold	140	90	140	90	140	85	140	90
Target goal	125	75	130	80	<140	<85	120–140	70–90

QOF, Quality and Outcomes Framework; NICE, National Institute of Health and Clinical Excellence.

and diastolic between 70 and 90 mmHg.[17] The Quality and Outcomes Framework CKD BP indicator is set at 140/85.

Multiple drug therapy is commonly required to achieve BP goals in CKD. Over-treatment of hypertension in CKD may be detrimental; diastolic hypotension and a wide pulse pressure may increase cardiovascular risk.[18]

Treatment should also be directed towards cardiovascular risk reduction, including smoking cessation and obesity management. In diabetes, treatment should focus on BP management and glycaemic control. A medication review is needed, to reduce or stop drugs likely to impair renal function.

Specialist referral and shared care

Most older patients with CKD can be managed in primary care. Referral planning can be complex, as poorly controlled heart failure or diabetes (associated with poor renal function) may be best initially referred to a cardiologist or diabetologist. Men with possible urinary tract obstruction and people with haematuria without signs of renal disease may be best referred to an urologist initially. A specialist renal opinion should be considered for older people who have CKD with:[17]

+ very poor kidney function (CKD stages 4 and 5: eGFR <30 ml/min/1.73 m²);
+ rapidly declining kidney function – progressive fall in eGFR >5 ml/min/1.73m² per year, or >10 ml/min/1.73 m² over 5 years;[17] repeated measures are required to demonstrate progression, as there is variability in eGFR estimations;
+ nephrotic syndrome;
+ treatment-resistant hypertension;
+ non-visible haematuria and proteinuria with clinical features suggesting a multisytem inflammatory disease;
+ renal anaemia, which typically develops in CKD stage 4, and sometimes earlier in diabetes.

Other causes of kidney disease in older people

Renovascular disease

Atheromatous renovascular disease (ARVD) is increasingly recognized as a cause of hypertension and CKD in older people. When ARVD causes critical renal artery stenosis (RAS), resistant hypertension and progressive CKD follow especially with bilateral disease.

ARVD should be suspected when there is poorly controlled BP, progressive renal failure, episodic pulmonary oedema with normal left ventricle function, or when there is deterioration in renal function with introduction of an ACEI or ARB. Suspected ARVD requires specialist evaluation. The great majority of patients with ARVD have clinically significant cerebral, coronary or peripheral arterial disease. A difference in renal size on ultrasound is suggestive, but may not be present with bilateral RAS. A renal bruit is not a reliable sign and there is typically little or no abnormality on urinalysis.

Not all patients with ARVD, even those with significant RAS, require angioplasty and stenting; indications include poorly controlled BP, progressive renal failure, and episodic pulmonary oedema.

Glomerular disease and multisystem disease affecting the kidneys

The commonest glomerular diseases are diabetic nephropathy, amyloid, and the various forms of GN. Proteinuria is the hallmark of these conditions. Most older people with proteinuria do not need a renal biopsy to define the glomerular disease; it is sufficient to know that proteinuria has a negative influence on renal and cardiovascular outcomes (see above: CKD). Renal biopsy should only be considered when there is a high likelihood that a precise diagnosis will alter treatment recommendations.

In diabetic nephropathy, renal biopsy is often unnecessary; it is usually appropriate to make a presumptive diagnosis based on a long history of diabetes, and on the presence of other microvascular complications (retinopathy, neuropathy).

Referral for specialist assessment including renal biopsy is required for suspected GN in some circumstances:

◆ When there is nephrotic syndrome (i.e. proteinuria of sufficient severity to cause a fall in serum albumin and oedema). Nephrotic syndrome can occur with a normal GFR. Nephrotic syndrome must be distinguished clinically from other causes of generalized dependent oedema, including congestive heart failure, and chronic liver disease.

◆ When the GN is rapidly progressive with renal failure developing in days or weeks. There is usually proteinuria *and* haematuria, and it is more common in association with multisystem disease (e.g. systemic vasculitis) so there may be general symptoms (fever, arthralgia, anaemia), as well as evidence of other organ involvement (most commonly skin and respiratory tract). This is uncommon but can be a medical emergency since delay in diagnosis even by a few days or weeks can result in ESRD, which is avoidable if immunosuppressive treatment is started early. Any patient with blood and protein in the urine suspected of having GN should have eGFR checked again within 1 week to see if the rate of change justifies urgent referral.

Myeloma

Myeloma increases in incidence with increasing age. It should be suspected in older people presenting with anaemia, bone pain, and hypercalcaemia. Renal involvement is due to amyloid (proteinuria is typical) or to myeloma kidney, in which casts of light chain obstruct renal tubules (there is often little or no dipstick urine abnormality, although free light chains in the urine will be detected by PCR but not ACR). If renal involvement is diagnosed early, active management of myeloma may prevent ESRD.

Renal cysts

Renal cysts are a common finding in older people undergoing ultrasound scan to investigate CKD, and are usually a coincidental finding, especially isolated simple cysts. Complex cysts (e.g. with septae and calcification) may be malignant and need evaluation by computed tomography.

Autosomal dominant polycystic kidney disease (PKD) is the commonest inherited kidney disease, and an important cause of CKD; there are multiple cysts in both kidneys. Renal failure typically develops in the fourth the sixth decades of life, but some older people with PKD may have normal renal function.

Even when there are multiple cysts in both kidneys, a diagnosis of PKD should not be made unless there is a typical family history of renal failure or sudden death, and the presence of liver as well as renal cysts. Correct identification of other rarer forms of cystic renal disease requires specialist evaluation.

Prescribing in kidney disease

Introduction

Many drugs should be avoided or used differently in people with kidney disease, which exacerbates the challenges of medicines management in older people. Many drugs or their metabolites are excreted by the kidney (see Chapter 4). Dose reductions or increased dosing interval are often needed; only one class of drug needs *increased* dosing–loop diuretics. Prescribers should always use an up-to-date drug dictionary and interactions table or a computerized decision support system; advice should be available from a nephrologist or specialist pharmacist. Prescribing guides have previously recommended dose changes according to creatinine clearance, but advice based on eGFR will gradually appear.

Angiotensin-converting enzyme inhibitors and angiotensin receptor blockers

Agents that block the renin–angiotensin system—ACEIs and ARBs—are the agents most likely to be protective in proteinuric CKD, but they also risk harm.

Deterioration in renal function and hyperkalaemia may occur when ACEI or ARB treatment is initiated or doses increased; this may occur in a few days if there is bilateral RAS. eGFR and serum potassium should be checked within a week of starting or altering dose. A 10% fall in eGFR over a period of 2 months after starting ACEIs or ARBs is acceptable, and may be associated with better long-term preservation of renal function. Serum potassium ≥5.6 mmol/l requires dose reduction or discontinuation of ACEIs or ARBs.

Medication review in the management of CKD

Medication, both prescribed and non-prescribed, is also an important factor in CKD development. Other than ACEIs and ARBs, the most problematic class of drugs is non-steroidal anti-inflammatory drugs (NSAIDs). NSAID prescribing, especially with high cumulative exposure, is associated with rapid decline in renal function and the benefits of prescribing should be carefully weighed up against the risk.[19]

Hypoglycaemic agents

Metformin can cause lactic acidosis and is contraindicated in CKD stages 4 and 5, but current practice in many clinics is to prescribe it in CKD stage 3.[20,21] Short-acting sulphonylureas (e.g. gliclazide) and glitazones can be used in CKD. Arcarbose should be avoided if eGFR <25 ml/min/1.73 m^2.

Antibiotics

Nitrofurantoin can accumulate with eGFR <50 ml/min/1.73 m^2 and may cause peripheral neuropathy. Trimethoprim dose should be reduced with eGFR <25 ml/min/1.73 m^2. Penicillins can accumulate with very low eGFR (<20 ml/min/1.73 m^2).

Bisphosphonates should not be prescribed in CKD stages 4 and 5

A number of drugs are usually initiated as part of specialist care for kidney disease, but primary care may have to be involved in prescribing and monitoring. These include phosphate binders, active vitamin D and other agents for bone metabolism; erythropoietin for renal anaemia; and immunosuppressive drugs for transplant recipients.

Urinary tract infection

UTI is very common in primary care, and only in a small minority is it a presenting feature of significant renal disease. Lower urinary tract symptoms are typical, and there may be visible haematuria. Upper urinary tract infection, i.e. acute pyelonephritis, is characterized by loin tenderness and systemic upset.

UTI in adults does not cause renal scarring but often causes transient deterioration in renal function, especially on a background of CKD, which usually improves with successful treatment of infection.

Use of dipstick urinalysis has refined management of UTI, reducing the necessity for urine culture. In the absence of nitrites and leukocytes on urine testing, the likelihood of UTI is very low, and urine culture is not necessary. In the presence of nitrites and leukocytes, empirical therapy can be started while awaiting the results of urine culture to guide antibiotic choice.

Indwelling bladder catheters

Bacteriuria is extremely common and urine should not be cultured unless there is a high clinical suspicion of symptomatic urinary tract infection.

Ileal conduit

Bacteriuria is virtually inevitable in drainage bag specimens. Urine should only be cultured and antibiotics given if there is strong clinical suspicion of urinary tract infection, usually fever, systemic upset, and loin pain.

Treatment of UTI

Antibiotic choice should always be consistent with local antibiotic policies. For uncomplicated lower UTI, a 3 day course of trimethoprim, a fluoroquinolone, or co-amoxiclav is usually sufficient. For complicated UTI (e.g. acute pyelonephritis) 10–14 days of treatment is needed.

Admission to hospital with UTI is required if systemic illness and vomiting prevent adequate administration of antibiotics, or if fever and loin pain continue after 48–72 h of active management.

In older people referral for specialist urological evaluation after UTI is recommended after treatment of UTI for:

- persistent or recurrent UTI;
- visible haematuria or persistent non-visible haematuria;
- persisting lower urinary tract symptoms suggestive of bladder outflow obstruction;
- abdominal mass consistent with urinary tract origin.

Prevention of acute kidney injury

Acute kidney injury describes sudden deterioration in renal function either with pre-existing CKD or with previously normal kidneys.

Development of acute kidney injury severe enough to require admission and specialist treatment is a life-threatening illness. Acute kidney injury referred to renal units has a 50% mortality, higher in older people because of associated co-morbidity. Preventable acute kidney injury is more common with increasing age. Medications commonly necessary in older people, particularly ACEIs, ARBs and NSAIDs, become nephrotoxic during episodes of intercurrent illness especially with fluid depletion, intercurrent infection, and also during the perioperative period for both elective and emergency surgery. Older people are especially prone to fluid depletion as impaired urine-concentrating ability (even when eGFR is preserved) makes them less able to compensate appropriately for fluid losses. Transient hypotension increases the risk of acute kidney injury even in the absence of fluid depletion, and is more likely in older people with cardiovascular disease.

Temporary withdrawal of ACEIs, ARBs, and NSAIDs should always be considered with inter-current illness, especially when there is infection, and when gastrointestinal problems increase the risk of fluid depletion. This simple strategy can prevent acute kidney injury and save lives.

Fluid and electrolyte disorders

Electrolyte abnormalities are common, and may often be incidental numerical findings.

Hypokalaemia

Moderate hypokalaemia (3.0–3.5 mmol/l) is asymptomatic; lower levels may cause muscle weakness. It most commonly follows prescription of thiazide and loop diuretics, or occurs with persistent vomiting and diarrhoea. If diuretics cannot be avoided, encourage high potassium foods (fruit, especially bananas, and chocolate) or give potassium supplements. It is especially important to keep potassium in the reference range for those taking digoxin.

Hypokalaemia occuring without drug treatment or gastrointestinal upset requires specialist referral.

Hyperkalaemia

Moderate hyperkalaemia (5.6–6.0 mmol/l) is asymptomatic; higher levels may cause life-threatening arrhythmias. Hyperkalaemia most commonly occurs in people with CKD stages 4 and 5, and in less severe CKD during treatment with ACEIs, ARBs, NSAIDs, or potassium-retaining diuretics such as spironolacotone. Discontinue all unnecessary drugs. If it is important to continue ACEIs or ARBs, advise the patient to avoid high potassium foods. If there is metabolic acidosis (serum bicarbonate <22 mmol/l) sodium bicarbonate supplements will lower serum potassium.

Hyperkalaemia without such drug treatment, or with normal eGFR, requires specialist referral.

Hyponatraemia

Hyponatraemia and hypernatraemia are confusing terms and often misinterpreted as indicating whether the patient is overall sodium depleted or sodium overloaded. Changes in sodium concentration in the blood must always be interpreted in the context of a clinical assessment of a patient's fluid status. For example, a patient with hyponatraemia associated with diuretic therapy may be severely sodium overloaded in heart failure.

Hyponatraemia is usually asymptomatic. Moderate hyponatraemia (125–135 mmol/l) is very common in heart failure, and is often aggravated by diuretics, which should be minimized where clinically possible, but no other action is usually necessary.

More severe hyponatraemia (<125 mmol/l) without diuretics or abnormal fluid status requires specialist evaluation. Diabetes insipidus and syndrome of inappropriate antidiuretic hormone secretion are commonly mentioned causes of hyponatraemia; both are rare. In the absence of major disturbances in fluid balance, hypernatraemia and hyponatraemia are uncommon and evaluation is less urgent.

Hypernatraemia

Moderate hypernatraemia (145–155 mmol/l) in the absence of fluid depletion is uncommon. Recommend an increased water intake, but if it persists, specialist referral is recommended.

Hypocalcaemia

With normal renal function, hypocalcaemia is almost always due to dietary deficiency of calcium and vitamin D, or malabsorption. If it does not respond to dietary advice and treatment with cholecalciferol, specialist gastroenterology referral should be considered if there are any other features of malabsorption.

Hypocalcaemia with CKD does not respond to vitamin D_3, and requires specialist referral.

Hypercalcaemia

Always exclude excess use of cod liver oil, and other over-the-counter preparations containing vitamin D, as a cause of moderate hypercalcaemia (2.7–3.0 mmol/l).

Patients with CKD are often prescribed calcium-containing preparations and vitamin D, in which case these are the commonest cause of hypercalcaemia, which often transiently reduces GFR; dose adjustment is required.

In the absence of drug therapy, malignancy is the commonest cause of hypercalcaemia; bone metastases, myeloma, or non-metastatic effects; severe hypercalcaemia (>3.0 mmol/l) is more common. If there is no evidence of malignancy consider sarcoidosis or hyperparathyroidism.

If the clinical evaluation provides no clear pointers, serum parathyroid hormone will help to discriminate; it will be very low in malignancy or sarcoidosis, but inappropriately high in hyperparathyroidism. Specialist referral is required for severe hypercalcaemia.

Advanced CKD and RRT

Although CKD is common, progression to ESRD is uncommon. This may be partly because many patients with CKD die prematurely from cardiovascular disease before they develop renal failure, and also because not all CKD progresses to ESRD particularly with modern management of BP and proteinuria (see above).

As GFR progressively falls, complications of CKD increase regardless of the cause of kidney disease. Anaemia, disordered calcium and phosphate metabolism, hyperkalaemia, metabolic acidosis, and nutritional problems are all common, and require specialist treatment.

Regular dialysis treatment will control fluid and acid–base problems, but issues of nutrition, anaemia, and calcium/phosphate metabolism continue, unless the patient has a successful transplant.

Anaemia

The majority of patients with CKD stages 4 and 5 (including those on long-term dialysis) receive erythropoetin (EPO) by subcutaneous injection (typically weekly). Intravenous iron supplementation is required for effective red cell production to be driven by EPO (oral iron is poorly tolerated and ineffective) and is usually given in the renal unit or at home under hospital supervision.

Calcium, phosphate and bone metabolism

Control of serum phosphate and calcium is needed to minimize metabolic bone disease, and also to avoid vascular calcification, an important contributor to cardiovascular disease. Control of phosphate is particularly challenging requiring specialist dietetic advice as well as phosphate binders (e.g. calcium carbonate, sevelamer). Active vitamin D preparations (alfacalcidol, calcitriol) are usually required.

Nutrition

Malnutrition is very common in patients with CKD stage 4 or 5, appetite may be poor and necessary dietary restrictions require specialist dietetic care.

Choice and preparation for RRT

About 30% of patients with ESRD will not be known to the local renal unit until they present urgently requiring immediate dialysis treatment. These patients are significantly disadvantaged being unable to prepare practically and psychologically for the enormous impact which renal replacement therapy has on their lives and those of their famies. The more fortunate remainder will have access to the multiprofessional specialist care needed to provide optimal preparation and delivery of RRT. Adequate preparation may take up to 12 months before RRT starts. Immunisation against influenza, pneumococcus, and hepatitis B is part of this preparation.

Patients receive much information and have to make major choices between different modalities of treatment which should all be regarded as part of a continuum of care. Patients' first-choice treatment modality is not necessarily the treatment on which they remain long term. The principles of choice of RRT are:

- Kidney transplant is the preferred treatment for anyone who is fit for such surgery, which will be only a minority of older people. Transplant from a living donor is preferable, and ideally this should be pre-emptive (i.e. before dialysis treatment is necessary).

- If transplant is not an option, independent dialysis in the community (haemodialysis or peritoneal dialysis at home) is preferred.

- If a transplant or community-based dialysis is not possible, haemodialysis in a hospital setting is required.

- For some older people it is an appropriate choice to have 'conservative' treatment, i.e. not to accept any form of RRT. With good care, older people choosing a conservative approach may maintain quality of life until very close to death. Even with optimal support, long-term dialysis can be a very challenging treatment for some older people with multiple co-morbidities, and may not increase either quantity or quality of life.

Dialysis access

Haemodialysis patients are critically dependent on vascular access, which is ideally provided by an arteriovenous fistula in the upper limb, but in some patients by a tunnelled venous catheter which carries an increased risk of infection. For patients on peritoneal dialysis (PD), peritonitis presenting with abdominal pain and cloudy PD effluent is an important complication. Dialysis access requires specialist care and patients are usually recommended to report directly to their renal unit when problems arise.

It is important for effective care that the relative roles of the multiprofessional specialist team and primary care are well defined by local agreement. Transplant patients and those dialysing in the community will typically interact with primary care more than those on hospital-based haemodialysis, who may often seek help for intercurrent medical problems while attending for dialysis.

Transplantation

Renal transplantation is now very successful. Up to 70% of transplants are still working after 10 years. Few older people receive a transplant, although many longstanding transplant recipients live into older age. Cardiovascular death is common and conventional cardiovascular risk factors should be actively managed. Although there is limited specific evidence in transplant patients, statins should be used to a total cholesterol target of 4 mmol/l. Risk of malignancy is also increased, especially skin malignancy. Testicular and breast self-examination are recommended.

It is critical that local arrangements provide easy access for primary care to specialist advice from a nephrologist or transplant surgeon. Transplant surgeons are typically involved in the first 3–12 months of transplant care only, and long-term follow-up is provided by nephrologists.

References

1. Stevens PE, O'Donoghue DJ, de Lusignan S, *et al.* Chronic kidney disease management in the United Kingdom: NEOERICA project results. *Kidney Int* 2007;72:92–9.

2. Chan MR, Dall AT, Fletcher KE, Lu N, Trivedi H. Outcomes in patients with chronic kidney disease referred late to nephrologists: a meta-analysis. *Am J Med* 2007;120:1063–70.

3. Navaneethan SD, Aloudat S, Singh S. A systematic review of patient and health system characteristics associated with late referral in chronic kidney disease. *BMC Nephrol* 2008;9:3.

4. Farrington K, Rao R, Gilg J, Ansell D, Feest T. New adult patients starting renal replacement therapy in the UK in 2005 (Chapter 3). *Nephrol Dial Transplant* 2007;22(Suppl 7):vii11–29.

5. Renal Association. http://www.renal.org

6. National Health Service. NICE (National Institute of Health and Clinical Excellence). http://www.nice.org.uk/

7. European Renal Association–European Renal Dialysis and Transplant Association (ERA-EDTA). http://www.era-edta.org/

8. Lin J, Knight EL, Hogan ML, Singh AK. A comparison of prediction equations for estimating glomerular filtration rate in adults without kidney disease. *J Am Soc Nephrol* 2003;14:2573–80.

9. National Kidney Association Kidney Disease Outcome Quality Initiative (NKF KDOQI). K/DOQI Clinical Practice Guidelines for Chronic Kidney Disease: Evaluation, Classification, and Stratification. Available at: http://www.kidney.org/professionals/KDOQI/guidelines_ckd/toc.htm

10. Archibald G, Bartlett W, Brown A, *et al.* UK Consensus Conference on Early Chronic Kidney Disease – 6 and 7 February 2007. *Nephrol Dial Transplant* 2007;22:2455–7.

11. New JP, Middleton RJ, Klebe B, *et al.* Assessing the prevalence, monitoring and management of chronic kidney disease in patients with diabetes compared with those without diabetes in general practice. *Diabet Med* 2007;24:364–9.

12. Lindeman RD, Tobin JD, Shock NW. Association between blood pressure and the rate of decline in renal function with age. *Kidney Int* 1984;26;861–8.

13. de Lusignan S, Chan T, Stevens P, *et al.* Identifying patients with chronic kidney disease from general practice computer records. *Fam Pract* 2005;22:234–41.

14. Elsayed EF, Sarnak MJ, Tighiouart H, *et al.* Waist-to-hip ratio, body mass index, and subsequent kidney disease and death. *Am J Kidney Dis* 2008;E-pub 28 May.

15. van Domburg RT, Hoeks SE, Welten GM, Chonchol M, Elhendy A, Poldermans D. Renal insufficiency and mortality in patients with known or suspected coronary artery disease. *J Am Soc Nephrol* 2008;19:158–63.

16. Hillege HL, Fidler V, Diercks GF, *et al.*; Prevention of Renal and Vascular End Stage Disease (PREVEND) Study Group. Urinary albumin excretion predicts cardiovascular and noncardiovascular mortality in general population. *Circulation* 2002;106:1777–82.

17. National Institute of Health and Clinical Excellence. *National Clinical Guideline for the Management of Adults with Chronic Kidney Disease in Primary and Secondary Care.* London; Royal College of Physicians, 2008. Available at: http://www.nice.org.uk/page.aspx?o=ChronicKidneyDisease

18. Peralta CA, Shlipak MG, Wassel-Fyr C, *et al.* Association of antihypertensive therapy and diastolic hypotension in chronic kidney disease. *Hypertension* 2007;50:474–80.

19. Gooch K, Culleton BF, Manns BJ, *et al.* NSAID use and progression of chronic kidney disease. *Am J Med* 2007;120:280.e1–7.

20. Shaw JS, Wilmot RL, Kilpatrick ES. Establishing pragmatic estimated GFR thresholds to guide metformin prescribing. *Diabet Med* 2007;24:1160–3.

21. Warren R, Strachan M, Wild S, McKnigh J. Introducing estimated glomerular filtration rate (eGFR) into clinical practice in the UK: implications for the use of metformin. *Diabet Med* 2007;24:494–7.

Chapter 15

Ear, nose, and throat

Shaun Jackson and Andrew Swift

Introduction

Increasing age brings with it particular ear, nose and throat (ENT) morbidities which can lead to marked decrease in quality of life, particularly as many of the special senses are affected. This brief overview will aim to highlight some of the commoner ENT problems which will be encountered by those dealing with an elderly population.

The ear

Deafness

Hardness of hearing is one of the commonest ENT complaints in older people. Many patients, whether suffering from an underlying deafness or not, will be found to have excessive or impacted ear wax. The external auditory canal has a self-cleaning mechanism which often starts to default in elderly people. This problem is usually worse in men who often have an increase in the hairs present in the lateral aspect of the canal which impedes the natural migration of the wax.

Often a softening agent is required prior to attempted removal of the wax; olive oil or sodium bicarbonate drops applied topically for ≥5 days is often helpful. Water has proved to be the most effective wax softener but is seldom used, possibly from a fear of it causing maceration of the skin and subsequent infection.

A history of previous ear problems should be taken prior to considering an ear syringing. If the patient gives a history of a tympanic membrane perforation then it is advised that the patient be referred to an appropriate clinician for manual removal of the wax and inspection of the tympanic membrane.

Occasionally, elderly patients develop a condition known as keratosis obturans where a build-up of hard impacted wax with underlying squamous debris occurs. The occluding mass can cause erosion of the underlying external canal. They are, characteristically, very difficult to remove and a general anaesthetic may be required. If wax cannot be removed by syringing after application of a softener then referral to a specialist clinic will be required. Regular follow-up is required to prevent recurrence.

The commonest cause of hearing loss in the elderly is presbyacusis or the degeneration of the sensori neural components of the hearing mechanism. The onset is usually insidious and often noticed by others prior to the patient realizing that they have a problem. The most difficult hearing loss to treat is due to low frequency hearing being markedly superior to that in the high frequencies, leading to speech discrimination problems as well as difficulties hearing high pitch sounds such as door bells and ringing telephones. Such hearing problems may not resolve with simple amplification alone. The advent of modern digital hearing aids, where selective amplification of selected frequencies can occur, has helped to solve this problem.

Various devices can also be installed in the home of an elderly person who suffers from hardness of hearing, for example doorbells attached to flashing lights, or loop systems which can be fitted into a room allowing the sound from a television to be fed wirelessly directly into the hearing aid.

It is far from unusual for those sent by family and friends for an assessment of hearing and, being found to have a significant loss, to refuse an aid on the grounds that they 'are not ready' or that it 'will make me look old'. It is also far from uncommon to ask a patient who is very obviously hard of hearing whether they would like a hearing aid, only to have a pristine aid, usually in its box, pulled from a pocket or handbag. It is important to encourage older people to use their hearing aids and reassure them that it may take them a period of time to adjust to using the devices.

Co-morbidities such as arthritis in the hands may cause some people to need help in placing the aids into the ears.

Tinnitus

Tinnitus is the perception of an internal noise either in the ears or the head and is often associated with presbyacusis. It is important to ask about the nature of the noise. Otological tinnitus is usually a constant high-pitched hum. A pulsatile tinnitus may be due to a carotid bruit or a vascular tumour in the temporal bone (glomus jugulare).

It is helpful for an audiogram to be obtained. If the tinnitus is unilateral, or audiogram reveals a unilateral sensorineural hearing loss, then, unless contraindicated, a magnetic resonance imaging of the internal auditory meati, to exclude an acoustic neuroma, should be obtained.

Most cases of tinnitus in elderly people are due to hearing loss, and the first line of treatment is reassurance that the patient does not have a serious underlying problem such as a brain tumour. It is also important to dispel the myth that the condition is untreatable. Reassurance that it usually fades into the background, given time, is helpful. The level of environmental sound is also important, as the louder the ambient noise the less the tinnitus is likely to be noticed. It often appears to be louder at night when the house is quiet. Equally, when the patient is distracted it is likely to drift into the background, whereas the noises often appear louder during periods of introspection and depression.

Many different treatments have been used to alleviate the problem including relaxation, distraction or masking. The latter technique uses extraneous sound to 'mask' out the tinnitus and can vary from the simple, such as a radio, to the complex, such as a masking device; usually a modified hearing aid which is programmed to create white noise in frequencies just above and below that of the tinnitus. The frequency of the tinnitus can usually be measured by an audiologist using a pure tone audiometer, allowing programming of the masking device.

The most effective masking device for the majority of patients is a hearing aid which will amplify the ambient noise and speech displacing the internal noises into the background.

For recalcitrant cases, group therapy or tinnitus retraining using psychological techniques has proved very useful. Sadly, in very severe cases (often associated with psychological or psychiatric problems) the tinnitus can lead to a patient committing suicide.

Tinnitus self-help groups and helplines can often give the time and support that busy professionals cannot. It is helpful to have contact numbers or leaflets to give to patients.

Vertigo

Vertigo and disequilibrium are common in older people. The symptoms can range from a sensation of unsteadiness to true rotatory vertigo when the world appears to spin around—a hallucination of movement. Many elderly patients with disequilibrium have multiple co-morbidities and are best served by referral to a falls clinic or care of the elderly clinic, rather than ENT. Blackouts are rarely, if ever, caused by vestibular problems and such patients deserve a more general medical opinion.

However, vestibular problems can occur at all ages and can benefit from specific therapy. The presentation is usually of the world appearing to rotate in a horizontal direction often associated with nausea and occasionally vomiting. Vertical rotation (oscillopsia) is much less common.

It is important to view the patient in motion as this can give vital clues as to general unsteadiness and balance. It is helpful to personally call them from the waiting area or watch them walk out of the consultation. If a woman wears high heels then this may be the cause of some imbalance or, conversely, a sign that there is little wrong with the balance system. In a woman who veers to one side it may be worth weighing her handbag, if she has one, they can be heavy enough to cause the problem.

Benign paroxysmal positional vertigo (BPPV) usually presents as a short-lived rotatory vertigo precipitated by turning to the affected side, often while in bed. The condition accounts for ~40% of cases of vertigo in the elderly population.

BPPV is easily diagnosed by performing the Dix–Hallpike manoeuvre. Patients are sat on a couch with legs extended and arms held loosely in their lap. The examiner holds the patient's head, rotated 45° to one side and briskly drops the patient back until the head is below the end of the couch.

Patients are held in this position for 10–20 s to see if they exhibit any nystagmus. They are then brought upright. Any vertigo should be allowed to settle before turning the head to the opposite side and repeating the procedure to confirm which is the affected ear. The BPPV sufferer will have a short-lived episode of vertigo on being dropped back with the head towards the affected side and often a further episode on being sat back up. The vertigo can be quickly settled by asking patients to keep their eyes fixed on a distant object, while turning the head from side to side.

The pathogenesis is thought to be a small otolith or piece of calcium 'floating' in the lateral semicircular canal which falls onto the cilia of the sensory organ during movement of the head in the appropriate direction, causing excessive impulses in the vestibular nerve compared to the normal side, resulting in vertigo.

The condition is usually self limiting, but can often be cured by using the Epley manoeuvre whereby the patient is manipulated in such a way that the otolith is repositioned in a part of the inner ear where it does not cause symptoms. The manoeuvre can be performed by a physiotherapist or clinician with the appropriate training. Medication is seldom of any benefit for this condition.

Vestibular neuronitis, commonly known as labyrinthitis, causes a sudden onset of rotatory vertigo which can last for several hours and leaves a patient feeling generally unwell for several days. The patient can develop similar but often less severe acute attacks over a period of several weeks. The acute phase is best treated using a prochlorperazine 3 mg buccal preparation, which can be used in the presence of nausea and vomiting. Once the rotation and nausea have resolved the medication is stopped, as being a sedative it often produces a sensation of unsteadiness which patients believe is part of the condition and may result in them using more of the medication causing a vicious circle.

Vestibular function tests allow assessment of the vestibular system indirectly by the effect on eye movement caused by various movements, and induce short-lived vertigo by caloric irrigation; these tests often reveal hypofunction of one of the vestibular organs following neuronitis. We all rely on the brain to compensate for the asymmetry in the vestibular responses to movement; as a general rule, compensation is less likely to occur if damage has occurred in more advanced age. This can lead to a degree of unsteadiness which, combined with the fear of the vertigo returning, can turn the patient into a recluse. Vestibular rehabilitation exercises undertaken by an appropriately trained physiotherapist can speed up recovery. Use of a walking stick can be far more effective than medication in restoring balance as sensory input to the non-otological neural pathways of the balance system is increased. As with hearing aids, some patients feel that they will look infirm if they use a walking stick, but may be amenable to one of the hiking poles used by ramblers and hikers.

It should also be remembered that vision has a major part to play in the balance system and, as such, visual problems are likely to further decrease the recovery from a vestibular insult. Patients who have had a vestibular insult should avoid getting out of bed in total darkness, as they will also lose the visual aspect of the balance system and risk a fall. This is particularly pertinent for men suffering from prostatism who may need to visit the toilet several times during the night. Many patients do not wish to turn a light on, as it may disturb their partners; in such a situation, a child's plug-in night light may prove useful to supply low level constant illumination.

Infections

Otitis externa is not uncommon in older people. It may be caused by people using cotton buds or other implements to clean away wax or 'scratch' a dry itchy external canal. Such manipulation can traumatise the delicate skin deep in the canal, causing a breach in the defences against the pathogens that are usually found as scanty commensal organisms, in particular *Pseudomonas aeruginosa*. This leads to an itch and discomfort which if untreated can develop into discharge, swelling of the external canal with obstruction, pain and in the worst cases facial cellulitis requiring admission to hospital for intravenous antibiotics.

If treated early in the infection, the condition will respond to ear drops often containing a mixture of aminoglycoside antibiotic, steroid and an antifungal. Astringents with a low pH are also useful at this stage as most of the micro-organisms cannot exist in an acid environment. Aluminium acetate drops can be prepared by a pharmacist. Oral antibiotics have little part to play in the majority of such infections.

If the condition is refractory to such simple measures then referral for aural toilet is usually required so that the ear can be mopped dry and a medication-soaked wick inserted for 24–48 h. Also useful when dealing with oedematous tissues are small tampon-type wicks which have a hollow centre and, after being inserted into the external canal, will expand when soaked with the antibiotic drops for 48 h. The wicks usually need to be removed by a clinician.

Hearing aid wearers should not use the aid while the infection is active as the mould may carry organisms causing reinfection. In cases of recurrent otitis externa it is useful for the patient to seek the audiologist's advice as to whether the mould can be ventilated to try to decrease humidity in the external auditory canal.

A rare but potentially fatal infection which occurs almost exclusively in elderly patients with diabetes is known as malignant otitis externa. It is caused by a pseudomonal infection which can spread to the temporal bone, or further, causing osteomyelitis and potentially damaging the facial nerve. Any patient with diabetes who develops an extremely painful discharging ear should be referred urgently to an ENT unit.

Throat

Presbyphonia

Swallowing and voice problems are quite common in older people and can be difficult to diagnose without access to endoscopes and special investigations.

Presbyphonia is due to weakening of the muscles controlling the vocal cords. When the larynx is visualized during phonation a small gap is seen between the cords during adduction. This can have quite subtle effects on the voice, and often the history describes intermittent fluctuations in the voice as well as hoarseness. Often elderly patients will complain of being unable to sing. They can be reassured that this is not a serious problem and speech therapy can be offered.

Swallowing difficulties

Dysfunction of the swallowing mechanism can occur in older age and be intensified by the loss of teeth and wearing of dentures. Such problems appear commoner in nursing homes.

The oral phase of swallowing, i.e. chewing, is under voluntary control but once a food bolus reaches the posterior tongue the mechanism is involuntary with a series of steps that should ensure that muscles contract and relax in a specific order, passing the bolus eventually through the relaxed cricopharyngeus muscle into the oesophagus. In older people this mechanism can become uncoupled resulting in the bolus hitting a section of the pharynx which may be contracting when it should relax, or vice versa. This can result in difficulty swallowing or aspiration into the airway.

Dysphagia and aspiration can occur in those patients who have had a stroke involving the lower cranial nerves or neurological conditions, such as dementia, Parkinson's disease and motor neurone disease.

Radiological examination using a contrast swallow can be helpful. Assessment of swallowing should be made by a speech and language therapist who can give advice on swallowing techniques or, in the presence of severe aspiration, suggest that the patient should be nil by mouth and fed enterally.

Pharyngeal pouches present almost exclusively in later life and develop over a period of many years. It is thought that, if a swallow takes place against a cricopharyngeus muscle that is not fully relaxed, then pressure is put on a small posterior pharyngeal dehiscence in the inferior pharyngeal constrictor muscle (Killian's dehiscence) which causes a posterior pouch to develop.

The patient classically has difficulty swallowing food and then regurgitates undigested food several hours later. Aspiration may occur. Diagnosis is usually confirmed by a radiological contrast swallow. The pouches are treated by endoscopic stapling or an external approach. Stapling is becoming increasingly common but, because the staple gun does not cut to its full length, a small shelf remains; although swallowing is usually much improved, a sensation of food 'catching' may remain and a further pouch can develop over a period of several years.

Laryngopharyngeal reflux

Laryngopharyngeal reflux involves overspill of gastric juices into the lower pharynx and larynx, often in the absence of indigestion or heartburn. It is common in patients who have a hiatus hernia. The commonest symptom is of a sensation of a lump in the throat which is intermittent and does not interfere with swallowing. Usually, the patients point to the level of the cricoid cartilage in the midline of the lower neck as the site of the sensation. Other symptoms include intermittent hoarseness, non-productive sensation of a post-nasal drip and a dry cough.

Treatment is as for oesophageal reflux, though often using a double dose of a proton pump inhibitor. The higher dose must be used with care in older people.

Anyone, particularly a smoker or ex-smoker, who has constant hoarse voice or difficulty swallowing for over 3 weeks should be referred urgently to an ENT surgeon to exclude malignancy. These symptoms, combined with sore throat and otalgia in the presence of clinically normal examination, are due to a pharyngeal carcinoma until proved otherwise.

The nose

Although the older patient will present with nasal symptoms similar to those in younger people, they may have tolerated their nasal complaints for a long time, and it is therefore important to identify the main reason for seeking medical attention. Diagnoses such as depression, anxiety, loneliness or cancer phobia may therefore be crucial to understanding the prime reason for seeking medical advice. Unfortunately, these can be easily missed in a short single consultation, and a high index of suspicion needs to be maintained. Failure to diagnose a significant underlying cause in an older patient will inevitably lead to ineffective treatments, repeated unsatisfactory consultations and, at worst, several ineffective operations.

It is crucial to take a comprehensive drug history from older patients presenting with sinonasal symptoms. Many commonly prescribed medications cause rhinitic symptoms, nasal obstruction or disturbance of smell. Such medications include antihypertensive and cardiovascular drugs such as beta-blockers, angiotensin-converting enzyme inhibitors (ACEIs) and angiotensin II receptor blockers (ARBs).

Nasal medication

Steroid nasal sprays are the mainstay of treatment in all forms of rhinitis, but in older people they may worsen the situation by inducing dryness and crusting of the nasal mucosa. A potential side-effect of steroid nasal sprays is to induce epistaxis: in this age group, these may be heavy, frequent or prolonged due to the fragility of the nasal mucosa and blood vessels.

Antihistamine nasal sprays such as azelastine are helpful for older patients with seasonal or perennial allergic rhinitis, but are generally less effective than topical steroid sprays. Oral antihistamines are sometimes helpful in older patients with allergic rhinitis, especially if they have associated allergic conjunctivitis and pharyngitis.

However, caution is required, particularly with the older generation oral antihistamines which are associated with sedation, drowsiness and antimuscarinic effects that may induce urinary retention and glaucoma. Oral antihistamines are also associated with other side-effects such as dizziness, confusion and sleep disturbance, which can all be extremely relevant in caring for older people. The newer generation non-sedating oral antihistamines are the preferred treatment of choice.

Senile rhinorrhoea

Some elderly patients present with profuse watery rhinorrhoea known as senile rhinitis. This is caused by a disturbance in the autonomic control of the nasal mucosa and in particular the production of nasal mucus from parasympathetic neural activity. Senile rhinorrhoea may also induce a complaint of a sensation of 'drowning' due to a true post-nasal drip, as opposed to the common sensation of catarrh where complaints are way in excess of any physically recognized anomalies. Watery rhinorrhoea whilst eating is known as gustatory rhinitis, and is due to similar causes.

The symptoms of senile rhinorrhoea can often be well controlled with an ipratropium bromide nasal spray. However, such treatment is not without risk and it may induce excessive dryness and/ or epistaxis. An ipratropium spray should also be used with care in older patients suffering from closed angle glaucoma, and care should be taken not to spray it directly into the eye.

Epistaxis

Epistaxis can occur at any age but is more likely to lead to hospital admission in elderly subjects. For bleeding points in the region of the anterior nasal septum, twice daily topical Naseptin® nasal cream (chlorhexidine hydrochloride, and neomycin sulphate) is often successful at preventing further bleeds. The treatment compares favourably to silver nitrate cautery which must be used with caution in elderly patients for fear of inducing local mucosal atrophy, ulceration and exacerbation of the bleeding problem. Naseptin cream should be avoided in all patients with peanut allergy, whatever the age. Topical vaseline is also widely used to prevent epistaxis but the evidence of efficacy is not as strong as for the use of Naseptin.

Older people are also more likely to be taking an anticoagulant or antiplatelet drug such as aspirin or clopidogrel, and these will exacerbate epistaxes in these patients. The effects of aspirin and clopidogrel cannot be easily reversed and stopping the drug is unlikely to have any significant effect during the acute stages of the nose bleed. However, warfarin can be stopped if necessary. This decision should be based upon the degree of warfarin control: if the international normalized ratio (INR) is within the normal therapeutic range, it is quite reasonable to continue with warfarin at the prescribed dose: if the INR is too high, the warfarin should be stopped temporarily, until the INR returns to an acceptable level.

Further reading

American Academy of Otolaryngology—Head and Neck Surgery. *Geriatric Care Otolaryngology*. Available at: http://www.entnet.org/geriatricotolaryngology.cfm

Burton MJ, Dorée CJ. Ear drops for the removal of ear wax. *Cochrane Database Syst Rev* 2003;(3):CD004400.

Guest JF, Greener MJ, Robinson AC, Smith AF. Impacted cerumen: composition, production, epidemiology and management. *Q J Med* 2004;97:477–88.

Kendall K. Presbyphonia: a review. *Curr Opin Otolaryngol Head Neck Surg* 2007;15:137–40.

Manohar B. Hearing and aging. *Can Med Assoc J* 2007;176:925–7.

Matthew L, Kashima W, Goodwin Jr J, Balkany T, Casiano Roy R. Special considerations in managing geriatric patients. In: Cummings CW, Haughey BH, Thomas JR, Harker LA (eds), *Cummings Otolaryngology: Head & Neck Surgery*, Vol. 1, 4th edition. St Louis: Mosby; 2004.

Murthy P, Nilssen EL, Rao S, McClymont LG. A randomised clinical trial of antiseptic nasal carrier cream and silver nitrate cautery in the treatment of recurrent anterior epistaxis. *Clin Otolaryngol Allied Sci* 1999;24:228–31.

Reginelli A, Pezzullo MG, Scaglione M, Scialpi M, Brunese L, Grassi R. Gastrointestinal disorders in elderly patients. *Radiol Clin North Am* 2008;46:755–71,vi.

Sen P, Lowe DA, Farnan T. Surgical interventions for pharyngeal pouch. *Cochrane Database Syst Rev* 2005;20(3):CD004459.

Chapter 16

Ophthalmic problems

Mark Batterbury and Nicholas Cowland

Introduction

The chief problems that elderly people present to their general practitioner (GP) are disturbance of vision, problems of the outer eye and chance findings on testing by an optometrist (optician).

The GP should have a sight test chart (a mirror can be used to create the 6 m testing distance), a pen torch with a blue filter, a direct ophthalmoscope and some basic drops (fluorescein and local anaesthetic such as oxybuprocaine). Fluorescein is used to look for corneal foreign bodies, abrasions and ulcers. Local anaesthetic helps to examine a sore eye! Its use will not be harmful.

The optometrist plays an increasingly important role in eye care, performing the sight test for glasses, detecting signs of possible disease, shared care roles for the management of glaucoma, diabetic retinopathy screening, and direct referral and postoperative care of cataract. People presenting to the GP with disturbance of vision, especially if not acute, can very reasonably be asked to attend the optometrist for a sight test before referral to an ophthalmologist. The so-called GOS18 is the form by which the optometrist records the sight test, identifies possible abnormality and recommends further management. If the optometrist identifies possible pathology, he/she is obliged to bring it to the attention of the GP and will usually also suggest investigation or referral. This chapter will help the reader manage patients who return from a sight test with a GOS18 or who present with one of the many common eye disorders that occur in older age groups.

Suspected glaucoma

There are three tests for glaucoma: measurement of intraocular pressure (IOP), examination of the optic disc and assessment of the visual fields. Abnormality of any one of these will prompt referral to the hospital eye service (HES). Although false positives are common, it is generally better to refer to the HES than ignore the presence of an asymptomatic disease. The outcome is shown in Figure 16.1.

Risk factors

High IOP is not the cause of glaucoma, in that ocular hypertension and low tension glaucoma conditions exist. Risk factors that may prompt treatment include thin corneal thickness, myopia, Black race, field loss close to central vision, family history of glaucoma, and high IOP. Although the symptom of headache often precipitates a sight test and suspicion of glaucoma, it is rarely caused by any eye disorder.

Treatment

The purpose of modern glaucoma management is to prevent symptomatic sight loss during the patient's lifetime so that treatment must be tailored to the needs of the individual and take into account the above risk factors, patient anxiety and compliance and quality-of-life issues.

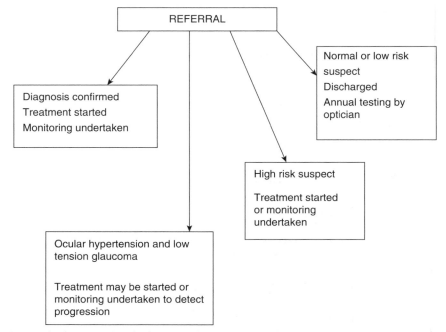

Fig. 16.1 Ocular hypertension: high intraocular pressure (IOP) without other abnormal feature. Approximate conversion to glaucoma: 10% in 5 years. Low tension glaucoma: features of glaucoma without elevated IOP. Approximately 50% do not progress.

Most patients require eye drop treatment only, usually only one or two medications. Prostaglandin analogues have become the first-choice treatment. They are effective and their IOP-lowering action is prolonged. Beta-blockers can impair exercise tolerance, especially elderly people, often unnoticed. Occasionally surgery (drainage surgery, trabeculectomy) is necessary. The commonly used medications are listed in Table 16.1.

Acute glaucoma

This is usually an acute onset, unilateral red eye with significant disturbance of vision and partly dilated pupil (Colour plate 1). Immediate referral is required.

Retinal changes and macular degeneration

During the sight test the optician may see a variety of colour changes, deposits and degeneration, and other possibly abnormal features.

- ◆ Pigment: most increases or decreases in pigmentation are insignificant, even if located in the macular part of the retina. If associated with symptomatic change in vision, referral is advised. Naevi should be referred.
- ◆ Haemorrhage: single isolated haemorrhage without disturbance in vision is rarely serious. It is sensible to exclude diabetes and measure the blood pressure.
- ◆ Haemorrhage in the macular area, especially if associated with symptomatic change in vision, should prompt referral.

Table 16.1 Glaucoma medications

Class	Names	Administration	Chief side-effects[a]	Potency
Prostaglandins	Latanoprost (Xalatan) Travoprost (Travatan) Bimatoprost (Lumigan)	Once daily in the evening	Red eye, iris darkening, eyelash lengthening, darkening of eyelid skin	+ + + + +
Beta-blockers	Timolol Levobunolol Carteolol Betaxolol	Twice a day (long-acting once daily in the morning formulations exist)	Contraindicated in pulmonary disease, caution in cardiac disease. Reduced exercise tolerance in the elderly (often goes unrecognized)	+ + +
Carbonic anhydrase inhibitors	Dorzolamide (Trusopt) Brinzolamide (Azopt)	Twice a day	Red eye, stinging, dry mouth, blurred vision	+ +
Alpha-agonist	Brimonidine (Alphagan)	Twice a day	Red, sticky, gritty eye, follicular conjunctivitis, dry mouth, taste alteration	+ +
Cholinergic agonist	Pilocarpine	Four times a day	Interferes with accommodation in young people, worse vision in the presence of cataract, small pupil for retinal assessment, headache	+ + +

Other formulations:

Prostaglandin + beta-blocker: Xalacom, Duotrav, Ganfort once a day in the evening.
Alpha-agonist + beta-blocker: Combigan twice a day.
Long-acting beta-blocker: Timoptol-LA, Nyogel once a day in the morning.
Long-acting Pilocarpine: Pilogel 4% at night.
Preservative-free drops: Timolol and Dorzolamide are the only medications available.

[a] When unwanted effects occur, switching between classes is recommended, rather than within class.

- Multiple haemorrhages occur most commonly in diabetes and retinal vein occlusion. Referral is necessary.
- Pale or white dots and particles: again, most are not significant. Exudates occur in diabetes and the 'wet' form of macular degeneration (see below).

Macular degeneration

Two chief forms of age-related macular degeneration (ARMD, or AMD) are recognized: 'wet' and 'dry'. These terms refer to the outcome of a degenerative process that inevitably occurs with longevity. The term 'wet' is used when there is an abnormal vascular growth (choroidal neovascular membrane) which leaks blood, fluid and lipoprotein, causing rapid loss of central vision (Colour plates 2 and 3). In the early stages of its development it can be treated to prevent further sight loss and even bring about visual improvement. Photodynamic therapy has been superseded by injection into the vitreous cavity of an inhibitor of vascular endothelial growth factor (anti-VEGF; Lucentis®, ranibizumab). Identification of 'wet' ARMD requires special imaging techniques including fluorescein angiography and optical coherence tomography. Injections have to be given every few weeks for ~2 years. There is a small risk of endophthalmitis (intraocular infection).

'Dry' ARMD in the fellow eye of 'wet' ARMD can later progress to 'wet'. The risk is ~10% per year.

'Dry' ARMD (Colour plates 4 and 5) is not a treatable condition. It is important to maximize remaining vision by using glasses, magnifying (low vision) aids and a good light.

Risk factors include smoking, hypertension, elevated cholesterol and myopia. There is also a genetic susceptibility. Dietary deficiencies are of uncertain significance.

Visual disturbance such as distortion and rapidly changing vision and features of haemorrhage and exudates at the macula suggest 'wet' ARMD so that urgent referral is required. Rapid access clinics are being set up, particularly now that anti-VEGF treatment is so effective.

'Dry' ARMD without symptoms does not need referral. If other problems are present (especially cataract and glaucoma) the relative contributions of these to the patient's overall disability may need to be assessed in the HES.

A healthy balanced diet should not need to be supplemented. There is some evidence that supplements can prevent progression of 'dry' to 'wet' ARMD in the fellow eye of a person with 'wet' ARMD.

The registration process for the Certificate of Visual Impairment has been modernized and patients can even be referred for social service assistance without formal registration.

Cataract

Modern cataract surgery, termed phacoemulsification ('phaco'), is performed under local anaesthesia, even sometimes eye drop anaesthesia only, using a sophisticated probe to remove the cataractous lens followed by placement of an artificial intraocular lens implant. The cataract pathway has undergone extensive modernization and is one of the chief beneficiaries of National Health Service investment (Figure 16.2).

Referral

The presence of cataract itself does not require referral. Surgical removal is required if there are symptoms, typically problems with reading, driving and undertaking hobbies and pastimes. Age and absolute level of visual acuity are rarely factors in deciding on surgery, but lack of co-operation and general health may be.

Outcomes

Ninety-five per cent of patients will undergo trouble-free surgery. Problems are usually related to pre-existing eye disease that limits visual recovery or predisposes to complicated surgery and uncommon sight-threatening complications, including infection, bleeding and posterior capsule rupture requiring vitrectomy, that affect the retina. About 10% develop late-onset posterior capsule opacification that diminishes vision. It can be cured by a simple YAG (yttrium–aluminium–garnet) laser capsulotomy. Despite implantation of an artificial lens implant, most patients will need reading glasses and many will require spectacles for optimum distance vision. Innovations in implant design are reducing this need for spectacles postoperatively.

A preoperative measurement called biometry permits choice of an implant of the appropriate focusing power for the visual needs of the individual. Thus short- and long-sighted persons can be made 'normally' sighted. However, this can lead to unequal focusing of the two eyes (anisometropia). Generally it is better to plan to operate on both eyes, one after the other, aiming for both to become 'normal', and put up with the short period of anisometropia.

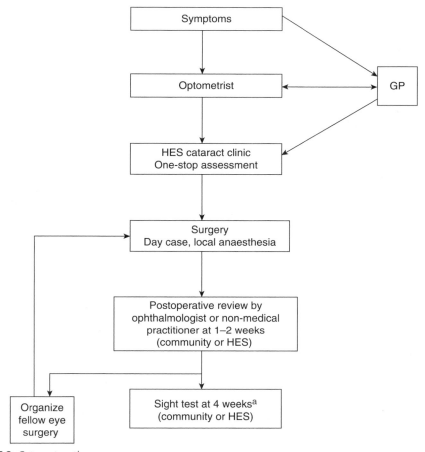

Fig. 16.2 Cataract pathway.
[a]Usually after each eye. Provision of spectacles may be delayed until after both eyes have had surgery. HES, hospital eye service.

Pre-existing disease

Conditions such as ambylopia, ARMD and retinal vascular disease, whether diagnosed preoperatively or not, can limit the success of cataract surgery. Cataract surgery rarely makes pre-existing disease worse. Glaucoma control can be impaired, but the chief difficulty is diabetic retinopathy: ischaemic retinopathy and maculopathy can be aggravated, requiring careful postoperative assessment and appropriate treatment.

Disorders of the outer eye

Red, gritty, sticky, sore, watery eyes are common problems (see Figures 16.3 and 16.4).

Dry eyes

Tears are a complex fluid of water, lipids, oils and proteins. Disturbance of the production of any one of these, such as occurs in blepharitis, causes a 'dry eye' state with symptoms of soreness, grittiness, foreign body sensation. Even paradoxical watering can occur!

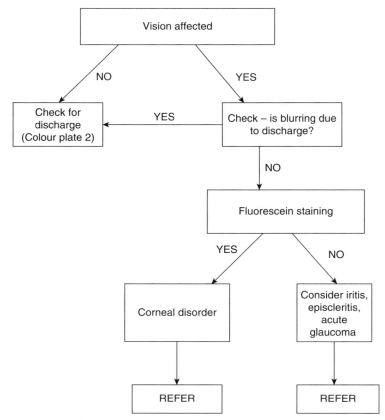

Fig. 16.3 Algorithm for referral of acute red eye.

A wide variety of artificial tears and lubricants are available and can be prescribed. These will rarely do any harm; none is superior to another, so any might be recommended for a treatment trial. In general, ointments give longer relief than gels which perform better than drops, but the longer-acting the formulation the greater the stickiness and disturbance of vision they cause. Occasionally the preservatives in eye medications can cause an allergic or mildly toxic effect so that preservative-free medications can be tried.

A true dry eye state rarely occurs. Rheumatoid arthritis is the commonest cause.

Blepharitis

This common condition can be intensely irritating to endure and frustrating to treat! Its cause is unknown. A set of symptoms that comprise bilaterality and chronicity with lid margin redness and swelling (Colour plate 6), intermittent red eye, eyelash crusts (Colour plate 7) and grittiness suggests the diagnosis.

The chief aspects of management are:

1) Warm compresses applied daily to the lid margins to unblock meibomian gland orifices (Colour plate 6). Firm pressure is required.

2) Antibiotic administration to reduce the load of bacterial flora, including normal commensals. Topical chloramphenicol ointment (or fusidic acid) is usually sufficient but is needed in 6–12 week courses. Occasionally systemic tetracycline used for a similar period is necessary.

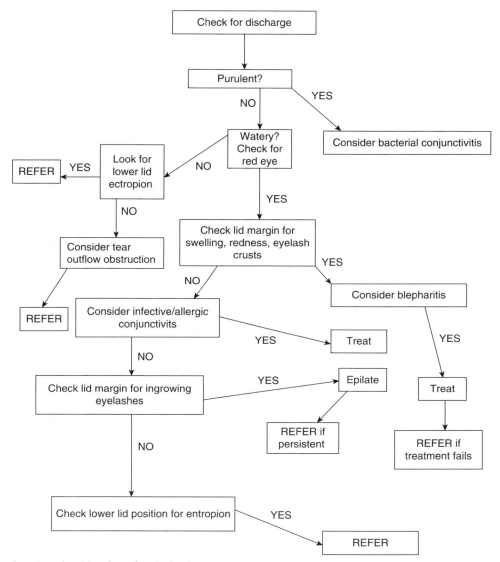

Fig. 16.4 Algorithm for referral of red or sore or gritty or sticky or watery eye(s).

3) Administration of artificial tears or lubricants for the irritation, even if there is watering, as often as required.

Ptosis

Most cases of ptosis are caused by an age-related loss of tissue tension. Corrective surgery is rarely necessary, usually only when the lid interferes with vision. The risk is overcorrection and corneal exposure, especially during sleep.

Blepharochalasis and dermatochalasis are similar problems that can mimic a ptosis, the upper lid skin hanging down. Surgery is only required if the field of vision is truly impaired.

Entropion and ectropion

Surgical correction is required, particularly for entropion, because of the risk of corneal damage. A single operation only is usually sufficient. Surgery comprises skin incisions plus deeply placed sutures to redirect the pull of muscles involved in eyelid position or to alter the position of the eyelid 'skeleton'. It takes about half an hour and is performed under local anaesthesia.

Tear outflow obstruction

Tears pass through the medially located upper and lower lid puncta into a canalicular system that drains into the lacrimal sac and thence into the nose via the nasolacrimal duct. Obstruction usually occurs due to a stenosed punctum or nasolacrimal duct. The former is simple to remedy; the latter requires major corrective surgery, (dacrocystorhinstomy) externally through the skin and nasal bones, or internally through the nose. Referral is only necessary if the patient wishes to have an operation.

Lumps and bumps

The eyelids are a common place for cysts, papillomas, horns and xanthelasma. Removal is cosmetic. Basal cell carcinoma is usually obvious and requires removal with a wide margin to prevent local spread.

Shingles

Herpes zoster of the eye is a common form of shingles. The typical skin affliction, in which tingling followed by erythema and then blistering up to but not beyond the midline, affects the eye itself in about half of cases of ophthalmic zoster. It is said that if the skin of the nose is affected then the eye is very likely to be affected. Eye involvement is always indicated by redness; absence of redness indicates that the eye is not involved. When the eye is affected, referral to an ophthalmologist is necessary. Complications include corneal ulceration, iritis and an acute secondary glaucoma. Otherwise referral is not necessary.

Styes and chalazion

A stye (Colour plate 8) is an acute folliculitis and is self-limiting. A chalazion (Colour plate 9) occurs in a meibomian gland, pointing anteriorly or posteriorly rather than towards the lid margin. The infective stage passes quickly, requiring a topical and rarely a systemic broad-spectrum antibiotic plus warm compresses to assist its resolution. Often the acute stage progresses into a chronic granulomatous phase of intermittent inflammation and swelling. If it has not resolved after 3 months, referral for removal by incision and curettage is appropriate.

Corneal ulcers and abrasions

Corneal abrasions are usually caused by trauma, though sometimes without a definite history. Fluorescein drops illuminated by a blue light should show the typical green lesion. Chloramphenicol ointment, with or without a patch to close the lids, should be used for a few days. Failure to show sign of improvement after 24 h requires referral.

The presence of a white patch on the cornea (Colour plate 10), loss of corneal clarity and loss of the mirror-like brightness of the cornea, suggest more severe pathology. Urgent referral is advised.

Dendritic ulcers (Colour plate 11) occur in both herpes simplex and zoster. Topical aciclovir for a week should be curative. Look out for the other features of severe corneal disease (above).

Diabetic eye disease

Whereas diabetic retinopathy is the most notorious ocular complication of diabetes mellitus, sufferers are also more likely to develop cataract, glaucoma and even some corneal epithelial disorders.

Optimization of diabetic control (HbA1c), cessation of smoking and reduction of elevated cholesterol are essential in helping to reduce the risk of sight loss from diabetic retinopathy.

The National Service Framework for diabetes sets out targets for retinopathy screening and treatment of retinopathy. Two screening systems are in operation. One uses trained and accredited optometrists, the other multifield photography and grading of images by trained and accredited graders. The screening process may result in referral to the HES for further assessment because diabetic retinopathy has been detected, because cataract prevents adequate retinopathy screening, or because of chance finding of another condition, especially glaucoma.

Criteria for treatment have been thoroughly elucidated. The two chief pathological processes of retinal vascular occlusion and leakage are responsible for the typical clinical features (Colour plate 12). Sight-threatening eye disease, in the form of maculopathy and proliferative retinopathy, require laser therapy.

Floaters and flashing lights

Most of us have floaters, usually most noticeable looking at a bright white wall or blue sky. However, a very sudden onset of a shower of floaters (likened to a net curtain or spider's web), often accompanied by a flashing light, indicates sudden 'detachment' (posterior vitreous detachment) of the vitreous gel from its adhesions to the retina. This degenerative process can result in a retinal tear and thence a retinal detachment. You should refer patients with such sudden onset of symptoms and warn the patient to look out for peripheral visual loss, a shadow or curtain blocking out part of the field of vision.

Chapter 17

Dermatology

Maggie Kirkup and Diana Bloss

Introduction

Skin problems are very common in elderly individuals. In addition to the unwelcome development of the visible signs of ageing, skin becomes dry and heals less well. Some of the commoner difficulties which can arise will be covered in this chapter. There are practical difficulties in applying topical agents to elderly skin. The skin may be thin and easily bruised. Co-morbidities, general weakness and reduced joint flexibility may render areas of the skin inaccessible to the owner. Impaired hearing and vision can make patient education about the use of these medicaments a particular challenge. Many dermatology units offer day care treatment facilities but this may require provision of transport which increases the cost and inconvenience, so management at home is ideal. There are sometimes disputes in the support services as to whether skin treatments are 'medical treatment' or 'personal care'. We should insist on the former being the rule. Sadly education about the use and method of application of topical treatment can be lacking in health professionals outside dermatology units. It is important that patients are supplied with adequate amounts of creams and ointments in order to treat themselves properly. As a rough guide, a single application of a cream to the whole body surface of an adult will require most of a 30 g tube. In this chapter we will consider some of the commonest skin symptoms, possible causes and management plans.

General assessment and treatment issues

In elderly patients, it is worthwhile taking time to obtain a detailed medical history, as the skin problems may relate to their past or current general disorders or to the drugs that they are taking. Discovering patients' understanding of their problem, taking account of their overall functionality, and reaching a shared understanding of their treatment will help in compliance and the overall management.

A history of the rash or lesion, together with any creams or ointments either prescribed or bought over the counter, or even borrowed from relatives or friends, may be important. Anything applied to the skin or used in washing the skin may have significance. Corroborative evidence from a relative or carer can be helpful here. The general practitioner (GP) needs to be aware of general medical conditions that may predispose patients to their skin problem, such as: diabetes in patients with infection, chronic renal failure in patients with pruritus, heart failure causing oedema and leg ulceration, and conditions that might make treatment more hazardous, e.g. hypertension when considering oral steroids, renal failure with certain disease-modifying agents.

A previous history of skin disease is important, as is a history of allergy to medication or to topical treatments. A detailed drug history is especially important, as many frequently prescribed drugs can cause rashes. Furthermore, patients may be concerned that the most recently prescribed drug is responsible for their rash and it may be important to eliminate this as a cause.

It is often helpful to examine the whole skin, noting the distribution of a rash or multiplicity of lesions in order to make the diagnosis. The time during which the patient undresses enables the practitioner to assess the patient's overall functional ability. Palpating lesions can help in determining their depth and induration. When assessing a patient with a blistering disorder it is important to check the mucous membranes too.

The patient's social circumstances and manual dexterity is an important consideration when prescribing topical agents. Those who live alone or have no social support from family members or carers may require the support of the community nursing team in order to treat their skin effectively. The patient's mental capacity and expectations of outcome need to be considered.

When prescribing topical therapy it is important that the patient fully understands how to use the preparations and in what quantities. Prepared written information is helpful, as is a personal tailored written management plan. Topical chemotherapy for premalignant conditions (see below) may rather alarmingly make the skin condition appear worse initially, and patients need to be made aware of this. The expectation and time taken for improvement needs to be stressed, as patients often have unrealistic expectations of the time taken for their rash to resolve and this ultimately affects compliance and their trust in the clinician.

Problem: pruritus

Itching can have a devastating effect on the quality of life and presents a challenge to the GP in terms of making a diagnosis and planning effective management, especially where no rash is obvious. The commonest itchy rashes are scabies, eczemas, psoriasis and drug eruptions. These are dealt with below. Diffuse skin damage due to chronic sun exposure can mimic a rash and can itch. The existence of 'senile pruritus' or pruritus of senescence as a disease entity is disputed and tends to be a diagnosis of exclusion. Prevalence of itching in the elderly population is not known with any accuracy but may be as high as 30–60%.[1–3] In a UK study of hospital outpatients, 2–12% of elderly individuals attending for non-dermatological reasons gave a history of chronic itch.[4] Those living in care homes appear to be particularly prone.[5] Dry, over-warm ambient air is believed to contribute.

Itching is an important symptom of some systemic disorders and these are listed in Box 17.1.

It is important to take a careful history at this stage. Examination must be done in a good light and subtle signs such as the burrows of scabies specifically looked for. This diagnosis should trigger treatment not only of the index case but all contacts which may include care home staff,

---

Box 17.1 Systemic causes of itching without a rash

Iron deficiency
Over- or underactive thyroid
Chronic renal failure
Biliary stasis
Sensory neuropathy
Psychological issues
Internal malignancy
Drugs (opiates, aspirin, B vitamins, retinoids)
HIV/AIDS
Dry skin (xerosis)
Senile pruritus?

Box 17.2 Treatment of scabies in elderly individuals

- Apply permethrin 5% cream or malathion 0.5% aqueous lotion all over, including nail folds and all skin creases. A paintbrush can be handy for applying.
- Reapply to area washed during treatment, e.g. after using toilet.
- Permethrin can be washed off after 8–12 h, malathion after 24 h.
- Change all bedding and underclothing after this time.
- Repeat 1 week later in severe cases but do not keep repeating.
- Treat all household and 'kissing' contacts including staff and visitors if in care home or other institution.
- Remember that itching can persist for 3–6 weeks after all the mites are dead.

patients and visitors. Remember that not all infested individuals itch. Scratching can lead to linear excoriations, nodules with ulceration and secondary scarring and lichenification. See Box 17.2 for treatment recommendations for scabies.

When there are no signs other than the results of scratching, the hunt for a systemic cause should include investigation for the conditions listed in Box 17.1 as guided by the history and general examination. If there is no obvious cause and a simple check of haematology and biochemistry draws a blank, it is worth considering referral to a dermatologist.

Where a cause is found, management of the condition will often result in relief from the itch. If there is no simple cause to correct, management is aimed at relief of symptoms. Unfortunately there is no panacea. Antihistamines are often used. First-generation antihistamines such as chlorphenamine and hydroxyzine are the most likely to give benefit but sedation may be unwelcome or dangerous.[6] Although there is no good research basis, avoidance of irritants including skin cleansers, soaps and bath products will often help. Most moisturising agents can be used as soap substitutes and application of emollients to the whole skin several times a day usually gives some relief. Antipruritic topical agents include crotamiton cream, the mode of action of which is unknown, doxepin cream which probably works via an antihistamanic effect, and lauramacrogols, found in many emollients which have some local anaesthetic properties. Addition of menthol 1–2% to a simple inexpensive emollient such as aqueous cream BP is a non-evidence-based but widely used measure. Pruritus is a cause of great misery and it can sometimes be worth referring to a dermatologist for consideration of more toxic drugs such as ciclosporin and thalidomide or use of UV phototherapy.

Problem: new onset of rash

The commonest causes of a new rash in elderly people are the eczemas, scabies, drug reactions, bullous pemphigoid and, more rarely, vasculitis. Chronic conditions such as psoriasis or eczema can of course persist into, or relapse in, old age. Indeed psoriasis can begin in mature adult life (see below). There are rare but important conditions such as subacute lupus erythematosus, paraneoplastic conditions, and cutaneous T-cell lymphoma which can present late in life. Gaining familiarity with common morphologies is important and any rash with an unusual appearance or which does not respond to treatment with good compliance should be referred to a dermatologist for diagnosis. Undressing the patient for examination is important as the distribution may give clues, e.g. is it in a light-exposed distribution? There may be areas of involvement not noticed by the patient or carer. Good lighting and magnification can help clarify the characteristics of the rash, such as whether there are macules, papules, blisters, pustules and whether there is scaling, crusting, excoriation or indeed burrows of scabies. Performing a skin biopsy without a clue as to the diagnosis is rarely helpful as the pathologist needs good clinical information. We shall deal here with the major features of the common problems and refer the reader to larger dermatological texts for details of the less common conditions.

Eczemas

Many types of eczema are seen in the elderly population (Colour plate 13). The rash of scabies is a papular eczema and must always be considered in the differential diagnosis. Many drug eruptions are also eczematous in nature (see 'Problem: drug eruptions' below).

The main features of eczemas are erythema, blisters (usually tiny and often have tops scratched off), scaling, and itch. Fissures are common on thick areas of skin. Summary of management is shown in Table 17.1.

Chronic atopic eczema may persist from childhood but can present at any age. In older people this can be related to increasing xerosis (dryness).

Seborrhoeic eczema typically appears on the scalp, eyebrows, creases of the face and neck, as well as the presternal region but can also be troublesome in any skin crease. The appearance is of a redness which has a subtle, rather greasy-looking, yellowish hue with scaling. On the scalp this can be mistaken for psoriasis.

Contact dermatitis can be allergic or irritant. Allergic contact dermatitis (ACD) in older people occurs most commonly to medicaments used on leg ulcers or lower leg eczema,[7] but many other substances such as plants can be implicated. Ideally this should be confirmed by patch testing done in dermatology units. The rash in ACD begins at the site of contact but can become more

Table 17.1 Guide to management of eczemas

Diagnosis	First-line treatments	Consider referring
Atopic eczema	Emollients and topical steroids of appropriate potency for site	Failure to respond to treatment with good compliance
Seborrhoeic dermatitis	Mild or moderately potent topical steroids and antifungal agents	Failure to respond to treatment with good compliance
Contact dermatitis (allergic or irritant)	As for atopic eczema plus avoidance of precipitating factors	For diagnosis
Discoid eczema	Moderately potent and potent topical steroids	Failure to respond to treatment with good compliance
Asteatotic eczema	Emollients and sometimes mild topical steroids	Failure to respond to treatment with good compliance
Stasis eczema	Improvement of venous return by compression and elevation having excluded significant ischaemia, topical steroids, and emollients	To vascular surgeon if clinical features and ABPI suggest arterial disease. To dermatologist if secondary contact dermatitis suspected
Nodular prurigo	As for atopic eczema, intralesional steroid, paste bandages	Failure to respond to treatment with good compliance

ABPI, ankle/brachial pressure index.

generalized. Irritant contact dermatitis of the hands is less common in elderly than working age people.[8] However, cleansing agents, soaps, shower and bath additives together with water can result in significant problems on any site. Irritants may contribute to intertrigo of the flexures which often has super-added yeast or bacterial infection (see below).

Discoid eczema presents as discrete areas, usually on limbs, of intensely inflamed skin which may be exudative and crusty (Colour plate 13a). It usually settles in time but does need intermittent use of relatively potent topical steroids. While there is often bacterial overgrowth, actual infection is rare and antibiotics are rarely helpful. Topical antibiotics, if used, should be limited to a few days only to prevent emergence of bacterial resistance.

Stasis eczema is primarily a condition of the lower legs where there has been chronic venous disease but can occur in a setting of lymphoedema and immobility (Colour plate 13b). Obesity also predisposes to lower leg problems. This too can generalize and can ultimately lead to ulceration (see Chapter 18).

Nodular prurigo is believed to be a form of eczema for which no cause is known but which results in irresistible drive to scratch vigorously, leading to nodules which can bleed, ulcerate and scar. It tends to persist for years and can be very difficult to manage.

Asteatotic eczema is very common in the older population. The typical appearance is rather like 'crazy paving' (Colour plate 13c). Tending to be worse in winter, the cause is thought to be dry skin plus low humidity, and it is very common in care homes and hospitals.

Topical steroid potencies are important. Fluorinated steroids are more potent and are more easily absorbed through the skin. It is worth getting used to using one or two products from each potency group. Examples of commonly prescribed agents are given in Box 17.3. Potent and supra-potent steroids must be avoided on the face, genitals and skin creases because of the risk of skin atrophy, infection and systemic absorption. Facial use can provoke rosacea and acne-like pustulation which will flare on stopping the steroid application. It is essential not to allow the patient to re-start the preparation because of this flare or it may prove impossible to stop completely. There are a few exceptions for specific conditions such as biopsy-proven lichen sclerosis of the genitals and discoid lupus erythematosus of the face, on advice of a dermatologist.

Blistering rashes

Elderly skin blisters relatively easily. The diagnostic possibilities depend on whether the blistering is localized or generalized. Common causes of localized blistering in older people are:

- Lower legs:
  - oedema
  - cellulitis
  - early bullous pemphigoid
  - vasculitis (uncommon)
  - drug eruptions (uncommon)
  - prolonged pressure.
- Hands and/or feet:
  - acute eczema
  - fungal infection (usually unilateral).
- Dermatomal distribution
  - herpes zoster (see below).

Box 17.3 Guide to topical treatment for eczemas

Steroids

- Low potency: 1% hydrocortisone acetate.
- Moderately potent: clobetasone butyrate.
- Potent: betamethasone valerate (available as 0.1% and diluted 1 in 4 as Betnovate®). Mometasone furorate is licensed for once daily use.
- Super-potent: clobetasol propionate.

Vehicle

- The base or vehicle used can be important.
- The more 'wet' the skin condition, the wetter the preparation which should be used. Thus lotions or creams can be used for acute exudative eczemas.
- Ointments usually give superior results if the eruption is dry and scaly.
- Over-the-counter hydrocortisone and clobetasone butyrate are only available as creams.

Quantities

- Emollients should be prescribed in large quantities, e.g. 500 g, and many are available in pump dispenser. This amount might be needed for a week's use as soap substitute and adequate application to the whole body.
- Topical steroids should be available in sufficient amounts for the area to be treated. 30 g will cover the body once only and is woefully insufficient for a generalized eruption.
- The fingertip unit is a useful guide to the patient as to how much to use (Bewley 2008).[9] Careful counselling can avoid under- as well as overtreatment.

Commonest causes of widespread blistering are:
- Bullous pemphigoid.
- Vasculitis (uncommon).
- Drug eruption (uncommon).
- Other immunobullous conditions (rare).

Bullous pemphigoid is by far the commonest reason for generalized blistering. The cause is not known. Recent research shows a rate of 4.3 per 100 000 person-years in the UK with average age at presentation being 80 years. There is a significant mortality.[10] Bullous pemphigoid may be preceded by the appearance of itchy, red, urticated plaques which then blister. Blisters can appear on previously normal skin and at least some of them are likely to be haemorrhagic. Mucous membranes are involved in ~10%. Confirmation of diagnosis requires biopsy of lesional and perilesional skin with direct and indirect immunofluoresence and is a secondary care technique. Patients should be referred urgently, usually by telephone to avoid delay in starting treatment. Management usually involves immunosuppressive therapies and often needs to be continued for 12–18 months with careful monitoring. Localized disease might be managed with super-potent topical steroids.[11] Pemphigus vulgaris is much less common and more difficult to manage. It usually presents with involvement of mucous membranes and skin erosions, the blisters being superficial and rarely seen before tops slough off.

Linear IgA disease is also uncommon. The classical presentation is of blisters around the margins of red or eroded areas described as a looking like a row of pearls.

Psoriasis

Psoriasis is a genetically based disorder which has two peaks of onset: youth and middle age. It rarely develops for the first time in old age. The classical appearance of well-defined, red plaques covered by silvery scales distributed on elbows, knees and scalp makes the diagnosis easy, but psoriasis can affect any area of the body including the nails. In older people nail changes, particularly on the feet, are common and there can be additional changes due to fungal infection and chronic pressure from footwear. Psoriasis variants which cause difficulties in diagnosis and management in the older population are flexural psoriasis and sebo-psoriasis. In the former, the skin in skin creases is a beefy red and shiny, lacking the scales seen in the classical form. Topical steroids work well but care must be taken to use appropriate potencies. Control can often be gained with moderately potent preparations, sometimes as a proprietary mixture with antimicrobials (e.g. Trimovate™). Once under control, reduction of the steroid potency is wise and addition of liberal quantities of emollient can be effective maintenance therapy.

In sebo-psoriasis, the condition appears in the same distribution as seborrhoeic eczema, i.e. areas where there is a high density of sebaceous glands including face, scalp, behind the ears, axillae, groins and upper trunk. It is unclear if this is a separate condition or co-incidence of psoriasis and seborrhoeic eczema. As far as treatment is concerned, mild topical steroids with coal tar (e.g. Alphosyl HC™) or with anti-yeast agents such as Daktacort™ can help.

Management of psoriasis proceeds along the standard lines as at any age but there may be a case for earlier referral to dermatology in the older patients for consideration of second-line therapies because of the difficulties in applying skin preparations adequately (see Box 17.4).

Vasculitis

Vasculitis is uncommon but important. The hallmark of small vessel cutaneous vasculitis is purpura which is palpable. Usually this will begin on the lower legs. Almost any rash on elderly lower

---

Box 17.4 Psoriasis management

- Chronic plaques: vitamin D analogues (e.g. calcipotriol, short-contact dithranol (Dithrocream™), topical steroids, salicylic acid, tazarotene, coal tar.
- Flexures and face: mild and moderately potent topical steroids with or without coal tar and antimicrobials, calcitriol.
- Scalp: topical steroid lotions (alcohol-based applications often sting), short-contact dithranol (Dithrocream), keratolytics with coal tar such as Cocois™ or SebCo™ (applied overnight and washed off next day.
- Nails: short trial of super-potent topical steroids locally.

Compliance is helped by careful explanation of how to use these agents, providing sufficient quantities and warnings, e.g. Dithrocream™, will cause temporary discoloration of skin and hair, SebCo™ and Cocois™ will stain clothes, etc. Emollients should be used in all cases.

legs can look purpuric but patients with vasculitis will complain of burning discomfort or pain rather than itching. If in doubt, referral for appropriate investigation including biopsy is advised. Blistering can also occur in more severe cases.

In vasculitis it is important to look for a cause and to determine whether any other organs are involved. The commonest causes are systemic infection, tumours and medication. In 50% no cause is found. If vasculitis is limited to the lower legs and there is no systemic involvement or serious underlying condition, it can be a relatively benign disease. The main risk is that large or blistered areas can result in necrosis, and these require careful nursing care.

History and examination may exclude many causes. Urinalysis looking for haematuria should always be done and repeated frequently. Laboratory investigations should include blood count, renal and liver function, inflammatory markers (erythrocyte sedimentation rate and C-reactive protein which can act as a guide to progress), autoantibodies, immunoglobulins, appropriate cultures/serology if infection is suspected. Biopsy can confirm both diagnosis and size of vessels involved.

Management of mild cases with no evidence of systemic involvement requires rest and analgesia. More severe involvement may require systemic steroids or other immune modulating drugs, usually under the guidance of a dermatologist. Colchicine is a relatively non-toxic drug which can be effective in small vessel vasculitis limited to the skin. The main side-effect of colchicine is diarrhoea which is dose dependent.

Intertrigo

Intertrigo is a term used for a flexural inflammation and is very common in older people, especially if overweight and immobile. It is commoner in women and can be very itchy or sore. Severe cases can ulcerate. There is no single cause for this condition and there may be a combination of sweat, under- or overwashing, eczema or psoriasis and yeast or dermatophyte infection.

Management should include:

◆ Sampling for microbiology (swab and scrapings from edge).

◆ Advice on washing with emollients.

◆ Avoidance of irritants.

◆ Application of combined low or moderately potent topical steroids with antimicrobials.

◆ Help to lose weight.

Consider referral if there is no response. However, many cases are very treatment resistant or recurrent.

Herpes zoster

There is a 50% lifetime risk of herpes zoster ('shingles') in anyone aged 80 years.[12] The presentation is usually obvious with dermatomal distribution of erythema and blistering which then crusts and may heal with scarring. There is an increased risk of post-herpetic neuralgia in elderly individuals and it is worth using systemic antiviral agents as soon as the diagnosis is suspected. Aciclovir is very safe with few interactions and should be used in the doses for immunosuppressed patients. Famcicolvir and valaciclovir have more convenient dosage regimens but are significantly more expensive.

Problem: drug eruptions

Drug eruptions are common in older people. Elderly patients are often on many drugs and it can require astute detective work to find the culprit. That said, there are some patterns of eruption

Box 17.5 Patterns of drug eruption with common culprit drugs

- Morbilliform or widespread eythematous eruptions: any drug, antibiotics, thiazides beta-blockers, allopurinol, non-steroidal anti-inflammatory drugs (NSAIDs), anticonvulsants.
- Urticaria: antibiotics, angiotensin-converting enzyme inhibitors, salicylates, opiates.
- Blistering: sulphonamides, penicillamine, captopril, furosemide, penicillin.
- Photosensitivity: thiazides, tetracyclines, amiodarone, NSAIDs.
- Peri-orifical or peristomal ulceration: nicorandil.
- Psoriasis: lithium, antimalarials, beta-blockers (rare).
- Fixed drug eruption: laxatives, paracetamol, tetracyclines, NSAIDs.
- Acne-like or rosacea: systemic steroids, androgens.
- Stevens–Johnson syndrome and toxic epidermal necrolysis: sulphonamides, anticonvulsants, NSAIDs, allopurinol.
- Skin infections: immune suppressants.
- Itching of upper body and face: opioids.
- Cholestatic or liver toxicity: oestrogens, captopril, chlorpromazine, anticonvulsants, paracetamol, isoniazid, erythromycin, minocycline, testosterones, phenothiazines,
- Dry skin: retinoids, beta-blockers, tamoxifen.

which suggest the cause, and common patterns with common causes are listed in Box 17.5. The onset is usually within a few weeks of beginning the drug but can rarely be months. Again, the distribution and morphology of the rash can help. Drug rashes are usually symmetrical and widespread. A fixed drug eruption is a localized area of rash which may blister and usually becomes pigmented between attacks. This is often due to a drug taken intermittently sometimes not considered by the patient to be a drug at all, e.g. paracetamol, aspirin and some old-fashioned laxatives containing phenolphthalein. Tetracyclines and sulphonamides can also cause fixed drug eruptions. This eruption always occurs at the same site. Remember to ask about over-the-counter medications and complementary therapies which may cause interactions and rashes.

Problem: new skin lesion

Discrete new skin lesions are very common in the elderly population. While many are benign, skin malignancies and premalignant conditions of all types are more common with increasing age. With visual impairment, asymptomatic lesions may not be noticed until they are at an advanced stage. History of change in a lesion is very important, malignancies usually enlarging slowly but relentlessly. Suspected malignant melanomas and squamous cell carcinomas should be referred by a fast-track route to a dermatologist or plastic surgeon and should never be tackled in primary care. Any skin lesion which is removed in primary care must be submitted to histological examination, the result noted and acted upon if necessary. While usually affecting the face, scalp and neck, many skin cancers appear on the backs of older men and it is a good practice to examine this area whenever an opportunity arises. Lower legs of ladies are also a site worth checking. The National Institute of Health and Clinical Excellence guidelines for improving outcomes in patients with skin cancer including melanoma recommend that GPs should only remove skin cancers in primary care if they have been specifically trained and accredited to do this work, and that they should treat only low-risk lesions.[13]

Malignant melanoma

Pigmented lesions give rise to most concern. It is unwise to subject suspicious pigmented lesions to diagnostic biopsy. They should always be removed completely in case of missing a malignant melanoma (MM) which are more common with advancing age (Box 17.6; Colour plate 14). These make up ~10% of the skin cancers seen in the UK.[13]

Superficial spreading malignant melanomas (SSMM) make up at least 50% of all melanomas and are flat or very slightly raised above the skin surface. Usually ≥6 mm in diameter at presentation, they have an irregular margin and variable pigmentation (Colour plate 14b). They may ulcerate and this worsens the prognosis. Very rarely melanomas are not pigmented (amelanotic). These are rarely diagnosed clinically and are a good reason for ensuring that all lesions removed are sent for histological examination. The prognosis for any melanoma survival depends on the thickness of the lesion measured by the pathologist (Breslow thickness).

Nodular melanomas make up ~20% of melanomas. These are raised and often ulcerate. These are sometimes found on sun-protected skin (Colour plate 14c). Generally the outcome is less favourable.

In situ MM or lentigo maligna is relatively common on the face or other sun-exposed sites in older people (Colour plate 14a). Whether or not these are treated depends on the general state of health of the individual. When in doubt, refer for a second opinion. Melanoma arising in a lentigo maligna is termed a lentigo maligna melanoma and these account for some 15% of melanomas.

Subungual melanomas (e.g. Colour plate 14d) are one type of acral lentiginous melanoma which is found on the palm or sole and can be very large before detection. These have a relatively poor prognosis but are quite rare. They are, however, the commonest form of melanoma in dark-skinned people.

The following is an aide-memoire for melanoma recognition which can also be taught to patients:

A. Asymmetry: half of the lesion does not look like the other half.

B. Border irregularity.

C. Colour variation: particularly new colour change.

D. Diameter >6 mm longest axis.

Differential diagnosis of pigmented lesions includes the very common and benign seborrhoeic wart (Colour plate 15). Often beginning flat and becoming raised, these usually have a rough, warty surface in which tiny keratin cysts may be visible on magnification. They can show colour variation and have irregular shapes. Some are rather 'stuck-on' looking and others are greasy and shiny (ancanthotic). Seborrhoeic warts can be removed surgically (remembering to send the tissue for histology), subjected to cryotherapy or left alone. They are often profuse and it is impossible to

Box 17.6 Differential diagnosis of malignant melanoma

Pigmented basal cell carcinoma
Seborrhoeic wart
Benign naevus
Solar lentigo
Haemangioma
Dermatofibroma
Pyogenic granuloma

remove all of them. If they become inflamed and itchy, simple emollients such as aqueous cream BP or 50% liquid paraffin in white soft paraffin may give relief. Failing that, non-fluorinated mild or moderately potent topical steroids such as 1% hydrocortisone or clobetasone butyrate (Eumovate™) may help. Sudden appearance of many seborrhoeic warts on the trunk has been termed the sign of Lesser–Trelat and may indicate a systemic malignancy. However, the evidence for this is not strong. Benign naevi often regress before late adult life and it is very rare for new naevi to develop in mature skin.

Solar lentigos are flat, rather angular, evenly brown macules up to 1 cm in diameter are very common on sun-exposed sites and indicate UV damage. These are sometimes illogically termed 'liver spots'. Purplish red papules varying from pinpoint to several mm in diameter appear in increasing numbers, especially in non-exposed fair skins. These are benign haemangiomas or Campbell de Morgan spots and do not require treatment or indicate any systemic disease. Pyogenic granulomas are a type of rapidly growing benign haemangioma, often arising at the site of minor injury. They bleed easily and can be difficult to differentiate from nodular MM without good history. Dermatofibromas are very firm and do not enlarge. Their pigmentation tends to be around the edge only. They are harmless and need not be treated unless the diagnosis is in doubt.

Non-melanoma skin cancers

Basal cell carcinoma

Skin-coloured skin lesions are more likely to be non-melanoma skin cancers or premalignant lesions, especially if located on sun-exposed skin. Basal cell carcinoma (BCC) is the commonest malignant neoplasm found in humans. Although they rarely metastasize, they continue to grow and cause tissue damage, bleeding, pain and even death if they infiltrate vital structures. The commonest finding is a pink nodule with surface telangiectases on close inspection. Some pigmentation may be seen. There are other clinical patterns (Colour plate 16).

The gold standard treatment is surgical excision with a 4 mm margin.[14] Those on the central part of the face, around the ears and temples are more likely to recur, as are morphoeic BCCs which can mimic an area of scarring while inexorably spreading in the dermis (Colour plate 16b). Although surgery is again likely to be curative, those which do recur may prove very difficult to manage.

However, superficial BCCs are often found on the trunk where they may behave differently. They can expand laterally to several centimetres in diameter before becoming nodular. They may be treated surgically but thorough cryotherapy using repeated freeze–thaw cycles could be used. There are two patient-applied topical agents used to treat superficial BCC, namely imiquimod and 5% fluorouracil cream. Both are also used for premalignant skin conditions (see below) and both cause considerable tissue inflammation. The patient and carers need to be carefully instructed in their use. Specialist training in recognition of these lesions and use of these treatment modalities for superficial BCC is recommended. Imiquimod was originally licensed for the treatment of genital warts.

Squamous cell carcinoma

Squamous cell carcinomas (SCCs) have a higher rate of metastasis than BCCs but are usually cured by excision with a generous margin of normal tissue.[15] They can be recognized as keratotic or scaly papules or nodules, often in a background of sun damage. They often ulcerate and can be painful. Like suspected MM, suspected SCC should always be referred under a rapid access system to a dermatologist or plastic surgeon. People with non-melanoma skin cancers often have multiple primary lesions. Cancer databases underestimate the true incidence which rises with age and is higher in men than women.

Premalignant skin conditions

In situ SCC may be termed Bowen's disease. This consists of a pink or red scaly plaque which slowly expands (Colour plate 17). Ladies' legs are commonly involved but any sun-exposed site can be affected. Rate of progression to SCC is reported to be 3–5%.[16] This can be a rather indolent condition. Differential diagnosis is an isolated patch of inflammation (eczema or psoriasis or even fungal infection). Referral should be considered to confirm diagnosis. Successful treatment depends on patient factors including age, site of lesion and co-morbidities including immune suppression as well as compliance. Cryotherapy, surgery, 5- fluorouracil topically and imiquimod cream are all used. The place of photodynamic therapy is yet to be established but success is reported and it is well tolerated in elderly patients.

Actinic keratoses (Colour plate 18) are usually multiple and can sometimes be very thick and scaly and difficult to differentiate from SCC. Thicker lesions are more likely to progress to SCC. Overall rate of progression is between 0.025% and 16%.[17] Most actinic keratoses are relatively thin with no induration and respond to adequate cryotherapy or application of diclofenac with hyaluronic acid gel (Solaraze™) used twice daily for 3 months, reported success rates of both being 75%.[18] Fluorouracil (5% cream) has a published success rate of ~80%. Studies have varied enormously in design, making it difficult to compare treatments.[19] The evidence that treatment prevents progression to SCC is lacking. If patients have >10 actinic keratoses they have a 14% risk of developing SCC over 5 years.[20]

Keratoacanthoma

Keratoacanthomas are rapidly growing, self-healing lesions which can closely resemble SCC (Colour plate 19). Usually appearing on sun-exposed skin, they develop within a small number of weeks and very slowly resolve with scarring. When in doubt these are best removed by complete excision as the differentiation from SCC by the pathologist depends on the morphology of the lesion which is destroyed by curettage.

References

1. Beauregard S, Gilchrest BA. A survey of skin problems and skin care regimens in the elderly. *Arch Dermatol* 1987;123:1638–43.
2. Yalcm B, Tanner E, Toy GG, Hayran M, Alli N. The prevalence of skin diseases in the elderly: analysis of 4099 geriatric patients. *In J Dermatol* 2006;45:672–6.
3. Thiapisuttikul Y. Pruritic skin diseases in the elderly. *J Dermatol* 1998;25:153–7.
4. McFadden N, Handke KO (1989). A survey of elderly new patients at a dermatology outpatient clinic. *Acta Dermatol Venereol* 1998;69:260–262.
5. Norman RA. Xerosis and pruritus in elderly patients, Part 1. *Ostomy Wound Manage* 2006;52:12–14.
6. Greaves M Antihistamines in dermatology, *Skin Pharmacol Physiol* 2005;18:220–9.
7. Machet L, Couhé C, Perrinaud A, Hoarau C, Lorette G, Vaillant L. A high prevalence of sensitization still persists in leg ulcer patients: a retrospective series of 106 patients tested between 2001 and 2002 and a meta-analysis of 1975–2003 data. *Br J Dermatol* 2004;150:292–35.
8. Patil S, Maibach HI. Effect of age and sex on the elicitation of irritant contact dermatitis. *Contact Dermatitis* 1994;30:257–64.
9. Bewley A, Dermatology Working Group. Expert consensus: time for a change in the way we advise our patients to use topical corticosteroids. *Br J Dermatol* 2008;158:917–20.

10. Langan SM, Smeeth L, Hubbard R, Fleming KM, Smith CJ, West J. Bullous pemphigoid and pemphigus vulgaris—incidence and mortality in the UK: population based cohort study. *Br Med J* 2008;337:160–3.

11. Joly P, Roujeau J-C, Benichou J, *et al.* A comparison of oral and topical corticosteroids in patients with bullous pemphigoid. *New Eng J Med* 2002;346:321–7.

12. Schmader KE. Epidemiology and impact on quality of life of postherpetic neuralgia and painful diabetic neuropathy. *Clin J Pain* 2002;18:350-4.

13. National Institute for Health and Clinical Excellence. Improving outcomes for people with skin tumours including melanoma. NICE Cancer Service Guidance; 2006. http://www.nice.org.uk

14. Telfer NR, Colver GB, Morton CA: British Association of Dermatologists. Guidelines for the management of basal cell carcinoma. *Br J Dermatol* 2008;159:35–48.

15. Motley R, Kersey P, Lawrence C: British Association of Dermatologists; British Association of Plastic Surgery. Multiprofessional guidelines for the management of the patient with primary cutaneous squamous cell carcinoma. *Br J Plast Surg* 2003;56:85–91.

16. Kao GF. Carcinoma arising in Bowen's disease. *Arch Dermatol* 1986;122:1124–6.

17. Gupta AK, Bowen J, Cooper E, Soon SL, Pierre P, Chen SC. Actinic keratoses and Bowen's disease. In: Williams H (ed.). *Evidence Based Dermatology*. London: Blackwell; 2008. p. 295.

18. Pirard D, Vereecken P, Melot C, Heenen M. Three percent diclofenac in 2.5% hyaluronan gel in the treatment of actinic keratoses: a meta-anlaysis of the recent studies. *Arch Dermatol Res* 2005;297:185–9.

19. Pierre P, Weil E, Chen S. Cryotherapy versus topical 5-fluorouracil therapy of actinic keratoses: a systematic review. *Allergologie* 2001;24:204–5.

20. De Berker D, Mc Gregor JM, Hughes BR: British Association of Dermatologists Therapy Guidelines and Audit Subcommittee. Guidelines for the management of actinic keratoses. *Br J Dermatol* 2007;156:222–30.

Chapter 18

Pressure ulceration and leg ulcers

Joseph Grey, Julie Stevens, and Keith Harding

Introduction

A pressure ulcer is a localized area of tissue damage, usually developing when an external surface compresses the skin and soft tissue over a bony prominence for a prolonged period of time (Box 18.1; Figure 18.1). Pressure ulcers may arise wherever there is compression between a bony prominence and an external surface (Figure 18.2).

In adults the majority of pressure ulcers develop around the pelvis and the lower limbs (Figure 18.3). In infants and children they are more likely to occur on the occipital area or ears. Elderly people, especially those aged >70 years, are most prone to pressure ulceration, 30% of whom will have had surgery to repair a hip fracture. Up to a third of individuals with spinal injuries will develop a pressure ulcer 1–5 years after initial injury. Whereas most pressure ulcers arise in the hospital setting, almost 20% develop at home with a further 20% occurring in nursing homes. The elderly person developing pressure ulceration faces a five-fold increase in mortality.

The damage leading to pressure ulceration is largely attributable to four extrinsic factors, usually acting together (Figure 18.4): Interface pressure (acting perpendicular to the tissue surface); shear (acting parallel to the tissue surface), friction (acting tangentially to the tissue surface) and moisture, which increases the effect of friction up to five-fold.

Many systems have been proposed to classify pressure ulcers; none is perfect. The European Pressure Ulcer Advisory Panel (EPUAP) has developed a four-grade classification (Box 18.2; Colour plate 20a–d). Difficulties arise when, for example, trying to distinguish grade 1 ulceration in people with darkly pigmented skin and accurately grading a pressure ulcer covered with Eschar (generally graded as grade 4 due to the uncertainties as to what lies beneath) (Colour plate 21). Undermining and sinuses commonly occur and may affect grading as well as healing (Colour plate 22).

Risk assessment

Holistic, regular, assessment of the at-risk individual should include the use of an established risk calculator that is suited to the individual patient. Combined with clinical judgement, this ensures systematic evaluation of individual risk factors. Several risk assessment scales have been developed (Gosnell, Knoll, Doyles Norton, Braden). Although some components form the basis of all, some scales are more comprehensive than others: they are all subject to inter-observer error. The Waterlow scale is commonly used in hospital and the community in the UK (Figure 18.5). The scale stratifies the patient into a risk level. Any scale is only of use if it is followed by appropriate intervention (mattress, cushion, etc.).

Risk factors

Many intrinsic risk factors (Box 18.3) have been associated with the development of pressure ulceration. Although pressure ulceration is more common in older individuals, age itself is not an

Box 18.1 Pressure ulcer definition (EPUAP[1])

A pressure ulcer may be defined as an area of localized damage to the skin and underlying tissue caused by pressure, shear, friction or a combination of these.

independent risk factor. Rather it is the concomitant problems associated with ageing that lead to the increased risk. Impaired mobility (the inability to reposition without assistance or limited mobility) due to physical illness, disability, medication or psychological states, is one of the most important risk factors.

Pressure ulceration is more common in those who have poor oral intake or are (protein-energy) malnourished. High risk malnourished patients experience more than twice the incidence of pressure ulceration compared with individuals who are adequately nourished.[3] The extent and severity of pressure ulceration is correlated with the degree of malnutrition.[4]

Pressure ulcer assessment

A comprehensive, holistic assessment of an individual with a pressure ulcer should include a detailed history and careful examination of the individual leading to identification of the contributory intrinsic and extrinsic risk factors (Figure 18.4; Box 18.3). Once identified these factors should be managed appropriately. Accurate assessment of the ulcer itself is also vital for appropriate management. Ulcer characteristics are listed in Box 18.4. Photography, if possible, is a valuable adjunct to ulcer assessment and documentation.

Other ulcer aetiologies should be differentiated, for example, ischaemia, vasculitis, radiation injury and pyoderma gangrenosum.

Management: pressure relief

Pressure relief (pressure reduction and/or pressure redistribution by increasing the surface area in contact with the support surface) is fundamental to the prevention and treatment of

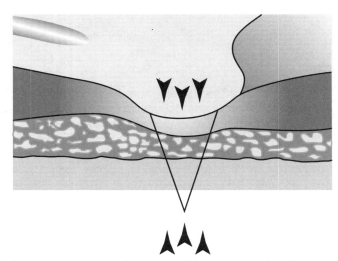

Fig. 18.1 Cone of pressure: pressure at the surface of the skin is translated into more diffuse higher pressure at the bone–tissue interface.

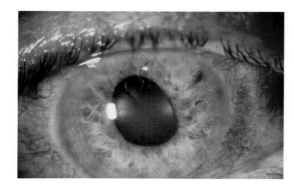

Colour plate 1 Acute angle closure glaucoma.

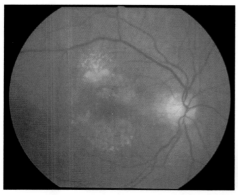

Colour plate 2 'Wet' age-related macular degeneration: exudate and oedema.

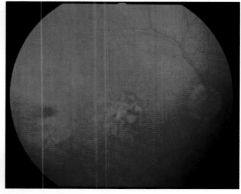

Colour plate 4 'Dry' age-related macular degeneration: drusen.

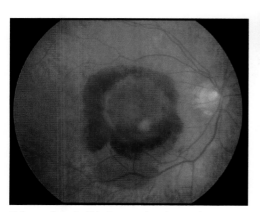

Colour plate 3 'Wet' age-related macular degeneration: haemorrhage.

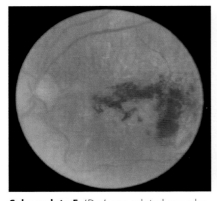

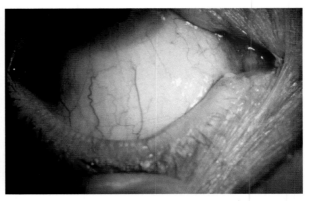

Colour plate 5 'Dry' age-related macular degeneration: hyper- and hypopigmentation.

Colour plate 6 Blepharitis: meibomian gland inflammation and plugging.

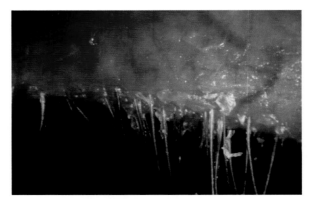

Colour plate 7 Blepharitis: eyelash crusts.

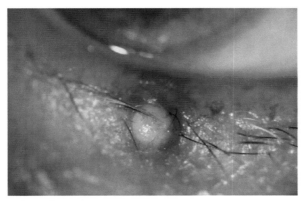

Colour plate 8 Stye.

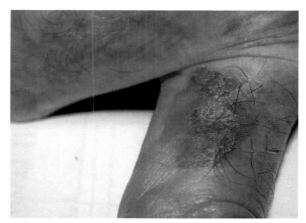

Colour plate 17 Bowen's disease (squamous cell carcinoma *in situ*) on a finger.

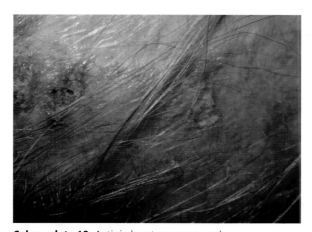

Colour plate 18 Actinic keratoses on a scalp.

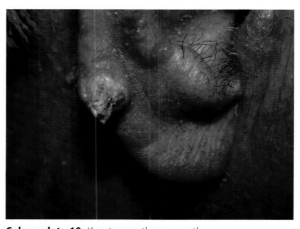

Colour plate 19 Keratoacanthoma on the ear.

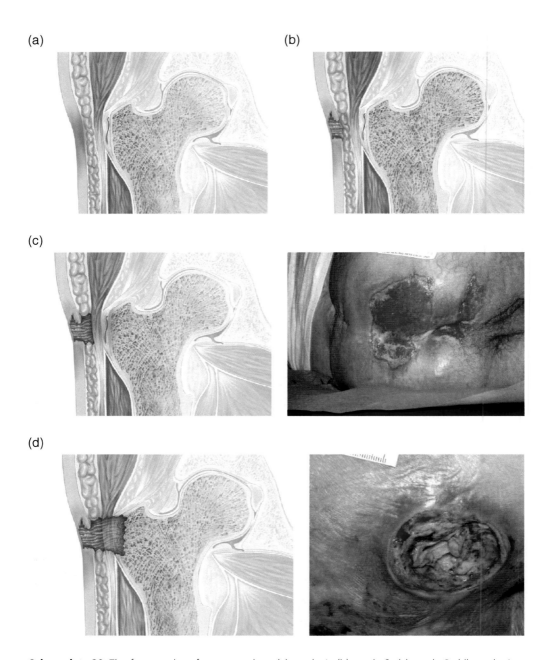

(a)

(b)

(c)

(d)

Colour plate 20 The four grades of pressure ulcer: (a) grade 1; (b) grade 2; (c) grade 3; (d) grade 4.

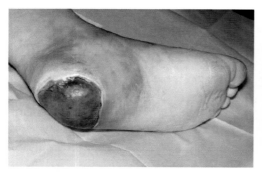

Colour plate 21 Eschar covering heel pressure ulcer: grade 4 pressure ulcer.

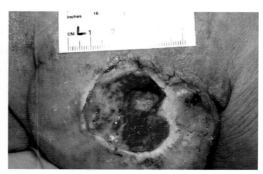

Colour plate 24 Local wound infection.

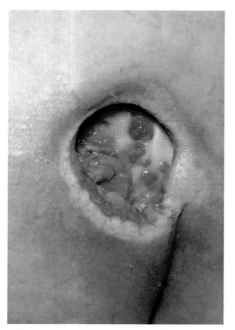

Colour plate 22 Undermining of grade 3 pressure ulcer.

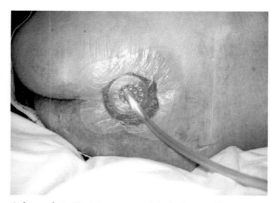

Colour plate 25 Vacuum-assisted closure therapy being used to treat sacral pressure ulcer.

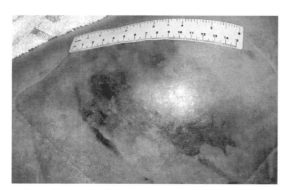

Colour plate 23 Cellulitis associated with grade 2 pressure ulcers.

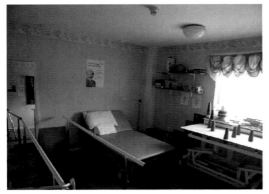

Colour plate 26 A physiotherapy room.

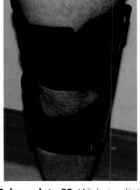

Colour plate 29 Wicket splint.

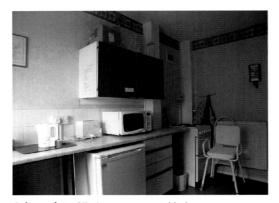

Colour plate 27 An assessment kitchen.

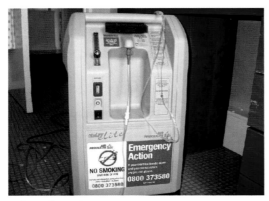

Colour plate 28 An oxygen concentrator.

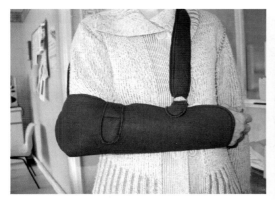

Colour plate 30 Lancaster arm sling.

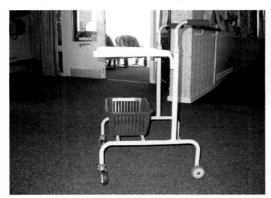

Colour plate 31 Trolley.

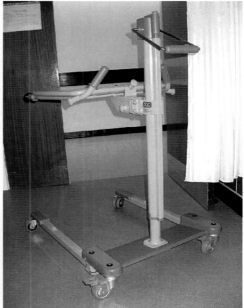

Colour plate 33 Pulpit frame.

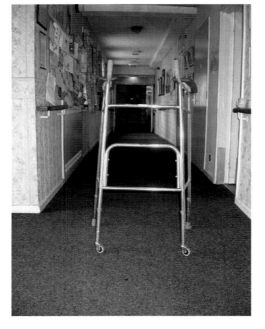

Colour plate 32 Elbow gutter frame.

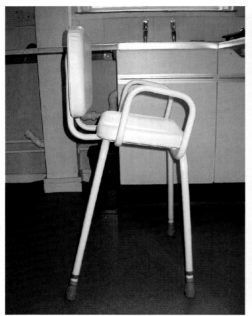

Colour plate 34 Perching stool.

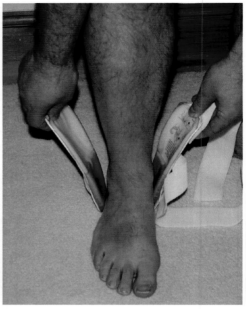

Colour plate 36 Ankle brace.

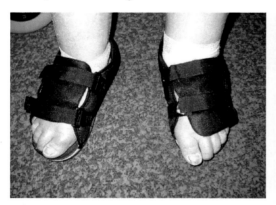

Colour plate 35 Post-op sandals.

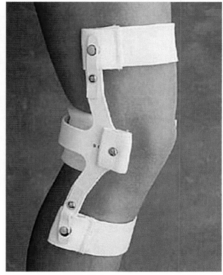

Colour plate 37 Swedish knee cage.

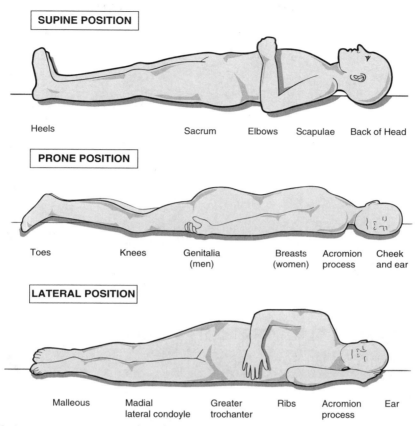

SUPINE POSITION

Heels   Sacrum   Elbows   Scapulae   Back of Head

PRONE POSITION

Toes   Knees   Genitalia   Breasts   Acromion   Cheek
                 (men)   (women)   process   and ear

LATERAL POSITION

Malleous   Madial   Greater   Ribs   Acromion   Ear
            lateral condoyle   trochanter   process

Fig. 18.2 Areas prone to pressure ulceration.

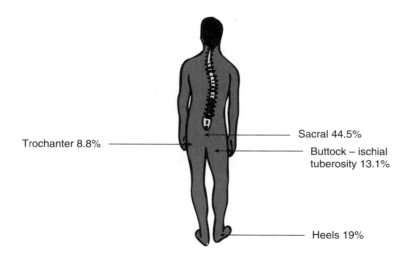

Trochanter 8.8%

Sacral 44.5%

Buttock – ischial
tuberosity 13.1%

Heels 19%

Fig. 18.3 Common sites of pressure ulceration.

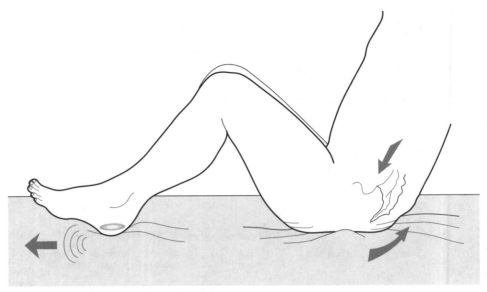

Fig. 18.4 Friction pressure at the heel and shear pressure at the sacrum.

Box 18.2 Classification of pressure ulcers according to pattern of tissue damage (EPUAP)

Grade 1

Non-blanchable erythema of intact skin. Discoloration of the skin, warmth, induration or hardness may also be used as indicators, particularly on individuals with darker skin.

Grade 2

Partial thickness skin loss involving epidermis, dermis or both. The ulcer is superficial and presents clinically as an abrasion or blister.

Grade 3

Full thickness skin loss involving damage to, or necrosis of, subcutaneous tissue that may extend down to, but not through, underlying fascia.

Grade 4

Extensive destruction, tissue necrosis or damage to muscle, bone or supporting structures with or without full thickness skin loss.

---

pressure ulceration. Individuals with pressure ulcers, as well as those at risk, should be nursed on appropriate pressure-relieving surfaces including mattresses, mattress overlays and cushions.

Such surfaces fall broadly into two categories: the continuous low pressure (static) system designed to redistribute pressure and; the alternating (dynamic) pressure system which relieves the pressure under different parts of the body in a sequential and cyclical manner. The surface

WATERLOW PRESSURE SORE PREVENTION/TREATMENT POLICY

RING SCORES IN TABLE, ADD TOTAL. SEVERAL SCORES PER CATEGORY CAN BE USED

BUILD/WEIGHT FOR HEIGHT	★	SKIN TYPE VISUAL RISK AREAS	★	SEX AGE	★	SPECIAL RISKS	★
AVERAGE	0	HEALTHY	0	MALE	1	TISSUE MALNUTRITION	★
ABOVE AVERAGE	1	TISSUE PAPER	1	FEMALE	2	e.g.:TERMINAL CACHEXIA	8
OBESE	2	DRY	1	14 – 49	1	CARDIAC FAILURE	5
BELOW AVERAGE	3	OEDEMATOUS	1	50 – 64	2	PERIPHERAL VASCULAR	
		CLAMMY (TEMP↑)	1	65 – 74	3	DISEASE	5
		DISCOLOURED	2	75 – 80	4	ANAEMIA	2
		BROKEN/SPOT	3	81+	5	SMOKING	1
CONTINENCE	★	MOBILITY	★	APPETITE	★	NEUROLOGICAL DEFICIT	★
COMPLETE/ CATHETERISED	0	FULLY	0	AVERAGE	0	e.g.:DIABETES, M.S, CVA, MOTOR/SENSORY	0
OCCASION INCONT	1	RESTLESS/FIDGETY	1	POOR	1		1
CATH/INCONTINENT OF FAECES	2	APATHETIC	2	N.G. TUBE/		PARAPLEGIA	4 – 6
DOUBLY INCONT	3	RESTRICTED	3	FLUIDS ONLY	2		
		INERT/TRACTION	4	NBM/ANOREXIC	3	MAJOR SURGERY/TRAUMA	★
		CHAIRBOUND	5			ORTHOPAEDIC - BELOW WAIST, SPINAL	5
						ON TABLE > 2 HOURS	5
						MEDICATION	★
						CYTOTOXICS, HIGH DOSE STEROIDS ANTI-INFLAMMATORY	4

SCORE	10+ AT RISK	15+ HIGH RISK	20+ VERY HIGH RISK

Fig. 18.5 Waterlow pressure sore prevention/treatment policy (redrawn).
NG, nasogastric; NBM, nil by mouth; MS, multiple sclerosis; CVA, cerebrovascular accident. © J. Waterlow 1991, revised March 1992.

Box 18.3 Risk factors for pressure ulceration[a]

Acute illness

- Increased metabolic rate and demand for oxygen compromising tissues.

Age

- Chronic disease.
- Stroke.
- Impaired nutrition.
- Bed- or chair-bound.
- Faecal incontinence.
- Fractured neck of femur.
- Confusion.

Level of consciousness

- Acute/chronic illness.
- Medication.
  - Sedatives.
  - Analgesics.
  - Anaesthetics.

Limited mobility/immobility

- Cerebrovascular accident.
- Spinal cord injury.
  - Hemiparesis.
  - Paraparesis.
  - Quadriplegia.
- Spasticity.
- Arthritis.
- Orthopaedic problems, especially fractured neck of femur.
- Bed- or chair-bound individuals.

Sensory impairment

- Neuropathies, e.g. diabetes.
- Decreased conscious levels.
- Medication.
- Spinal cord injury.

Severe chronic or terminal disease

- Diabetes.
- Chronic obstructive pulmonary disease.
- Chronic cardiovascular disease.
- Terminal illness.

Box 18.3 Risk factors for pressure ulceration *(continued)*

Vascular disease

- ◆ Smoking.
- ◆ Diabetes.
- ◆ Peripheral vascular disease.
- ◆ Anaemia.
- ◆ Antihypertensives.

Malnutrition/dehydration

- ◆ Weight loss.
- ◆ Lymphopenia.
- ◆ Low albumin, prealbumin, transferrin.

History of pressure damage

[a] Based on NICE guidelines for pressure ulcer prevention.[2]

---

should not be able to 'bottom out', i.e. the mattress (or overlay) or any part of it providing <2.5 cm of support.

The National Institute for Health and Clinical Excellence (NICE)[5] recommends that individuals with grade 1 or 2 pressure ulcers should be managed on a high specification foam mattress, but if there is any deterioration this should be changed to a high specification continuous low pressure or alternating pressure system. Individuals with grades 3 or 4 ulceration should be managed on an alternating pressure system. Liaison with local wound-healing specialist or tissue viability nurses will help define the appropriate surface.

Individuals should be encouraged to change position regularly. However, patients' general mobility and bed mobility are often compromised; appropriate pressure relief should include

---

Box 18.4 Pressure ulcer characteristics

- ◆ Cause of ulcer.
- ◆ Site/location.
- ◆ Dimensions of ulcer.
- ◆ Stage or grade.
- ◆ Exudate amount and type: purulent, serous, sero-sanguinous.
- ◆ Local signs of infection.
- ◆ Pain.
- ◆ Wound appearance.
- ◆ Surrounding skin.
- ◆ Undermining/tracking (sinus or fistula): including measurements.
- ◆ Odour.
- ◆ Involvement of clinical experts: e.g. tissue viability nurse.
- ◆ Ulcer bed: type of tissue; healthy, necrotic, bone visible/palpable.

a regular repositioning schedule (at least 2-hourly is generally recommended). The frail, immobile and ill elderly patients are at increased risk of pressure ulceration when seated due to reduced muscle bulk around the pelvis and reduced skin elasticity. As such, the tissues over the ischial tuberosities are subject to higher than normal pressures.

Individuals at risk of pressure ulceration should also be assessed for appropriate pressure-relieving surfaces. Risk assessment scales are employed as a tool in identifying at-risk individuals. They should, however, not be a substitute for clinical judgement. Ring, 'doughnut', cushions must not be used as they may cause rather than prevent pressure ulceration. Foam wedges or pillows may be used to avoid direct contact of bony prominences such as ankles or knees.

Nutrition

Adequate nutrition is essential both in the prevention and healing of pressure ulcers. The serum albumin concentration is often used as a marker of nutritional status. However, given its relatively long half-life (>3 weeks) this can be misleading. Other markers of malnutrition include weight loss, reduced lymphocyte count and decreased prealbumin and ferritin levels. In any event, individuals with pressure ulceration should be under regular review by a dietician. The person's diet should be optimized with increased protein-energy and fluid intake: dietary supplements may be helpful. Severely malnourished people who are unable to take sufficient diet orally may require supplementary nasogastric feeding. A small number of individuals may benefit from temporary percutaneous endoscopic gastrostomy (*PEG*) tube feeding, though this is a controversial area.

Wound cleansing

Gardner and Frantz[6] have defined wound cleansing as 'a process, which removes less adherent inflammatory molecules (such as cytokines and matrix metalloproteins) from the wound surfaces and renders the wound less conducive to microbial growth'.

The EPUAP[1] has developed guidelines for cleansing pressure ulcers (Box 18.5). Tap water suitable for drinking may be used to cleanse pressure ulcers. Sterile saline (0.9% sodium chloride), though more commonly used, is more expensive. Antiseptics should not be routinely used to cleanse an ulcer as they are toxic to non-bacterial cells found in the wound including fibroblasts and macrophages.

Showering with large amounts of water helps with wound cleansing and improves the quality of life of the individual. Gentle irrigation of the wound in this way helps to reduce the bacterial burden on the wound surface.[7,8]

Box 18.5 Guidelines for cleansing pressure ulcers (EPUAP[1])

1. Cleanse wounds as necessary with tap water or with water which is suitable for drinking, or with saline.
2. Use minimal mechanical force when cleansing or irrigating the ulcer. Showering is appropriate. Irrigation can be useful for cleaning a cavity ulcer.
3. Antiseptics should not routinely be used to clean wounds but may be considered when bacterial load needs to be controlled after clinical assessment. Ideally, antiseptics should only be used for a limited period of time until the wound is clean and surrounding inflammation reduced.

Wound debridement

Removal of moist necrotic tissue (yellow or grey 'slough'), dry eschar (thick, hard, black, leathery necrotic tissue; Colour plate 21) and debris is important to promote wound healing, reduce bacterial load and for accurate pressure ulcer staging. High levels of proinflammatory cytokines and degradative proteases found in chronic wound exudate may prevent wound healing.[9–11] Debridement and wound cleansing help to remove this exudate and further promote wound healing.

There are various methods of debridement (Box 18.6). Generally pressure ulcers will be managed through a mixture of sharp debridement and use of appropriate modern dressings promoting autolysis.

Infection

The presence of bacteria in a pressure ulcer does not necessarily indicate infection. Many pressure ulcers will simply be colonized with bacteria that are not causing problems for the individual or harm to the wound. For this reason, random sampling ('swabbing') of the ulcer is not appropriate: it is costly, wasteful, and adds nothing to the management of the ulcer.

Swabs should be taken from ulcers that are obviously infected and those that are not healing despite optimal treatment. Indicators of wound infection, which are sometimes subtle, are listed in Box 18.7. Swabs containing transport media and charcoal are preferred as they help to preserve bacteria.

The treatment of infection should be guided by, not based solely upon, the results of microbiological investigations. Systemic, empirical antibiotic therapy is warranted for infections associated with systemic illness, deep invasion or cellulitis (Colour plate 23) while awaiting culture results. The flora of pressure ulcers is typically polymicrobial and is influenced by the site of the ulcer. Aerobic bacteria are common: methicillin-resistant *Staphylococcus aureus* (MRSA) is not uncommon. Enterococci and Enterobacteria may be present in ulcers close to the anus.

Topical antibiotic therapy is not advocated: there is inadequate penetration to treat deep skin infections; antibiotic resistance may develop, as may hypersensitivity reactions and local irritation which may in turn delay wound healing. However, topical metronidazole (0.75%) gel is sometimes used to control odour from anaerobic and pseudomonal infections.

Box 18.6 Debridement methods

- Sharp: removal of necrotic tissue at the bedside or in the treatment room using a scalpel, scissors or curette.
- Surgical: in the operating theatre; may be necessary for extensive grade 3 or 4 pressure ulcers.
- Autolytic: use of the body's mechanisms through the maintenance of a moist wound environment facilitated by the use of modern dressings.
- Enzymatic: removal of necrotic tissue with various enymes usually applied topically as an ointment, though may be injected.
- Mechanical: wet to dry technique, usually using woven cotton gauze. May lead to damage of healthy tissue when the dressing is removed. Not widely used in the UK.
- Myiasis: sterile maggot therapy may be considered a form of enzymatic therapy with a component of mechanical debridement.

Box 18.7 Signs of pressure ulcer infection

- Warmth.
- Redness.
- Pain.
- Swelling.
- Odour.
- Increased wound exudate: serous, sero-sanguinous, purulent.
- Contact bleeding.
- Poor healing.
- Epithelial bridging.
- Tissue breakdown.
- Increasing ulcer size.
- Unhealthy granulation tissue.
- Systemic illness in the absence of other focus of infection.

Local wound infection (Colour plate 24) may be amenable to treatment with topical therapies, including silver or iodine preparations. This also avoids the potential side-effects of systemic antibiotics, including *Clostridium difficile* diarrhoea, and the development of organisms resistant to antibiotics.

Osteomyelitis may develop as a result of ulcer infection and should be considered if a pressure ulcer is not healing. Investigations should include plain X-ray, though often a bone scan or magnetic resonance imaging is required to aid the diagnosis. However, differentiating osteomyelitis from chronic soft tissue infection may be difficult. Prolonged antibiotic therapy may be required, in consultation with the local microbiologist. Devitalized bone may need to be surgically debrided.

Topical ulcer therapy: dressings

Dressings are one of the mainstays of treatment for pressure ulceration. Modern dressings promote a moist environment facilitating debridement, granulation, proliferation and re-epithelialization. They also may help to reduce associated pain, cool and sooth and provide a barrier against bacteria. There is a bewildering array of dressings available. A simple schema of dressings for different grades of pressure ulcer is shown in Table 18.1.[12] Their use should be guided by the characteristics of the wound (Box 18.4): cost, availability, ease of application, patient preference and local and national guidelines may also need to be considered.[13,14]

Vacuum-assisted closure

A non-invasive, negative-pressure healing device can be used to treat deep, cavitating wounds with large amounts of exudates, including pressure ulcers (Colour plate 25). Removal of excess wound fluid leads to improved local oxygenation and blood flow, promotion of angiogenesis and granulation tissue formation. Vacuum-assisted closure (VAC) dressings may only need to be changed twice or three times per week, reducing patient discomfort and cost. Duration of treatment with the VAC is dependent on clinical improvement, patient compliance and resources. Average length of use is three to four weeks. The therapy often does not lead to complete healing but fills the wound considerably with healthy tissue. Conventional dressings are then used to manage the ulcer.

Table 18.1 Dressings suitable for pressure ulcers[12]

Dressing type	Pressure ulcer grade	Advantages/disadvantages
Semipermeable film	1 Minimally exuding 2	Promote moist environment. Adheres to healthy skin but not to wound. Allows visual checks. May be left in place several days. No cushioning. Not for infected or heavily exuding wounds.
Foams	Low to moderately exuding, non-infected 2–3	Degree of cushioning. May be left in place 2–3 days. Needs secondary dressing.
Hydrogels	Low to moderately exuding 2–4	Supplies moisture to low exudate wounds. Useful for cavities and sinuses. May be left in place several days. Needs secondary dressing. May cause maceration.
Hydrocolloids	Low to moderately exuding 3–4	Absorbable. Conformable. Good in 'difficult areas'—heel, elbow, sacrum. May be left in place several days. May cause maceration.
Hydrofibres	Moderate to highly exuding 2–4	Useful in cavities, sinuses, undermining wounds. Highly absorbent. Non-adherent. May be left in place for several days. Needs secondary dressing.
Alginates	Moderate to highly exuding 2–4	Useful in cavities, sinuses, undermining wounds. Highly absorbent. Needs secondary dressing. Needs to be changed daily.

Myiasis

Sterile maggots, usually of the 'green bottle' fly (*Lucilia* or *Phaenicia* species), may be used to treat sloughy and infected ulcers without damaging the surrounding healthy tissue. As well as secreting degradative enzymes, beneficial cytokines, antiseptic substances and proteases have also been demonstrated in the fluid secreted by maggots. Maggots have also been shown to ingest and kill bacteria.[15] Between 100 and 200 sterile maggots are used to debride wounds and are left in place for 2–3 days. Increased pain in the wound, psychological and aesthetics issues may lead to concordance issues.

Growth factors and tissue engineering

Initially promising results from small scale trials into the use of recombinant growth factors to treat pressure ulcers has not translated into large scale clinical use. Basic fibroblast growth factor (bFGF) and platelet-derived growth factor BB (PDGF-BB) have had some success in the treatment of stage III and IV pressure ulcers. Similarly tissue-engineered skin substitutes using allogeneic cultured grafts (e.g. Dermagraft, Apligraf) have been used to treat stage III and IV pressure ulcers in trials but are not in wide clinical use in the UK. When used, these modalities should complement the basics of good wound care—wound debridement and exudate management.

Surgical treatment

Surgical intervention for grade 3 or 4 pressure ulcers may be appropriate when attempts at healing through conservative management do not lead to healing, despite optimal holistic management. Durable muscle flaps are fashioned to close the tissue defect. Such surgery may be suitable in those individuals with underlying osteomyelitis; the devitalized and infected bone is excised and the ulcer filled with highly vascularized muscle. Immobilization on a pressure-relieving mattress for 2–4 weeks is required after surgery. A high level of vigilance is required to identify complications which may lead to failure of the graft, including infection, necrosis, seroma formation and dehiscence.

Palliative care

Skin 'failure' presenting as pressure ulceration may occur as part of the multisystem problems faced by individuals with terminal illnesses. Healing of the ulcer in these instances may be impossible and aggressive interventions wholly inappropriate. The person's dignity and quality of life should be paramount, with management plans reflecting these. Issues including comfort, pain relief and odour management may be the desired goals in such individuals. Keeping family and friends involved and informed in such decisions is also very important (see Chapter 25).

Leg ulcers

Leg ulcers are a common, painful, debilitating condition that affect the sufferer's quality of life and cause considerable morbidity.[16] The prevalence of venous ulceration varies according to the population surveyed. The prevalence ranges from 1.2 to 3.2 per 1000 population.[17] However, this can rise to 8.5% in those aged >85 years.[18]

With the prospect of an ageing population, more patients with long-term conditions and multiple co-morbidity such as peripheral vascular disease and diabetes, will require expert care for associated tissue viability problems, including leg ulceration, in the community.[19,20]

Leg ulcer services

Leg ulcer services across the UK vary in their provision, but some nurse-led community clinics have proved a successful cost-effective innovation, especially when linked to a hospital vascular surgical unit, or specialist wound care centre.[21–23] Patient outcomes in terms of quality of life, social isolation and healing are anecdotally thought to benefit from a community leg ulcer clinic environment where a client-centred approach, peer group support, and therapeutic nurse–patient relationships can be developed.[24,25] The use of one-stop diagnostic vascular services and telemedicine to plan patient care by accessing specialist advice is often necessary in more rural areas, where access to these services can be inadequate.[26] Staff education is vital to whatever model of service is provided, and support in the planning care of more complex leg ulcers needs to be provided by a tissue viability specialist nurse and closely linked to a specialist wound centre, vascular and/or dermatology unit.

Aetiology

A leg ulcer may be defined as: 'An open lesion between the knee and the ankle joint that remains open for at least 4 weeks'.[27] The early assessment of pre-tibial lacerations and treatment with compression therapy often results in rapid healing. Box 18.8 lists the main causes of leg ulcers.

Box 18.8 Main causes of leg ulceration

◆ Chronic venous hypertension   59–70%
◆ Mixed arterial/venous   15–20%
◆ Arterial   10%
◆ Secondary to systemic diseases and unusual causes   5%

Venous ulcers

The majority of venous ulcers are caused by persistently high venous pressure in the veins of the leg as a result of incompetent valves in the deep, perforating and superficial veins of the legs. If the valves are damaged through ageing or trauma from a deep vein thrombosis, backflow can occur on relaxation of the calf muscle. This results in high pressure in the superficial veins, leading to venous hypertension. This high pressure causes leakage of proteins, haemosiderin (from red blood cells), fibrin and water into the tissues, causing oedema, itching, eczema, staining, induration and loss of nutrients to the tissue. Any trauma to these affected tissues can result in a venous ulcer, infection, or cellulitis.

Arterial ulcers

Arterial ulcers are caused by insufficient arterial blood supply to the lower limb, either in the major arteries or in small distal capillaries, leading to tissue ischaemia and necrosis. Reduced arterial flow starves the tissues of oxygen and nutrients, making them vulnerable to trauma and breakdown. Diseases such as diabetes, rheumatoid arthritis and vasculitis can lead to arterial insufficiency in the major arteries and in distal capillaries, leading to tissue ischaemia.

Mixed venous/arterial

In 15–20% of cases the patient will present with a mixed venous/arterial ulcer; this percentage is likely to increase as the population ages. Mixed aetiology ulceration can present management problems. The aim is to achieve sufficient compression pressure from the bandages to control the venous hypertension, without compromising arterial blood flow to the leg. Severe damage can be caused by the inappropriate use of high compression in patients with arterial and small vessel disease, common in patients who have diabetes or rheumatoid arthritis. The patient may have a normal ankle/brachial pressure index (ABPI >0.8) indicating an adequate arterial supply for compression. However, application of high levels of compression (40 mmHg) may lead to micro-circulatory tissue damage if any dysfunction of the microcirculation exists.

Primary care practitioners can suspect microcirculatory dysfunction by taking a comprehensive history. Patients with rheumatoid arthritis, diabetes and other autoimmune diseases suffer from vasculitis of the microcirculation. The best method of treatment in patients with an ABPI >0.8, but coexisting disease, is to start with low reduced compression <25 mmHg and monitor closely for signs of ulcer deterioration and rapid tissue necrosis, due to microcirculatory occlusion. If the ABPI is <0.8, refer for duplex scan especially if the patient has diabetes, before applying any compression (see Boxes 18.9 and 18.11).

1) If possible the procedure should be performed in a quiet, warm room.
2) Reassure the patient and explain the procedure. Ensure that the patient is comfortably rested for 20 min, and is lying flat so that there is no pressure on the proximal vessels.

The sphygmomanometer should be at the same level as the heart. Check that the correct cuff size is being used, normally an adult alternative cuff.

3) Locate the brachial pulse and apply ultrasound contact gel. Angle the Doppler probe at 45 degrees and move it to obtain the best signal.

4) Inflate the cuff until the signal has disappeared. Then deflate the cuff slowly and record the pressure at which the signal returns, being careful not to move the probe from the line of the artery. Record the brachial systolic pressure in both arms. Check twice and record the higher reading. Use the higher of the two recordings to calculate the ABPI. A difference of ≥15 mmHg between brachial pressures may suggest the presence of arch vessel or upper limb arterial disease.

5) Cover the ulcerated area with a sterile towel or cling film and place the sphygmomanometer cuff around the leg just above the malleoli.

6) Examine the foot, locating the dorsalis pedis pulse and apply contact gel. Record the pressure.

7) Repeat on the posterior tibial, peroneal and anterior tibial arteries.

8) Use the highest reading obtained to calculate the ABPI for that leg.

9) Repeat for the other leg.

10) Use a calculator to calculate the ABPI for each leg using the formula below or look up the ABPI using a pressure index grid.

Box 18.9 Procedure for recording ankle/brachial pressure index (ABPI)[a]

In order to effectively treat patients suffering with leg ulcers, a differential diagnosis using objective methods must be carried out. Up to 50% of ulcer patients aged >70 years suffer with a degree of arterial disease, and it is important to assess this in order to exclude those for whom the use of high compression would be dangerous.

For this purpose a resting pressure index is recorded using Doppler ultrasound. This compares the brachial systolic to the ankle systolic and determines the percentage of blood flow to the feet. Before commencing a regime of high compression it is essential that an ABPI is recorded. Failure to do this could lead to tissue necrosis and possible amputation.

A differential diagnosis should never be made on Doppler readings alone. A thorough holistic assessment should be conducted first.

The nurse performing the Doppler assessment should be competent in the measurement of an ABPI and should understand the principles behind Doppler readings.

Procedure

Pedal pulses should be checked by palpation. Oedema may make this difficult.

Patients with normal arterial circulation will have an ankle systolic pressure equal to or higher than the brachial systolic pressure. Any deficit in the ankle pressure indicates a degree of arterial disease.

The results of the systolic recordings are expressed as a ratio (Table 18.2):

$$\text{ABPI} = \frac{\text{Highest pressure recorded at the ankle for that leg}}{\text{Highest brachial pressure obtained from both arms}}$$

[a] Adapted from Vowden.[28]

Uncommon causes

Approximately 5% of ulcers arise as a result of other causes and therefore require more specialist management (Box 18.10).[29] Any unusual or abnormal-looking leg ulcer that fails to progress or heal within 3 months should be referred for a specialist opinion to exclude malignancy.

Box 18.10 Unusual causes of leg ulceration[a]

+ Neuropathy, e.g. diabetes, paralysis, spina bifida, leprosy.
+ Vasculitis, e.g. rheumatoid arthritis, polyarteritis nodosa.
+ Blood disorders, e.g. anaemia, sickle cell, thalassemia.
+ Malignancy, e.g. squamous cell carcinoma, melanoma, basal cell carcinoma, Kaposi's sarcoma.
+ Lymphoedema, e.g. may be associated with infection.
+ Infection, e.g. cellulitis, fungal, tuberculosis, syphilis, leprosy.
+ Iatrogenic, e.g. bandage damage, plaster cast damage, self-inflicted.

[a] Adapted from King.[29]

Assessment and differential diagnosis

A new assessment may take an hour or more and this poses difficulties if timed appointments are too short to complete them adequately.[30]

Table 18.2 Pressure index ratio guidelines

ABPI	Pressure index ratio bandaging guidelines	Actions
1.0–1.3	Indicates normal arterial blood flow. 100% arterial blood flow to the foot. High compression bandaging is the first line of treatment.	Ensure readings are accurate. Document if the pulse sounds are monophasic, biphasic, or triphasic.
0.8–1.0	Indicates that the patient is receiving between 80% and 100% arterial blood flow to the foot, which although indicates mild arterial disease is still adequate for high compression bandaging.	Ensure readings are accurate. Document if the pulse sounds are monophasic, biphasic, or triphasic.
0.5–0.8	Indicates moderate arterial impairment. Intermittent claudication may be present on walking. **HIGH COMPRESSION MUST NOT BE USED**.	Following appropriate investigations a trial of **reduced compression therapy giving 15–23 mmHg** may be used on the advice of specialist leg ulcer/vascular services. Referral for vascular opinion required. Possible arterial imaging/Duplex scan or angiogram.
0.3–0.5	May have rest pain, necrotic or gangrenous tissue/ulcer. Indicates critical ischaemia. Risk of losing the limb. **NO COMPRESSION SHOULD BE USED**.	**Critical ischaemia: urgent referral to vascular emergency on-call team**. Surgical intervention, possible amputation.

ABPI, ankle/brachial pressure index.

Table 18.3 Differential diagnosis

	Venous ulcer	Arterial/ischaemic ulcer
Cause/medical history	Chronic venous hypertension. History of varicose ulcers, deep vein thrombosis, thrombophlebitis, poor calf pump muscle function.	Arterial disease. Ischemic heart disease. Cerebrovascular accident (stroke and transient ischaemic attack). Peripheral vascular disease, Rheumatoid arthritis. Diabetes. Autoimmune diseses.
Site	Gaiter area between malleolus and beginning of the calf. Lateral or medial malleolus.	Usually toes, foot ankle and back of the calf.
Size/duration	Varies. Slow, steady development, may be discrete or circumferential.	Small to variable. Rapid progression especially when infection present.
Oedema	Increasing oedema as day progresses, legs heavy and swollen.	Minimal oedema—may be pitting.
Foot pulses	Present, may be triphasic, biphasic or monophasic.	May be diminished or absent Doppler ultrasound or duplex scan necessary. Pulse sounds usually monophasic if present.
Skin changes	Leg warm to the touch, staining of skin brown from breakdown of red blood cells. Eczema from proteins and enzyme leakage resulting in itching, weeping, and erythema. Atrophie blanche, white fibrotic areas with poor blood flow. Ankle flare in the inner malleolus area. Lipodermatosclerosis.	Shiny, pallid, cold to the touch. Foot may be dusky pink when hung down and blanch white on elevation. Nails rough and thickened, hair loss due to lack of oxygenation to hair follicles.
Exudate levels	Generally high	Generally low except when infected.
Pain	Can be severe particularly when associated with gross oedema or infection.	Pain level dependant on amount of peripheral vascular disease present. May be severe requiring opiates.
Appearance	Shallow, flat and some evidence of granulation tissue and some sloughy areas.	Deep punched out ulcer. Presence of sloughy, necrotic tissue. Underlying bone, tendon or muscle may be seen.
Contributory factors	Family history of venous ulceration. Patient is tall. Stands for long periods for job.	Smoker. Hyperlipidaemia.

Examination includes excluding arterial disease by palpating the peripheral pulses and using the Doppler ultrasound (Figure 18.4) to determine the ankle/brachial pressure index.

The importance of holistic assessment, which includes physical, medical, emotional, cognitive, and environmental factors to determine the aetiology of the ulcer, is crucial in establishing a diagnosis (Table 18.3). Any underlying pathology and potential barriers to wound healing should be identified, including the patient's values, beliefs and their understanding of their condition.[18] Concordance with treatment may be affected by many factors such as pain and lack of carer support.

Aims of management

+ Determine aetiology of the ulceration.
+ Where possible treat the underlying cause, e.g. surgery for superficial varicose veins or arterial reconstruction to improve arterial blood supply.
+ Control oedema and reverse venous hypertension if present, using graduated high compression therapy/intermittent pneumatic therapy.
+ Control excessive exudates.
+ Control odour from the wound.
+ Control pain.
+ Treat any infection and prevent secondary infection.
+ Provide a wound environment that promotes healing.
+ Treat surrounding skin condition, e.g. eczema, dermatitis.
+ Provide social and psychological support to the patient and carers.

Compression therapy

Graduated high compression therapy providing 40 mmHg pressure is the treatment of choice for venous ulceration.[31] If appropriate, optimal compression uses a four-layer elastic bandage system (e.g. Profore®, K-Four®), which can remain in place for up to a week. This regime significantly reverses venous hypertension and has been found to be associated with greater health benefits and lower long-term costs than its alternatives.[32]

The patient's ankle circumference needs to be measured before initial application and a week later when oedema may have reduced. This gives an indication of the combination of bandages to be used to effect a 40 mmHg pressure, according to the law of La Place (Box 18.11 and Table 18.4).[33]

Research has demonstrated that if the 10 cm width multilayer bandages are applied according to the guidelines following training, at 50% stretch and 50% overlap in a spiral or figure-of-8 as recommended, you will achieve ~40 mmHg tension to the leg.[34] Pressure monitors have proven unreliable. The key is training!

Short-stretch bandages, particularly those with cohesive properties (e.g. Actico™ (Activa Healthcare)) or inelastic non-cohesive (e.g. Comprilan™ (Beiersdorf)) are useful when there are

Box 18.11 Sub-bandage pressure calculation

$$P = \frac{T \times N \times 4630}{C \times W}$$

P = sub-bandage pressure
T = bandage tension
N = number of layers
C = limb circumference
W = bandage width
The bandage is applied in the same technique, at 50% stretch tension, with 50% overlap using a 10 cm width bandage. The only thing in the equation that differs is the ankle circumference.

Table 18.4 Bandage combinations

Ankle circumference	Bandages	Pressure
>18 cm	≥2 orthopaedic wool layers to protect the shin and bulk out the ankle circumference, e.g. Softban™ (BSN). 1 cotton crepe. 1 elastic conformable bandage, e.g. Litepress™ (Smith & Nephew). 1 cohesive elastic bandage, e.g. Coban™ (3M) or Co-Plus™ (Smith & Nephew).	Provides 17 mmHg Provides 23 mmHg = 40 mmHg
18–25 cm	1 or more orthopaedic wool layer. 1 crepe. 1 elastic conformable bandage. 1 cohesive elastic bandage.	= 40 mmHg
>25 cm	1 or more orthopaedic wool layer. 1 elastic single-layer high compression bandage, e.g. Surepress™ (Convatec), Tensopress™ (Smith & Nephew). 1 cohesive elastic bandage.	35–40 mmHg 23 mmHg =40 mmHg

Adapted from Moffatt.[33]
The bandage combination is determined by the ankle circumference. This should be measured on the first assessment and repeated 1 week later when the oedema has reduced.

high levels of oedema, or patients or carers need to re-apply the bandage themselves. It is applied in a simple spiral at full stretch generally but other techniques may be applied. Short-stretch inelastic bandages are also an alternative, if four-layer elastic bandaging is not well tolerated by the patient, as it tends to give a lower resting pressure at night and cause less pain.[35]

Other long-stretch bandages, tubular bandages, are sometimes used but research has shown them to be less effective in respect of healing rate.

Information regarding removal of the bandages needs to be given in case the patient develops numbness, tingling in the toes or discoloration of the foot during treatment. Pneumatic compression (e.g. Flowtron™) may be useful in reducing oedema in patients who are unable to tolerate compression.

Dressings

At any one time in the UK, it is estimated that 200 000 people will be suffering from chronic wounds.[36] Open leg ulcers affect up to 190 000 people at a cost of £198 million per year. These costs include the number of nurses, doctors and hospital visits, dressings and bandages.

Most venous ulcers will heal with compression therapy regardless of primary dressing, but more complex interactive dressings (Box 18.12) may be required to address the problems associated with wound bed preparation and are considered to be cost-effective, e.g. infection, exudate management, non-viable tissue, non-healing ulcers.[37]

Dressings are estimated to cost £373 million per year and this burden is mainly met by community practices and Primary Health Care Trusts as more people are nursed at home. Despite this huge economic burden there are significant gaps in clinical evidence recommending one dressing over another. It is important for the practitioner to have in-depth knowledge of the properties and interactions of individual dressings.

A recent wound care audit was conducted in a London Primary Care Trust with a population of 250 000. For a period of a week district nurses undertook 496 dressings on 489 patients.

Box 18.12 Interactive wound dressings for leg ulcers

Necrotic (black)

Action: debride.

Hydrogel, e.g. Intrasite® gel, Purilon® gel.

Hydrocolloid, e.g. Comfeel®, Granuflex®.

Surgical/sharp debridement (conducted by trained clinician).

Infected (green, grey/black or dull red)

Action: antibacterial treatment and absorption.

Pseudomonas (green): silver sulphadine cream. Silver dressings.

Anaerobes (grey/black): metronidazole gel MRSA—sustained release iodine/silver.[b]

Cadexomer SR iodine:[b] e.g. Iodosorb, Iodoflex.

Sustained release iodine-impregnated dressing:[b] e.g. Inadine® (contraindications: thyroid disorders, pregnancy).

Silver dressing: Acticoat®, Acticoat Absorbant®, Aquacell AG®.

Honey: e.g. Activon Tulle.

Sloughy (yellow/grey)

Action: debride and absorb.

Hydrogel, e.g. Intrasite gel, Purilon gel, Granugel®.

Hydrocolloid, e.g. Comfeel Plus®.

Biosurgery, e.g. larvae.[a]

Hydrofibre, e.g. Aquacell®.

Polyurethane foam, e.g. Allevyn®, Mepilex®.

Alginate, e.g. Sorbsan®, Kaltostat®.

Malodorous/high exudate

Action: protection, absorption, treatment.

Charcoal dressing, e.g. Clinisorb®—odour; Carboflex®—absorption.

Silicone low adherent dressing, e.g. Mepitel®, Mepilex Transfer®.

Polyurethane foam, e.g. Allevyn Plus®, Mepilex.

Alginate, e.g. Kaltostat (Haemostat), Aquacell.

Charcoal dressing, e.g. Clinisorb, Carboflex.

Antibacterial, e.g. metronidazole gel[a] (may be useful to control odour by topically treating the underlying infection).

Granulating (red)

Action: protection, non-adherence.

Low adherent dressing, e.g. NA®, NA Ultra®.

Hydrocolloid, e.g. Comfeel.

Polyurethane foam, e.g. Allevyn Lite®, Mepilex Lite®.

Box 18.12 Interactive wound dressings for leg ulcers (*continued*)

Non-healing

Action: stimulate healing using protease inhibitors, e.g. Aquacell, Flaminal®, Oxyzme®, Promogram®, hyaluronic acid (Hyaff®).

Epithelializing (pink)

Action: protection.
Low adherent dressing, e.g. NA.
Film, e.g. Tegaderm®.
Surrounding skin, e.g. no-sting barrier film, zinc paste strips, or silicone strip.

[a] General practitioner to prescribe only.
[b] Always read product data sheet prior to use.
SR, slow release.

They used 1935 pieces of dressing and took 264 h to do them; 152 of these patients had open leg ulcers.[38]

Infection

Venous ulcers often become infected, although the presence of colonized bacterial contamination is not an indication of infection. Routine swabs should not be taken unless infection is suspected and the ulcer or leg shows signs of clinical infection, i.e. odour, pain, heat, erythema or cellulitis; a swab should then be sent for culture and microscopy.

The most common infections are caused by *Pseudomonas aeruginosa*, beta-haemolytic streptococci and anaerobes, although MRSA and fungi may also be present. A 2 week course of a broadspectrum antibiotic should be started and adjusted according to definitive microbiological results. Always treat if beta-haemolytic streptococcus A is found, as this can rapidly cause devastation to tissue.

Topical antibiotic creams should not be used, but topical antibacterial dressings and gels are very useful in treating infection or heavy colonization that is impairing healing.[39]

Exudate control

Wound exudate plays a major role in normal healing, providing essential nutrients for cell metabolism, assisting autolysis and migration of tissue-repairing cells. However, excess fluid/exudate can cause problems particularly in chronic leg ulcers, leading to maceration of the surrounding skin and leakage through the dressing ('strikethrough'). Changes in the volume, odour, and consistency of the exudate may indicate underlying problems such as infection or low protein levels.[40]

Protection of surrounding skin can be enhanced by using non-sting barrier films or creams (e.g. Cavilon™). The wound bed exudate can be controlled by use of absorbent alginate dressings and foams. In some cases topical negative-pressure therapy (e.g. VAC™) or fluid collection devices may be deployed to collect the exudate.

It may be necessary to remove devitalized tissue to encourage granulation using sharp debridement. This can be conducted in the community by an appropriately trained practitioner.

Skin care is very important and a simple emollient should be used at every dressing change and applied in a downward motion to avoid disturbing the hair follicles, reducing the likelihood of folliculitis. Venous eczema should be treated with topical steroids and emollients for 2 weeks, then gradually reduced to avoid rebound eczema.

Emollients for washing legs

A mild emollient should be used to wash legs (Table 18.5). Paraffin based emollients are commonly used and are safe and effective, although theoretically flammable.

Steroidal creams

Steroidal creams are useful for varicose eczema. Commence treatment with a 2 week application of moderate potency, e.g. Betnovate® (betamethasone 0.1%). Once under control reduce potency to maintenance cream, e.g. Eumovate® (clobetasone butyrate 0.05%, before diluting it with an emollient to wean the patient off the steroid and prevent a rebound effect.

Pain

Significant numbers of leg ulcer patients experience severe pain that affects their quality of life.[41,42] It is one of the main issues raised by leg ulcer sufferers and is often poorly managed in the community.[16]

Table 18.5 Emollients, creams, and ointments

Emollients		
First line	Aqueous cream	Emulsifying ointment 30%, phenoxyethanol 1%, in freshly boiled and cooled purified water.
	Liquid and white soft paraffin	Liquid paraffin 50%, white soft paraffin 50%.
Second line	Hydromol emollient	Isopropyl myristate 13%, light liquid paraffin 37.8%.
Third line	Dermol 500	Liquid paraffin 25%, isopropyl myristate 25%, benzalkonium chloride 0.5%: 600 ml. For washing infected skin to reduce colonisation of bacteria.
Creams		
First line	Cetraben emollient cream	White soft paraffin 13.2%, light liquid paraffin 10.5%, 500 g pump pack.
Second line	Diprobase cream	7.2% liquid paraffin, 6% white soft paraffin, 15% water-miscible basis, 500 g pump pack.
Third line	Dermol 500	Benzalkonium chloride 0.1%, chlorhexidine hydrochloride 0.1%, liquid paraffin 2.5%, isopropyl myristate 2.5%. Has antiseptic properties and can be used as a moisturiser for infected skin.
Ointments		
First line	Hydromol ointment	Isopropyl myristrate 39%, light liquid paraffin 37.8%. Price yellow soft paraffin 30%, emulsifying wax 30%. No allergens. If warmed in the hands, this ointment softens and spreads more easily.

Box 18.13 Pain stages

Stage 1: asymptomatic

Doppler recordings may reveal a low ankle/brachial pressure index with significant impairment of blood flow but no pain.

Stage 2: intermittent claudication

Cramp-like pain in the calf, thigh or buttocks, exacerbated by exercise and relieved by standing still to rest. Good predictor of arterial disease. (In immobile patients, nocturnal or rest pain may be the first indication of arterial disease.)

Stage 3: nocturnal/rest pain

May occur simultaneously with rest pain. Changes in blood pressure at night result in reduced peripheral perfusion leading to ischaemic neuritis—a constant intractable ache. This is relieved by hanging the affected leg out of the bed. The pain is often felt in the foot, particularly the toes and heel.

Stage 4: critical limb ischaemia

Severe persistent rest pain, often associated with ulceration, indicates extensive arterial disease. Clinically at risk of gangrene. Patient sits with affected limb dependent to facilitate perfusion in an attempt to relieve continuous pain. May need opiates. The incidence of amputation is higher in smokers and diabetics.

Compression therapy has been found to reduce pain in venous ulcers over time by rapidly reducing the oedema.[35] Night pain in venous disease caused by venous stasis in the calf may present as an aching leg. Rising from bed, analgesia, and walking around often settles the pain.

Arterial pain is often felt in the foot or toes regardless of where the ulcers are located and is often described as 'shooting'. Severe arterial pain is caused by tissue ischaemia. Patients often hang their leg out of bed at night: opiate analgesia is often required. Such patients require fast-track referral to a vascular surgeon (Box 18.13).

Pain is often caused by dressing procedures (e.g. changing dressings which have become adherent to the wound) and is generally poorly recognized and managed.[45–46] Pain relief may need to be taken before dressing procedures are conducted. Opiates, and sometimes Entonox in clinics, administered prior to dressing changes are sometimes required. A dressing with a silicone-based contact layer that is easy to remove without sticking may help to reduce pain and trauma (e.g. Mepilex Foam, Allevyn Gentle).

Prevention of recurrence

Once a venous ulcer has healed, the patient should be measured for compression hosiery (class 2) or socks to prevent recurrence. Many European grade levels of hosiery are now available on prescription (e.g. Medi, Actico).

For those unable to remove and replace their own stockings, some clinics offer a social 'healed leg ulcer clinic' where, weekly, the stockings are removed, legs checked, creamed and the stockings replaced. Recurrence rates are generally reported to be as high 20%[45] but in 'healed leg clinics', where patient adherence and health promotion is supported by health care assistants, it can be as low as 4%.[46]

References

1. European Pressure Ulcer Advisory Panel. *Pressure Ulcer Prevention Guidelines.* Available at: http://www.epuap.org.uk

2. National Institute for Health and Clinical Excellence. *Guideline on pressure ulcer management. Pressure Ulcers: the Management of Pressure Ulcers in Primary and Secondary Care.* 2005. Available at: http://www.nice.org.uk

3. Thomas DR, Goode PS, Tarquine PH, Allman RM. Hospital-acquired pressure ulcers and risk of death.
   J Am Geriatr Soc 1996;44:1435–40.

4. Allman RM, Laprade CA, Noel LB, *et al.* Pressure sores among hospitalized patients. *Ann Intern Med* 1986;105:337–42.

5. National Institute for Health and Clinical Excellence. Guideline on Pressure Relieving Devices. The Use of Pressure relieving Devices for the Prevention of pressure Ulcers in Primary and Secondary Care. London: NICE; 2003. Available at: http://www.nice.org.uk

6. Gardner SE, Frantz RA. Wound bioburden. In: Baranoski S, Ayello EA (eds), *Wound Care Essentials: Practice Principles.* Springhouse: Lippincott Williams & Wilkins, 2004, p. 91–116.

7. Bauer C, Geriach MA, Doughty D. Care of metastatic skin lesions. *J Wound Ostomy Continence Nurs* 2000;27:247–51.

8. Ayello EA. Cleansing and cleaners. In: Teot L, Banwell PE, Ziegler UE (eds), *Surgery in Wounds.* Springer: Berlin; 2004.

9. Harris IR, Yee KC, Walters CE, *et al.* Cytokine and protease levels in healing and non-healing chronic venous leg ulcers. *Exp Dermatol* 1995;4:342–9.

10. Schultz GS, Mast BA. Molecular analysis of the environment of healing and chronic wounds: cytokines, proteases and growth factors. *Wounds* 1998;10(Suppl F):1F–11F.

11. Grinnell F, Zhu M. Fibronectin degradation in chronic wounds depends on the relative levels of elastase, alpha1-proteinase inhibitor, and alpha2-macroglobulin. *J Invest Dermatol* 1996;106:335–41.

12. Grey JE, Harding KG. Pressure Ulceration. In: Pathy J et al. (eds), *Principles and Practice of Geriatric Medicine.* New York: Wiley; 2006. p. 1605–30.

13. Mulder GD, LaPan M. Decubitus ulcers: update on new approaches to treatment. *Geriatrics* 1988;43:37–9, 44–5, 49–50.

14. Eaglstein WH. Moist wound healing with occlusive dressings: a clinical focus. *Dermatol Surg* 2001;27:175–81.

15. Fleischmann W. Maggot debridement. In: Teot L, Banwell PE, Ziegler UE (eds), *Surgery in Wounds.* Berlin: Springer; 2004.

16. Franks P, Moffatt CJ, Connolly M, *et al.* Community leg ulcer clinics: effects on quality of life. *Phlebology* 1994;9:83–86.

17. Graham ID, Harrison MB, Nelson EA, Lorimer K, Fisher A. Prevalance of lower-limb ulceration: a systematic review of prevalence studies. *Adv Skin Wound Care* 2003;16:305–316.

18. Moffatt CJ. Factors that affect concordance with compression therapy. *J Wound Care* 2004;13:291–4.

19. Stewart S, MacIntyre K, Capewell S, McMurray JJV. Heart failure and the aging population: an increasing burden in the 21st century. *Heart* 2003;89:49–53.

20. Office of National Statistics. London; 2006. http://www.statistics.gov.uk

21. Moffatt CJ, Franks PJ, Oldroyd M, *et al.* Community clinics for leg ulcers and impact on healing. *Br Med J* 1992;305:1389–92.

22. Stevens JM, Franks P, Harrington M. A community/hospital leg ulcer service. *J Wound Care* 1997;6:61–8.

23. Morrell CJ, King B, Bereton LML. Cost effectiveness of community leg ulcer clinics: randomised control trial. *Br Med J* 1998;316:1487–91.

24. Lindsay E. Compliance with science: benefits of developing community leg clubs. *Br J Nurs* 2001;10:(Suppl):66–74.

25. Brown A. Does social support impact on venous ulcer healing or recurrence? *Br J Community Nurs* 2008;13:S6, S8, S10 *passim*.

26. Dodds R. Shared community-hospital care of leg ulcers using an electronic record and telemedicine. *Int J Lower Extremity Wounds* 2002;1:260–70.

27. Scottish Intercollegiate Guidelines Network. *The Care of Patients with Chronic Leg Ulcer: a National Clinical Guideline*. SIGN Publication, No. 26; 1998.

28. Vowden KR. Hand-held Doppler assessment for peripheral arterial disease *J Wound Care* 1996, No. 3.31.

29. King B. Is this leg ulcer venous? Unusual aetiologies of the lower leg ulcers. *J Wound Care* 2004;13:394–6.

30. Schofield J, Flanagan M, Fletcher J, Rotchell L, Thomson S. The provision of leg ulcer services by practice nurses. *Nurs Stand* 2000;14;54–6, 58, 60.

31. Stacey M, Falanga V, Marston W, *et al*. The use of compression therapy in the treatment of venous leg ulcers: a recommended pathway. *Eur Wound Mngmt Assoc J* 2000;2:3–7.

32. Iglesias CP, Nelson EA, Cullum N, Torgerson DJ. Economic analysis of VenUS1, a randomised trial of two bandages for treating leg ulcers. *Br J Surg* 2004;91:1300–6.

33. Moffatt CJ. *Compression Therapy in Practice*. Wiltshire: Wounds UK Publishing; 2007. p. 58.

34. Blair SD, Wright DD, Backhouse CM, Riddle E, McCollum CN. Sustained compression and healing of chronic venous ulcers. *Br Med J* 1988;297:1159–61.

35. European Wound Management Association (EWMA). *Position Document: Understanding Compression*. London: Medical Education Partnership; 2003.

36. Posnett J, Franks PJ. The costs of skin breakdown and ulceration in the UK. In: *Skin Breakdown, The Silent Epidemic*. Hull: Smith & Nephew Foundation; 2007. p. 6–12.

37. European Wound Management Association (EWMA). *Position Document: Wound Bed Preparation in Practice*. London: MEP; 2004.

38. Stevens JM, Murphy F. *Wound Audit Report*. Hounslow Primary Care Trust; 2007.

39. European Wound Management Association (EWMA). *Position Document: Management of Wound Infection*. London: MEP; 2006.

40. World Union of Wound Healing Societies (WUWHS). *Principles of Best Practice: Wound Exudate and the Role of Dressings. A Consensus Document*. London: MEP Ltd; 2007.

41. Cullum N, Roe B. *Leg Ulcers: Nursing Management. A Research-Based Guide*. Harrow: Scutari Press; 1995.

42. Lindholm C, Bjellerup M, Christiansen OB, Zederfeld B. Quality of life in chronic leg ulcers. *Acta Derm Venerol* 1993;73:440–443.

43. Briggs M, Torra I, Bou JE. *Pain at Wound Dressing Changes: a Guide to Management. EWMA Position Document*. London: MEP; 2002. p. 12–17.

44. Price P, Fagervik-Morton H, Mudge EJ, *et al*. Dressings-related pain in patients with chronic wounds: an international perspective. *Int Wound J* 2008;5:159–71.

45. Moffatt CJ, Dorman MC. Recurrence of leg ulcers within a community ulcer service. *J Wound Care* 1995;4:57–61.

46. Lewis C. Hounslow & Spelthorne community leg ulcer clinics: 1 year recurrence rate audit. *Leg Ulcer Forum J* 1999;Summer:11–12.

Chapter 19

Incontinence

Brenda Roe and Asangaedem Akpan

Introduction

Urinary and faecal incontinence have the highest prevalence in older people, apart from those with specific neurological disorders. As populations age, the number of older people globally who experience incontinence will increase.[1] With the focus of governments and health and social services on enabling older people to remain independent or supported in their own homes and communities, as opposed to institutional care, the prevention, management and treatment of urinary and faecal incontinence remains the responsibility of the primary health care team supported by clinical specialists. No matter how older or elderly populations are defined, their heterogeneity ranges from 'active, community-dwelling, working, healthy nona-generians to bed-bound, chronically ill, functionally and cognitively impaired people in their late 60s'.[2] Awareness that the former, healthier, group is closer in physiology and phenotype to middle-aged people than to frailer older people meant that the International Consultation on Continence has a separate panel for considering incontinence as it relates to frail older people aged ≥65 years.[2] As such, aetiologies and treatment specific to frail older populations should be considered along with quality of life, burden, disability, altered response to drug therapies, the role of caregivers, as well as the organization, delivery and goal of care. By contrast with healthier populations, urinary and faecal incontinence in frail older people tends to be multifactorial and includes factors beyond bladder and bowel physiology alone. This chapter comprises two sections—urinary and faecal incontinence—and includes information and evidence to guide and support assessment, diagnosis and management, along with aspects of prevention and lifestyle modification.

Urinary incontinence

Background

The International Continence Society (ICS) defined urinary incontinence as the complaint of any involuntary leakage of urine.[3] It has also been defined as 'the involuntary or inappropriate passing of urine (and/or faeces) that has an impact on social functioning or hygiene' and includes 'nocturnal enuresis or bed wetting'.[4] There is ample evidence that urinary incontinence is troublesome and has a major impact on quality of life,[5] although there is a paucity of research specific to frail older people on effectiveness and outcomes.[2,5] Frail older people usually have chronic co-morbidities, take multiple medications and need help to perform all or some of their activities of daily living (ADLs) which include bathing, dressing, toileting and ambulation. Care is usually provided by family, friends, neighbours, informal carers or professional staff, and often requires organized packages of care.

Epidemiology of urinary incontinence and impact on quality of life

Urinary incontinence (UI) affects 20% of older people living in the community and 30–71% in care home settings, with a higher prevalence in women than men.[6,7] Sufferers do not always present to medical services, cope in silence and do not receive effective care.[8–10] Caring for someone with UI can also have a detrimental impact on the quality of life of the carer.[11]

Incidence of UI in people aged ≥ 65 years has been associated with a two-fold increased risk of impairment in personal and instrumental ADLs and poor performance in physical tests, suggesting that UI is an early marker for frailty,[12,13] UI is a risk factor for care home admission, especially for older men and people in rural areas,[12,14] although there appears to be no association between UI and higher mortality.[12] The costs of UI to sufferers, carers and health and social care services are considerable.[15,16]

Government policy in the UK has recognized the need for proper assessment and management of UI, equitable access to services and the establishment of integrated continence services for older people underpinned by regular audit.[4,17]

Assessment and diagnosis of urinary incontinence

A basic and comprehensive assessment must first be undertaken to inform diagnosis and treatment (Figure 19.1). The first step is to treat potentially reversible conditions that can cause transient incontinence. Conditions include the following:

- Irritation or inflammation of the lower urinary tract, such as urinary tract infection (UTI), atrophic vaginitis, prolapse and faecal impaction.

- An increase in urine production due to excess fluid intake or caffeine consumption or medical conditions that cause osmotic diuresis or volume overload.

- Medication side-effects, i.e. sedative hypnotics, diuretics, anticholinergic agents, alpha-adrenergic antagonists, alpha-agonists, caffeine or alcohol—whereby medications can be discontinued or the dosage reduced.

- Impairment in the willingness or ability to toilet, such as functional impairments of cognition or mobility.

These conditions can be remembered by the use of the mnemonic DIAPPERS: delirium, infection (of the urinary tract), atrophic vaginitis, pharmaceuticals, psychological, excess fluid (in/out), restricted mobility, and stool impaction (including constipation).[18]

Causes of incontinence have been classified as being due to physiological bladder dysfunction presenting as urge, stress or mixed incontinence, factors influencing bladder function and factors affecting people's ability to cope with the bladder. Urge incontinence can present as urgency, frequency, nocturia, enuresis or nocturnal enuresis and is due to destrusor instability, overflow incontinence (due to obstruction such as an enlarged prostate) or an underactive bladder (due to peripheral nerve damage). Stress incontinence occurs as an involuntary loss of urine in the absence of a detrusor contraction due to coughing, exercise or exertion. It is common in women and related to injury at childbirth. Mixed incontinence refers to a combination of symptoms of stress and urge incontinence. Type and severity of incontinence (amount and frequency) are important to assess. Increased severity of incontinence and psychological distress are significantly associated with urge incontinence in women due to its unpredictable nature and social and hygienic consequences.[19] People with severe incontinence are significantly more likely to seek help from a health professional.[20] It is essential that a standardized single assessment form and frequency–volume bladder chart are completed, as this will help to determine the type and cause of incontinence and form the basis for subsequent treatment.[2] Typical questions about lower urinary

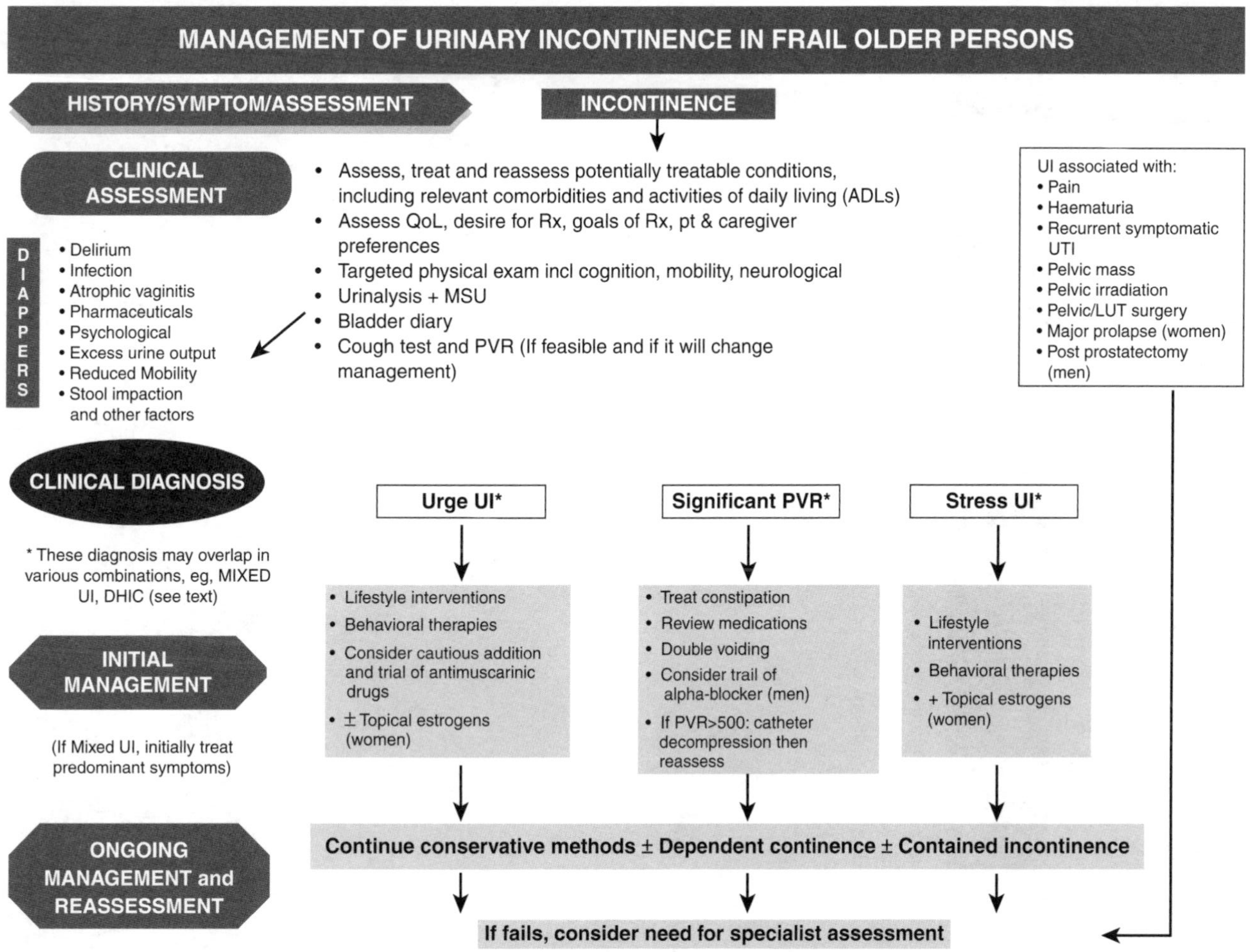

MANAGEMENT OF URINARY INCONTINENCE IN FRAIL OLDER PERSONS

HISTORY/SYMPTOM/ASSESSMENT

INCONTINENCE

UI associated with:
- Pain
- Haematuria
- Recurrent symptomatic UTI
- Pelvic mass
- Pelvic irradiation
- Pelvic/LUT surgery
- Major prolapse (women)
- Post prostatectomy (men)

CLINICAL ASSESSMENT

- Assess, treat and reassess potentially treatable conditions, including relevant comorbidities and activities of daily living (ADLs)
- Assess QoL, desire for Rx, goals of Rx, pt & caregiver preferences
- Targeted physical exam incl cognition, mobility, neurological
- Urinalysis + MSU
- Bladder diary
- Cough test and PVR (If feasible and if it will change management)

D • Delirium
I • Infection
A • Atrophic vaginitis
P • Pharmaceuticals
P • Psychological
E • Excess urine output
R • Reduced Mobility
S • Stool impaction and other factors

CLINICAL DIAGNOSIS

*These diagnosis may overlap in various combinations, eg. MIXED UI, DHIC (see text)

Urge UI*

- Lifestyle interventions
- Behavioral therapies
- Consider cautious addition and trial of antimuscarinic drugs
- ± Topical estrogens (women)

Significant PVR*

- Treat constipation
- Review medications
- Double voiding
- Consider trail of alpha-blocker (men)
- If PVR>500: catheter decompression then reassess

Stress UI*

- Lifestyle interventions
- Behavioral therapies
- + Topical estrogens (women)

INITIAL MANAGEMENT

(If Mixed UI, initially treat predominant symptoms)

Continue conservative methods ± Dependent continence ± Contained incontinence

ONGOING MANAGEMENT and REASSESSMENT

If fails, consider need for specialist assessment

Fig. 19.1 Algorithm for urinary incontinence (UI) in older people. Reproduced with permission of Health Publications Ltd, from Fonda et al.[2], p. 1229. UTI, urinary tract infection; LUT, lower urinary tract; PVR, post-void residual volume of urine; DHIC, detrusor hyperactivity with impaired contractility.

symptoms are included in the Leicester Urinary Symptom questionnaire (Box 19.1).[21] The assessment should also include history, physical examination, urinalysis and a post-void residual volume as well as assessment of cognitive function, mobility and environmental factors, which can cause or contribute to incontinence. Post-void residual volume of urine can be assessed by intermittent catheterization following voiding or use of a portable ultrasound. Referral to the local continence service may also be required. Where indicated, carefully selected patients should be referred for specialized urological or gynaecological examinations or urodynamics (Figure 19.1; Chapters 20 and 21).[2]

Box 19.1 Typical questions about common urinary symptoms from the Leicester Urinary Symptom Questionnaire[a]

These questions ask about some common urinary symptoms. Think about the symptoms you have experienced in the last six months.
Do you leak any urine/water when you don't mean to? That means anything from a few drops to a flood during the day or night.
  Yes
  No
Do you leak urine when you do any of the following? Please tick all that apply.
  Sneeze
  Exercise
  Cough
  Laugh
  Walk
  Bend
  Stand up
When you get the urge to pass urine, does any leak before you get to the toilet? Tick one only.
  Most of the time
  Sometimes
  Occasionally
  Or never
If you leak urine are you usually: (Tick one only.)
  Soaked
  Wet
  Damp
  Almost dry
  Do not leak urine
How often do you leak urine usually? (Tick one only.)
  Continuously
  Several times a day/night
  Several times a week
  Several times a month
  Less often
  Never

Box 19.1 Typical questions about common urinary symptoms from the Leicester Urinary Symptom Questionnaire[a] (continued)

When you first feel the need to pass urine how strong is the urge to go usually? Is it: (Tick one only.)

Overwhelming
Very strong
Strong
Normal
Weak
No sensation

Do you have difficulty holding your urine once you feel the urge to go? (For example what would happen if you needed the toilet and it was occupied, would you have difficulty in holding on?). Tick one only.

Yes, most of the time
Sometimes
Occasionally
No, never have difficulty holding urine

How often do you *usually* go to the toilet to pass urine during the daytime? Tick one only.

About every half an hour (or more often)
About every hour
About every hour and a half
About every two hours
Less often

How often do you *usually* get up at night to pass urine? Tick one only.

Not usually
Less often than once a night
Once a night
Twice a night
Three times a night
Four times or more a night

[a] Developed by the Leicestershire MRC Incontinence Study Team.[21]

Management of urinary incontinence

On deciding how to manage or treat urinary incontinence, it is important to involve the patient—and if appropriate the carer—to establish what they would like as the outcome. While for younger healthy people a minority will achieve dryness, frail older people may aim for a reduction in frequency of urination and incontinent episodes, and 'social continence' whereby they manage and avoid wet episodes detectable by other people. A paradigm for the management of incontinence in older people has four dimensions:

◆ Incontinent (wet).

◆ Independent continence (dry, not dependent on ongoing treatment).

◆ Dependent continence (dry with toileting assistance, behavioural treatment, and/or medications).

◆ Contained incontinence (urine contained in pads or appliances).[22]

The treatment goals and outcomes should be regularly reviewed, taking into account patient preference and quality of life. A range of techniques are available that can assist with promoting continence or managing incontinence. Conservative approaches are recommended before pursuing more interventionist treatments such as drug therapy or surgery.

Lifestyle

There has been no research on modifying lifestyle behaviours and continence outcomes for older people, and caution should be adopted before advocating major changes.

Significant associations between urinary incontinence and lifestyle behaviours in general populations have been found, and in women these include parity, increased baby birth weight, obesity and increased body mass index;[23,24] in both men and women, impaired mobility, disturbed sleep,[24] caffeine consumption,[25] alcohol consumption,[26] and smoking.[23] are also related to urinary incontinence. Other studies found that fluid intake, caffeine consumption, and diet were not associated with urinary incontinence when age and gender were controlled for.[24] There is general concern that older people, particularly those in care homes, do not get sufficient oral hydration[2] and so the effects of increasing oral fluids and reducing caffeine should be assessed on their voided volumes and frequency of incontinence. Smoking cessation or weight loss should be reviewed and may be indicated in conjunction with other health concerns or co-morbidities.

Behavioural interventions

A range of behavioural techniques are available to manage incontinence with some evidence of effectiveness. They include pelvic floor muscle exercise (PFME), traditionally for stress incontinence,[27] bladder training (BT),[28] prompted voiding (PV),[29] habit retraining (HT)[30] and timed voiding (TV).[31] PV, HT, and TV are categorized as toileting programmes and are aimed at older people with cognitive and physical impairments reliant on carers. There is some evidence of effectiveness for PV in the short term for managing urinary incontinence in both care home and community populations,[2,29] but insufficient evidence is available for HT and TV. PFME and BT are beneficial in the short term with some evidence for a longer-term benefit if sustained, but long-term follow-up studies are still required, particularly for older people. A recent meta-study synopsis of the four Cochrane systematic reviews on BT, PV, HT and TV found overlap in some of the operational definitions used and that BT was combined with PFME as well as lifestyle modification in some complex combined trials.[32,33] Research on combining PFME and BT or toileting programmes for older populations with or without specific co-morbidities, such as post stroke, is warranted. A trial that investigated the clinical and cost-effectiveness of a nurse-led continence service in primary care for people aged ≥40 years (with 45% aged ≥60 years) delivered an 8 week combined intervention of dietary and fluid advice, BT, PFME awareness and lifestyle advice with outcome measures collected at 3 and 6 months post randomization. An 11% improvement rate (95% CI: 7, 16; $P < 0.001$) and 10% cure rate (95% CI: 6, 13; $P = 0.001$) compared to standard care was found with the difference maintained at 6 months.[34] Long-term follow-up of the cohort between 3 and 7 years found a reduced cure rate of 5%,[34] which indicates the need for reinforcement of the intervention package over time. Behavioural interventions are useful conservative approaches to be adopted for the promotion and management of urinary incontinence in older, more frail, adults. Written information for health professionals and patients on behavioural interventions is available from national organizations Appendix 1, local continence services and community nursing services.

Drug treatments

A detailed review of trials and assessment of the levels and grades of evidence for the use of medications in frail older people was undertaken as part of the 3rd International Consultation on Incontinence,[2] and practical management recommendations are summarized here (Figure 19.1 and Chapter 20). Drug therapy has a role in the treatment of UI in older people and should be combined with behavioural therapy and treatment of other precipitating and confounding factors. Advanced age or frailty is not a contraindication for drug therapy, although co-morbidity, side-effects and polypharmacy need to be taken into account when prescribing (Chapter 4).

Antimuscarinic agents such as oxybutynin, tolterodine and solifenacin, which block the action of acetylcholine on detrusor muscarinic receptors, are available for urgency or mixed incontinence. These should be considered for people who have had other co-morbid factors addressed, who are able to toilet independently or with assistance, who do not become agitated when toileting, who have had a trial of behavioural intervention but have not achieved their goal and who have no contraindications. However, as no data are available for their long-term efficacy or tolerability (beyond 2–6 months) and as there is high morbidity and mortality within this particular population, regular monitoring and re-evaluation of efficacy and tolerability with continued drug therapy is necessary.

Immediate release oxybutinin can be considered for additional benefit where behavioural therapy has been found feasible. Extended-release antimuscarinic agents should only be prescribed with regular monitoring of their efficacy and tolerability. Regular monitoring for side-effects and adverse events are recommended for people taking antimuscarinic agents, in particular those causing increased confusion and tachycardia. Muscarinic receptors are present throughout the body. Choosing a drug with specificity for the bladder and using an extended-release formulation tends to reduce the impact of side-effects such as dry mouth, blurred vision, constipation and reflux. Using a non-oral route such as transdermal also reduces side-effects.[35] This group of drugs comprises the most commonly used but for older adults using either the extended-release formulations or the transdermal patch is recommended. Combinations of antimuscarinic agents are not recommended.

Tricylic antidepressants such as imipramine, calcium channel blockers, flavoxate, antidiuretics, and desmopressin are of limited benefit in older adults and should be reserved for use in specialist clinics.

Oral osterogen is not recommended, although topical oestrogen in the form of cream, tablet or ring may be used as an adjunctive treatment for women with atrophic vaginitis. Drug therapy is not recommended for the treatment of stress UI or isolated impaired detrusor contractility (underactive detrusor). Bladder relaxants should be used in frail older men only where there is experienced supervision and follow-up to monitor efficacy, tolerability and post-void residual volume of urine. The drug treatment of voiding disorders, which is more of an issue in males, is discussed in Chapter 20.

Surgical interventions

There is little evidence available on the outcomes of surgery for UI in frail older people and this reflects the focus on conservative management. There is some evidence for gynaecological surgery in women, and evaluation of surgical outcomes for post prostatectomy in frail older men barely exists.[2] Surgery for healthier older people for UI and other related conditions is included in Chapters 20 and 21. Figure 19.1 provides a guide for surgical referral based on assessment and diagnosis. Age is not a contraindication for referral for surgical treatment of UI, and morbidity and mortality rates are similar to those of other non-cardiac surgical procedures. Operative mortality is not consistently associated with age and many studies do not uniformly control for co-morbid conditions. Functional and quality-of-life outcomes remain to be investigated. For patients where surgery is being considered, preoperative risk should be assessed and urodynamic evaluation should be undertaken before surgical treatment of UI is undertaken.

Aids and appliances

Based on the management paradigm, people with 'dependence continence' and 'contained incontinence',[22] some older people will require the use of aids and appliances to contain their incontinence and provide 'social continence'. Generally these fall into two categories; containment products (disposable or reusable body worn pads/pants or pads for bedding and furniture) or conduction products (penile sheaths, indwelling urethral or suprapubic catheters and intermittent catheters).

A range of disposable and reusable pad and pant products is available and their selection depends upon frequency and quantity of urine loss, patients' mobility, dexterity and preference. These products can be bought over the counter or provided by community nursing services. Referral to the local continence service or community nurses for a thorough assessment of which products to use and for support on self-care is recommended.[36]

Penile sheaths and drainage bags can be used to manage intractable UI in physically dependent male patients who do not have urinary retention. For people with chronic urinary retention, intermittent catheterization may be useful and they can be taught to self-catheterize or their caregiver taught the technique. Intermittent catheterization may also be useful for people undergoing bladder training following acute urinary retention. Long-term indwelling urethral catheters and drainage bags or valves are indicated where urinary retention cannot be corrected or intermittent catheterization proves impossible, or where skin wounds or pressure sores may be contaminated with urine. They are also useful to care for people who are terminally ill or severely impaired for whom bedding or clothing changes are disruptive or cause discomfort to them or their caregiver.[2] Conduction equipment can be prescribed and selection will depend upon careful assessment and patient preference. Referral to the community nursing service or local continence service for advice on prescribing, fitting and management of equipment, teaching self-care and ongoing support is recommended. Suprapubic catheters are an alternative to indwelling urethral catheters, and referral to a urologist would be required (see Chapter 20).

PFME for stress incontinence may also be undertaken using vaginal cones and these have been used as alternatives to electrical stimulation or non-invasive PFME exercise (see Chapter 21). Outcome of PFME using vaginal cones in older women remains to be fully investigated but are a consideration in primary care.[37]

Faecal incontinence

Background

Faecal incontinence is the involuntary or inappropriate passing of faeces that has an impact on social functioning and hygiene.[38] There are several other definitions that have been used, and as a consequence the prevalence of faecal incontinence varies between most studies to date. From a patient's perspective, it is soiling of one's underwear, clothes or beddings that appears to be of most concern to the person or carer. Mere staining or infrequent episodes of faecal incontinence appear not to be of major concern.[39]

Epidemiology of faecal incontinence and impact on quality of life

The prevalence of faecal incontinence in the elderly in the UK ranges from 3 to 37% depending on the study population. Lower prevalence figures were obtained in a study of older adults aged ≥65 years living in their homes. The definition was very broad, allowing for all degrees of faecal incontinence to be included.[40] Higher prevalence rates were obtained in hospitalized patients and those in 24 h care.

Faecal incontinence is an embarrassing subject for discussion for both the health professional and the person with the condition. It is therefore not a surprise that studies have documented reluctance of those with the condition to discuss it, as well as health professionals being unaware that their patients have the condition.[41] This discomfort and reluctance stems from our attitude that faeces are dirty, unhygienic and disgusting and that voluntary defecation is expected to be done in private. Where this is not possible, for whatever reason, both the person carrying out the act of defecation and the observer are very likely to be at the very least uncomfortable, but more commonly will be embarrassed and ashamed. This is especially so where defecation occurs involuntarily or inappropriately.

This condition restricts the social activity of older people, with most too worried about the smell that would result following an episode of incontinence. There is a tendency even for those who go out to locate or be near the toilet just in case something happens. Some feel unhealthy, anxious and depressed about it all.

Where the condition has been identified, enough time should be given in a consultation and the issue discussed in a sensitive and empathic manner to encourage the person to open up.[42] Older dependent adults were less likely to have privacy during defecation, and certainly those who were both dependent and incontinent had to bear the embarrassment of being cleaned up.[43]

Assessment and diagnosis of faecal incontinence

Like any other condition that presents with signs and symptoms, faecal incontinence is not the end but the beginning of a process of finding out the underlying contributing factors and causes (Figure 19.2). Once these factors are elicited, a management plan including investigations and treatment can be implemented.[2,44] About 50% of patients with faecal incontinence also have urinary incontinence. Lax anal sphincters are found in adults of all ages with faecal incontinence. It is not associated with ageing and is usually more likely to be an issue in those with previous genitourinary surgical procedures and females who have had vaginal deliveries. In older people, the commonest contributory factors are frailty (co-morbidity), cognitive impairment (dementia and behavioural disturbances), impaired mobility, faecal loading and loose stools.[45]

Apart from faecal loading, loose stools and impaired mobility, the other factors are irreversible but being aware of them would enable one to implement measures to reduce their impact. Depending on where the person with faecal incontinence is, the distribution of these varies. Faecal loading, impaired mobility and cognitive impairment are commoner in hospital and nursing home settings whereas loose stools are commoner in patients in hospital and those living in their own homes.[46]

Assessment includes taking a comprehensive history to elicit possible contributing factors, rule out inflammatory bowel disease and symptoms suggestive of bowel cancer and then carrying out a general physical examination with particular emphasis on abdominal and rectal examinations. A cognitive and psychosocial assessment where indicated should be performed.

Management of faecal incontinence

The management outlined here should be applied to all in whom contributory factors are found following the above assessment (Figure 19.2).

Faecal loading, if present, is treated by prescribing enemas and thereafter regular laxatives until normal bowel movements are restored for that individual. Identify the cause of loose stools by reviewing medications, sending a stool sample for microscopy culture and sensitivity studies including *Clostridium difficile* testing if antibiotics have been prescribed recently. Once these

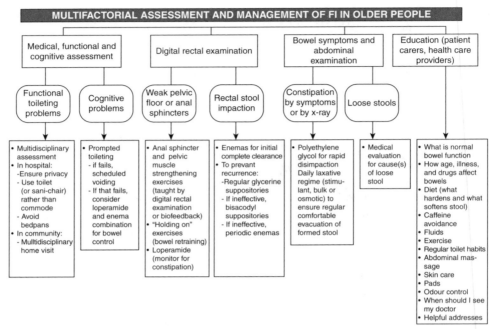

Figure 19.2 Algorithm for faecal incontinence in older people. Reproduced with permission of Health Publications Ltd, from Fonda et al.[2], p. 1222.

reversible causes have been excluded, if the incontinence persists the following issues should be addressed:

♦ Diet: recommend a combination of foods to achieve a stool consistency that is not too hard or too soft.

♦ Encourage bowel emptying after a meal and at regular intervals, especially for those with cognitive impairment.

♦ If toilet facilities are suboptimal, refer to an occupational therapist and social worker for adaptations to be made or a commode provided for ease of access. Encourage the use of a footstool when defecating to avoid straining. Where the person is dependent on assistance with toileting, the carer should be advised to aim for regular toileting, usually after each meal.

♦ If the above measures fail, antidiarrhoeal drugs can be prescribed (loperamide, codeine phosphate or co-phenetrope). Drugs should be avoided in those with hard or infrequent stools, acute diarrhoea and exacerbation of inflammatory bowel disease.

♦ Referral to the local continence service for advice and information on continence products and for support is essential.

♦ Arrange to review the person and, if the above measures have failed to resolve the condition, onward referral to a physician or surgeon with an interest in faecal incontinence is recommended.

Summary tips for managing faecal incontinence in older adults

♦ Obtain a history including all medications being taken.

♦ Physical examination including an abdominal and rectal examination.

- ◆ Resolve reversible factors.
- ◆ Put in measures to reduce the impact of irreversible factors.
- ◆ Contributory factors vary depending on setting.

Summary

There is an increased prevalence of both urinary and faecal incontinence in older people which impacts on individuals' and their carers' quality of life.[46] A range of treatments and interventions are available to promote continence and manage incontinence. Comprehensive assessment, diagnosis and conservative therapeutic approaches can be instigated within primary care and should involve patients and carers in decision-making and identifying achievable outcome goals and choices.

References

1. Baltes PB, Smith J. New frontiers in the future of aging: from successful aging of the young old to the dilemmas of the fourth age. *Gerontology* 2003;49:123–25.
2. Fonda D, DuBeau CE, Harari D, Ouslander JG, Palmer M, Roe B. Incontinence in the frail elderly. In: Abrams P, Cardozo L, Khoury, Wein A (eds), *Third International Consultation on Incontinence*, Monaco, 26–29 June 2004. Plymouth: Health Publications Ltd; 2005. Chap. 18. p. 1165–1239.
3. Abrams P, Cockburn L, Fall M, *et al*. The standardization of terminology of lower urinary tract function: Report from the Standardisation Sub-committee of the International Continence Society. *Neurourol Urodynam* 2002;21:167–78.
4. Department of Health. *Good Practice in Continence Service*. London: DoH; 2000. Available from: http://www.continence-foundation.org.uk/campaigns/goodpracticecontinence.pdf Accessed 28 March 2008.
5. Payne C, Blaivas J, Brown J, *et al*. (2005) Research methodology. In: Abrams P, Cardozo L, Khoury, Wein A (eds), *Third International Consultation on Incontinence*, Monaco, 26–29 June 2004. Plymouth: Health Publications Ltd; 2005. Chap. 3, p. 99.
6. Perry S, Shaw C, Assassa P, *et al*. An epidemiological study to establish the prevalence of urinary symptoms and felt need in the community: The Leicestershire MRC Incontinence Study. *Public Health Med* 2000;22:427–34.
7. Roe B, Doll H. Prevalence of urinary incontinence and its relationship with health status. *J Clin Nurs* 2000;9:178–87.
8. Button D, Roe B, Webb C, Frith T, Colin-Thome D, Gardner L. Consensus guidelines for the promotion and management of continence by primary health care teams: development, implementation and evaluation. *J Adv Nurs* 1998;27:91–9.
9. Roe B, Wilson K, Doll H. Public awareness and health education: findings from an evaluation of health services for incontinence in England. *Int Nurs Stud* 2001;38:79–89.
10. Teunissen TA, de Jonge A, van Weel C, Lagro-Janssen AL. Treating urinary incontinence in the elderly—conservative therapies that work: a systematic review. *J Fam Pract* 2004;53:25–30.
11. Cassells C, Watt E. The impact of incontinence on older spousal caregivers. *J Adv Nurs* 2003;42:607–16.
12. Thom DH, Haan MN, Van Den Eeden SK. Medically recognized urinary incontinence and risks of hospitalization, nursing home admission and mortality. *Age Ageing* 1997;26:367–74.
13. Holroyd-Leduc JM, Mehta KM, Covinsky KE. Urinary incontinence and its association with death, nursing home admission and functional decline. *J Am Geriatr Soc* 2004;52:712–8.
14. Coward RT, Horne C, Peek CW. Predicting nursing home admissions among incontinent older adults: a comparison of residential differences across six years. *Gerontologist* 1995;35:732–43.

15. The Continence Foundation (2000) *Making the Case for Investment in an Integrated Continence Service.* London: Continence Foundation.

16. Hu TW, Wagner TH, Hawthorne G, Moore K, Subak LL, Versi E (2005) Economics of incontinence. In: Abrams P, Cardozo L, Khoury, Wein A (eds), *Third International Consultation on Incontinence,* Monaco, 26–29 June 2004. Plymouth: Health Publications Ltd; 2005. Chap. 2, pp. 75–95.

17. Department of Health. *National Service Framework for Older People.* London, Department of Health; 2001.

18. Resnick NM. An 89-year-old woman with urinary incontinence. *J Am Med Assoc* 1996;276:1832–40.

19. Sandvik H, Kveine E, Hunskaar S. Female urinary incontinence-psychosocial impact, self care and consultations. *Scand J Caring Sci* 1993;7:53–6.

20. Roe B, Doll H, Wilson K. Help seeking behaviour and health and social services utilisation by people suffering from urinary incontinence. *Int J Nurs Stud* 1999;36:245–53.

21. Shaw C, Matthews RJ, Perry SI, *et al.* Validity and reliability of an interviewer-administered questionnaire to measure the severity of lower urinary tract symptoms of storage abnormality: the Leicester Urinary Symptom Questionnaire. *Br J Urol* 2002;90:205–15.

22. Fonda D. Improving management of urinary incontinence in geriatric centres and nursing homes. Victorian Geriatricians Peer Review Group. Aust Clin Rev 1990;10:66–71.

23. Burgio KL, Matthews KA, Engel BT. Prevalence, incidence and correlates of urinary incontinence in healthy, middle aged women. *J Urol* 1991;146:1255–9.

24. Roe B, Doll H. Lifestyle factors and continence status: comparison of self-report data from a postal survey in England. *J Wound Ostomy Continence Nurs* 1999;26:312-3, 315–319.

25. Creighton SM, Stanton SL. Caffeine: does it affect your bladder? Br J Urol 1990;66:613–14.

26. Ouslander JG. Diagnostic evaluation of geriatric urinary incontinence. *Clin Geriatr Med* 1986;2:715–30.

27. Hay-Smith EJ, Dumoulin C. Pelvic floor muscle training versus no treatment, or inactive control treatments for urinary incontinence in women. *Cochrane Database Syst Rev* 2006;(1):CD005654.

28. Wallace SA, Roe B, Williams K, Palmer M. Bladder training for urinary incontinence in adults. *Cochrane Database Syst Rev* 2004;(1):CD001308.

29. Eustice S, Roe B, Paterson J. Prompted voiding for the management of urinary incontinence in adults. *Cochrane Databse Syst Rev* 2002;(2):CD002113.

30. Ostaszkiewicz J, Johnson L, Roe B. Habit training for urinary incontinence in adults (Cochrane Review). In *The Cochrane Library.* Issue 2. Update Software. Chichester: Wiley; 2004.

31. Ostaszkiewicz J, Johnson L, Roe B. Timed voiding for the management of urinary incontinence in adults. *Cochrane Database Syst Rev* 2004;(1):CD002802.

32. Roe B, Milne J, Ostaszkiewicz J, Wallace S. Systematic reviews of bladder training and voiding programmes in adults: a synopsis of findings from data analysis and outcomes using metastudy techniques. *J Adv Nurs* 2007;57:15–31.

33. Roe B, Ostaszkiewicz J, Milne J, Wallace S. Systematic reviews of bladder training and voiding programmes in adults: a synopsis of findings on theory and methods using Metastudy techniques. *J Adv Nurs* 2007;57:3–14.

34. Williams KS, Assassa RP, Cooper NJ, *et al.* Clinical and cost-effectiveness of a new nurse-led continence service: a randomised controlled trail. *Br J Gen Pract* 2005;55518: 696–703.

35. Majmudar T, Slack M. Current drug treatments for female urinary incontinence. *Prescriber* 2006;1723:23–33.

36. Cottenden A, Bliss D, Fader M, *et al.* Management with continence products. In, Abrams P, Cardozo L, Khoury S and Wein A (eds), *Third International Consultation on Incontinence,* Monaco, 26–29 June 2004. Plymouth: Health Publications Ltd; 2005. p. 149–253.

37. Wilson PD, Hya-Smith J, Nygarrd I, *et al.* (2005) Adult conservative management. In: Abrams P, Cardozo L, Khoury, Wein A (eds), *Third International Consultation on Incontinence,* Monaco, 26–29 June 2004. Plymouth: Health Publications Ltd; 2005. Chap. 15, p. 857–964.

38. DH. *Good Practice in Continence Services*. London: Department of Health; 2002. Available from: http://www.continence-foundation.org.uk/campaigns/goodpracticecontinence.pdf (Accessed 28 March 2008).

39. Perry S, Shaw C, McGrother C, *et al*. Prevalence of faecal incontinence in adults aged 40 years or more living in the community. *Gut* 2002;50:480–4.

40. Edwards NI, Jones D. The prevalence of faecal incontinence in older people living at home. *Age Ageing* 2001;30:503–7.

41. Akpan A, Gosney MA, Barrett JA. Psychological impact of faecal incontinence on older adults. *Age Ageing* 2005;34:S2:26.

42. Royal College of Physicians. *Report of the Pilot of the National Audit of Continence Care for Older People*. England. London: Royal College of Physicians; 2004.

43. Akpan A, Gosney MA, Barrett JA. Privacy for defaecation and faecal incontinence in older adults. *J Wound Ostomy Continence Nurs* 2006;33:536–40.

44. National Institute for Health and Clinical Excellence. *CG49. Faecal Incontinence: Full Guideline*. London: NICE; 2007. Available at: http://www.nice.org.uk/nicemedia/pdf/CG49FullGuideline.pdf

45. Akpan A, Gosney MA, Barrett JA. Factors contributing to fecal incontinence in older people and outcome of routine management in home, hospital and nursing home settings. *Clin Interv Aging* 2007;2:139–45.

46. Akpan A, Gosney MA, Barrett JA. Impact on quality of life of faecal incontinence on older adults living at home. *Res Pract Alzheimer's Dis* 2007;12;178–183.

Appendix 1: Organizations providing advice and information on incontinence and products

Association for Continence Advice (ACA): http://www.aca.uk.com
Enuresis Resource Information Centre (ERIC): http://www.eric.org.uk
InContact: http://www.incontact.org
International Continence Society: http://www.icsoffice.org
The Continence Foundation: http://www.continence-foundation.org.uk

Chapter 20

Urology

Peter Malone and Christopher Blick

Introduction

Urology, as a discipline, covers the urinary tract of both genders and the male genital tract. As incontinence is dealt with separately (see Chapter 19), the main aspects of Urology for the purpose of this chapter can be divided into infection, obstruction and malignancy.

Infection

Urinary tract infection (UTI) is one of the most common pathologies in old age.[1] The basic principles of treatment are not influenced by age with the exception that underlying pathology is more common in elderly individuals. Asymptomatic bacteriuria is common but patients most frequently present with the classical symptoms of frequency, urgency, dysuria and strangury. It must be remembered, however, that urinary infection in an older person may present with incontinence or entirely non-specific symptoms of malaise or confusion as a result of bacteraemia.[2]

UTIs can be divided into simple and complex, and the diagnosis and treatment of each is different. The main distinction between them is in the history and examination. Patients with a simple UTI are usually female, complaining of frequency or dysuria, and are apyrexial. Patients with complex UTIs are of either gender, pyrexial or with a history of rigors. They may have pain, renal angle tenderness or are known to have an abnormality of their urinary tract making them more prone to infection.

Whereas simple UTIs can be dealt with by a short course of antibiotics, complex UTIs require investigation and more lengthy and considered treatment.

Kidney infections

Pyelonephritis is a common complaint in young women, but it is unwise to make the diagnosis too readily in an elderly person. The combination of flank pain and pyrexia should raise the possibility of pyonephrosis where the kidney is blocked by a stone, tumour or pelvi-ureteric junction obstruction. Pyonephrosis is potentially fatal and loss of renal function is rapid, therefore urgent ultrasound is required and the presence of hydronephrosis requires immediate referral.[3] In some patients the infection is chronic and causes few localizing symptoms, mimicking malignancy with weight loss and malaise (see Chapter 14).

Bladder infections

Stasis, stones and tumour are the main predisposing causes. In the ageing man this is most commonly due to prostatic enlargement.

Lower urinary tract symptoms in women

In the absence of signs of malignancy and infection, other diagnoses to consider are interstitial cystitis and detrusor instability or overactive bladder.

Interstitial cystitis

This is caused by bladder inflammation of unknown cause and symptoms are similar to UTI except that the mid-stream specimens of urine (MSSUs) are negative. The main feature is bladder pain which increases as the bladder fills and is relieved by passing urine.

Detrusor instability

The main symptom is urgency with or without incontinence. Anticholinergics usually produce a significant improvement if the side-effects of dry mouth, etc. can be tolerated.[4]

Other causes

Women too can have obstructive causes such as urethral stenosis, vulval fusion or severe prolapse, but detrusor failure is a more common pathology.

Prostate infections

UTIs in men are, almost by definition, more complex because men have prostates. As reflux down prostatic ducts is common during micturition, a man with urinary infection frequently also has bacterial prostatitis.[5] This has major implications for treatment as not all antibiotics penetrate well into the prostate. Inadequate treatment usually results in recurrent infection as, although the urinary infection clears, a nidus lingers in the prostate and recurs. Some serious infections require 4–6 weeks of antibiotics to eradicate the infection but 10 days to 2 weeks is usually enough. Quinolone antibiotics penetrate best but are implicated in the rise of meticillin-resistant *Staphylococcus* and *Clostridium difficile* infection, so are best reserved for those infections resistant to trimethoprim, which also achieves good prostatic tissue levels.[6] Bacterial prostatitis is usually accompanied by a raised prostate-specific antigen (PSA); a level of up to 50 ng/ml should be expected and should not trigger referral for biopsy but should be monitored in the expectation that it will normalize in 6–12 weeks.[7]

UTIs in patients with permanent indwelling catheters

The presence of a urinary catheter makes infection inevitable. It is impossible to eradicate the infection as long as the catheter remains. Treatment of infection, therefore, is limited to those that cause systemic illness to the patient. Constantly trying to eradicate the infection only produces resistant bacteria.[8]

Investigation of UTIs

Examination

Feel for a palpable kidney or bladder. Examine the foreskin in men and the vulvae in women and the external urinary meatus in both sexes. Examination of women while standing occasionally shows a severe prolapse.

Urine testing

The presence of blood and protein in urine is non-specific. Leukocytes are the body's reaction to infection but are also found with urinary tract stones, malignancy, and after urinary tract surgery (e.g. transurethral resection of the prostate). Nitrites are the breakdown products of bacteria and are most specific. In complex UTIs an MSSU is mandatory.[9]

Imaging

Urinary tract ultrasound is the most useful, non-invasive tool. When urinary lithiasis is suspected, computed tomography without contrast is the most effective. Flexible cystoscopy should be performed in patients with haematuria or persistent UTI. The combination of urinary tract ultrasound and urine cytology is powerful in excluding bladder and renal cancer but should not replace cystoscopy where the level of suspicion is high.

Urinary obstruction

Renal obstruction

Renal colic due to a ureteric calculus can occur at any age but is more common in young and middle-aged men. In the elderly population, therefore, one must consider alternative diagnoses. Obstruction from malignancy, shingles or ruptured aortic aneurism can all present with flank pain. In elderly women one must be particularly suspicious of the combination of obstruction and infection; pyonephrosis.

Bladder outflow obstruction

Benign prostatic hyperplasia

The cause for benign prostatic hyperplasia (BPH) has not been identified precisely but appears to be hormonally mediated. BPH leads to gradual occlusion of the urethra causing poor flow, hesitancy and incomplete bladder emptying.[10] Most patients, however, do not complain of these symptoms but more of the irritative symptoms of urgency, frequency and nocturia due to the secondary result of the obstruction on the detrusor muscle. The prostate is not always the cause so infection, detrusor instability and nocturnal polyuria should be considered.

Detrusor instability

The overactive bladder is a very common cause of lower urinary tract symptoms in both women and men. In men this is a diagnosis particularly common after a stroke or other neurological pathology such as Parkinson's disease.[11] It is generally distinguished from bladder outflow obstruction by ascertaining the urine flow rate (see Figure 20.1).

Nocturnal polyuria

The kidneys normally concentrate the urine at night to allow a good night's sleep but in some patients the reverse can be true. With advancing age this is an increasing problem and many

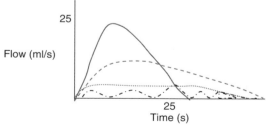

Fig. 20.1 Urine flow rate.
Solid line: normal; dashed line: obstructed; dotted line: stricture; dotted/dashed line: detrusor failure.

patients pass nearly all their 24 h output in the twilight hours.[12] The key to this diagnosis is to be made by simply keeping an output chart over a 48 h period.

Investigation of lower urinary tract symptoms in men

In order to secure a firm diagnosis, urine analysis, flow rate and post-micturition residue and a urinary output chart are completed. Many consider it wise to arrange a urinary tract ultrasound and PSA.

Treatment of bladder outflow obstruction

Many men with mild symptoms are managed conservatively by education, reassurance and lifestyle changes such as voiding before sleep and reducing alcohol intake.

Medical treatment

First-line therapy for patients with proven moderate-to-severe symptoms consists of alpha-blockers which relax smooth muscle in the bladder neck and prostate, hence easing the passage of urine. Side-effects associated with alpha-blockers include postural hypotension and retrograde ejaculation.[13] In patients with large prostates (40–50 cc or more), 5-alpha-reductase inhibitors, which block the production of dihydrotestosterone cause a reduction in prostate volume.[14] The best results are achieved by a combination of both of these medications.

Retention of urine

Urinary retention can be acute and chronic.

Acute urinary retention

This is when patients suddenly cannot pass urine. It is very painful and the immediate treatment is catheterization. This process, like UTI, usually results in a significant rise in the PSA.[15]

Chronic urinary retention

Chronic retention is generally painless, often presenting with enuresis. The post-micturition residual gradually increases as the bladder tires, contracting against the resistance caused by the prostate. As it does so the pressure in the system rises and eventually produces sufficient back pressure on the kidneys to produce renal failure. After relief of the retention, by catheterization, the bladder remains stretched and weak and complete recovery is not inevitable. All patients in chronic retention will either require surgery or have to accept permanent or intermittent catheterization. Trial without catheter in a patient with a painless palpable bladder will not be successful and should not be attempted. In addition, the initial catheterization carries some risks as it can be accompanied by profound diuresis, particularly when the patient is in renal failure, causing dehydration and electrolyte imbalance. Generally this should be done in a hospital setting.

Surgery

Transurethral resection of the prostate remains the mainstay of treatment in many centres. Laser vaporization does not provide histology but provides an alternative for those with significant co-morbidity due to lower intraoperative bleeding and a shorter hospital stay.[16]

Urological oncology

Cancer in the urinary tract is common and prostate cancer is very common.

Prostate cancer

Prostate cancer is rare below the age of 45 years, but the incidence rises rapidly thereafter. It is usually a silent cancer, although patients may present with lower urinary tract symptoms. Local invasion of prostate cancer can cause haematuria and impotence, and those with metastatic disease may present with bony pain, weight loss or malaise. Patients presenting with these symptoms should have a digital rectal examination (DRE) and be offered a PSA test after counselling, but the only way to reliably detect prostate cancer at an early stage is for regular PSA testing.[17]

PSA screening for prostate cancer

The current view of the government and the majority of the UK medical profession is that patients should not be refused a PSA test if they request it but, in the absence of symptoms, the request should come from the patient rather than the doctor. The general practitioner will undoubtedly be faced with patients with a raised PSA. How to deal with these patients becomes a vexed issue as patients become more elderly and infirm. Patients who are fit enough to undergo radiotherapy and likely to live long enough to benefit from it should be referred under the 2 week wait rule. The same applies to those who have a significant risk of extracapsular or metastatic spread as judged by a frankly malignant DRE, symptoms of dissemination or a PSA >20 ng/ml. In the frail patient with significant co-morbidity without these criteria, judicious monitoring seems a reasonable choice.[18]

Age-specific threshold PSA measurements are:

♦ 50–59 years: ≥3.5 ng/ml

♦ 60–69 years: ≥4.5 ng/ml

♦ ≥70 years: ≥6.5 ng/ml.

Treatment of prostate cancer

Prostate cancers are staged into three categories:

1) *Localized to the prostate.* The main treatment of this group is radical radiotherapy (given external beam or implanted seeds—brachytherapy) or surgery. Hormone treatment at this stage does not offer a survival advantage.

2) *Locally advanced but not metastatic.* It has become clear that early hormone treatment offers a survival advantage in this group and is frequently given in conjunction with external beam radiotherapy.

3) *Metastatic prostate cancer.* Early hormone treatment in this group does not offer a survival advantage but does reduce the risk of serious complications of the cancer such as paraplegia due to spinal cord compression.[17]

Bladder and renal cancers

Renal cancer is rare in people aged <35 years and bladder cancer in those aged <50 years; both increase in incidence over time and are more common in males. Patients of any age or gender who present with painless macroscopic haematuria even on one occasion, or microscopic or dipstix haematuria on two occasions in patients aged >40 years, should be referred under the 2 week wait, as should any patient with an abdominal mass identified clinically or on imaging that is thought to be arising from the urinary tract.[19,20]

Testicular cancer

Testicular cancer can occur at almost any age, but is most common in those aged 25–40. Germ cell tumours are rare in elderly men and lymphoma is the commonest testicular tumour in this age group. Be aware that the commonest causes of swelling confined to the scrotum (one cannot get above a hernia) in this age group are hydrocele, epididymal cysts (both transilluminate) and epididymitis secondary to a UTI. Ultrasound is excellent at distinguishing between these conditions.[21]

Penile cancer

Penile cancer is rare and an urgent referral should be made for any patient presenting with symptoms or signs of penile cancer. These include progressive ulceration or a mass on the glans or prepuce particularly, but can involve the skin of the penile shaft.[19] Lumps within the corpora cavernosa not involving glans or penile skin are usually not cancer but may indicate Peyronie's disease.

References

1. Lutters M, Vogt N. Antibiotic duration for treating uncomplicated, systematic lower urinary tract infections in elderly women. *Cochrane Database Syst Rev* 2001;(3):CD001535.

2. Mouton CP, Bazaldua OV, Pierce B, Espino DV. Common infections in older adults. *Am Fam Physn* 2001;63:257–268.

3. Watson RA, Esposito M, Richter F, Irwin RJ Jr, Lang EK. Percutaneous nephrostomy as adjunct management in advanced upper urinary tract infection. *Urology* 1999;54:234–9.

4. Patel AK, Chapple CR. Medical management of lower urinary tract symptoms in men: current treatment and future approaches. *Nat Clin Pract Urol* 2008;5:211–9.

5. Grabe N, Bishop MC, Bjerklund-Johansen TE, *et al. Guidelines on Urinary and Male Genital Tract Infections*. Arnhem: European Association of Urology; 2001 (latest edition 2008).

6. Deshpande A, Pant C, Jain A, Fraser TG, Rolston DD. Do fluoroquinolones predispose patients to *Clostridium difficile* associated disease? A review of the evidence. *Curr Med Res Opin* 2008;24:329–33.

7. Palou J, Morote J. Elevated serum PSA and acute bacterial prostatitis. *Urology* 1990;35:373.

8. Tenke P, Kovacs B, Bjerklund Johansen TE, Matsumoto T, Tambyah PA, Naber KG. European and Asian guidelines on management and prevention of catheter-associated urinary tract infections. *Int J Antimicrob Agents* 2008;31(Suppl 1):S68–78.

9. Yoshikawa TT, Nicolle LE, Norman DC. Management of complicated urinary tract infection in older patients. *J Am Geriatr Soc* 1996;44:1235–41.

10. Anderson JB, Roehrborn CG, Schalken JA, Emberton M. The progression of benign prostatic hyperplasia: examining the evidence and determining the risk. *Eur Urol* 2001;39:390–9.

11. Gades NM, Jacobson DJ, Girman CJ, Roberts RO, Lieber MM, Jacobsen SJ. Prevalence of conditions potentially associated with lower urinary tract symptoms in men. *Br J Urol Int* 2005;95:549–53.

12. Kujubu DA, Aboseif SR. An overview of nocturia and the syndrome of nocturnal polyuria in the elderly. *Nat Clin Pract Nephrol* 2008;4:426–35.

13. Djavan B, Marberger M. Meta-analysis on the efficacy and tolerability of alpha1-adrenoceptor antagonists in patients with lower urinary tract symptoms suggestive of benign prostatic obstruction. *Eur Urol* 1999;36:1–13.

14. Gormley GJ, Stoner E, Bruskewitz RC, *et al.* The effect of finasteride in men with benign prostatic hyperplasia. The Finasteride Study Group. *N Engl J Med* 1992;327:1185–91.

15. Polascik TJ, Oesterling JE, Partin AW. Prostate specific antigen: a decade of discovery—what we have learned and where we are going. *J Urol* 1999;162:293–306.

16. Heinrich E, Schiefelbein F, Schoen G. Technique and short-term outcome of green light laser (KTP, 80W) vaporisation of the prostate. *Eur Urol* 2007;52:1632–7.

17. Heidenreich A, Aus G, Abbou CC, *et al. Guidelines on Prostate Cancer*. Arnhem: European Association of Urology; 2007.

18. De Koning HJ, Liem MK, Baan CA, Boer R, Schroder FH, Alexander FE. ERSPC. Prostate cancer mortality reduction by screening: power and time frame with complete enrolment in the European Randomized Screening for Prostate Cancer (ERSPC) trial. *Int J Cancer* 2002;98:268–73.

19. National Instititue for Health and Clinical Excellence. *Referral for Suspected Cancer. A Clinical Practice Guideline.* London: NICE; 2005. Available at: http://www.nice.org.uk/guidance/index. jsp?action=byID&o=10967

20. National Institute for Health and Clinical Excellence. *Guidance on Cancer Services: Improving Outcomes in Urological Cancers.* London: Department of Health; 2002.

21. Richie JP, Birnholz J, Garnick MB. Ultrasonography as a diagnostic adjunct for the evaluation of masses in the scrotum. *Surg Gynecol Obstet* 1982;154:695–8.

Chapter 21

Gynaecological problems

Rajesh Varma

Introduction

The upper and lower female genital tract undergoes age-related changes that increase the risk of symptomatic dysfunction. 'Benign' conditions such as urinary incontinence and genital tract prolapse are common. However, primary care practitioners should be vigilant for genital tract malignancy that can be underlying in such conditions or even present insidiously as minimal postmenopausal bleeding, abdominal discomfort and increasing abdominal size.

Assessment

A systematic approach is helpful. This involves a comprehensive history and detailed physical examination; the key issues are highlighted in Tables 21.1 and 21.2. Furthermore, special consideration should be given to the following:

◆ The gynaecological history should be considered in context with women's quality of life and co-morbidities, as such factors impact on symptom presentation and definitive management.

◆ Polypharmacy should not be neglected, as drug interactions and side-effects commonly present as urogenital or abdomino-pelvic disorders.

◆ Any important omissions while acquiring the history should be rectified by taking supplementary 'witness' history from carers or family.

◆ Consider and evaluate risk factors for genital tract malignancy (Table 21.3).

◆ For many women, the prospect of a pelvic examination may be frightening and the need for it to be performed should be carefully considered.

◆ Identify and act on 'red flag symptoms and signs' suggestive of malignancy (Table 21.4).

Importance of prompt referral for suspected malignancy

Elderly women are at increased risk of cancer. General practitioners (GPs) should be vigilant for genital tract malignancy that can be underlying many of the specific conditions discussed below. Identifying risk factors for genital tract malignancy (Table 21.3) may increase the pre-test likelihood of developing malignancy and therefore impact on the necessity for secondary care referral given the findings obtained on history and clinical examination.

In the UK, women aged >65 years experience and account for 60% of cancers and 69% of cancer deaths.

Cervical, endometrial, ovarian and vulval cancers have a mean age of diagnosis of 52, 61, 50 and 65 years, respectively; however, their age-specific incidences peak at 50, 70, >70 and >80 years of age. In particular, cancer can present insidiously as minimal postmenopausal bleeding, abdominal discomfort and increasing abdominal size (Table 21.4).

Table 21.1 Gynaecological history-taking in elderly women

Generic history	Characteristic
Gastrointestinal (GI) tract	GI function: urgency, constipation and faecal incontinence Increased abdominal size/persistent bloating Faecal incontinence Abdominal or pelvic pain
Genitourinary Urinary incontinence	Haematuria, urinary tract infections (UTIs) *Asking her to complete a 3 day bladder diary* Fluid input Amount voided Frequency of leaks Number of pads used Symptoms of hesitancy, stress, urge, or continuous leakage Nocturia Any delay in voiding
Uterus/vulva Genital tract	Final menstrual period Postmenopausal bleeding Vaginal discharge Prolapse (dragging sensation or vaginal swelling) *Results of last cervical smear*
Menopause	Vasomotor: hot flushes, night sweats Urogenital atrophy: vaginal dryness, dyspareunia, UTIs CNS: depression, agitation, insomnia, concentration Libido and sexual activity Osteoporosis
Breast	Nipple discharge, bleeding Breast lumps *Results of mammography*
Systemic	Cardiac, vascular, neurological, or endocrine disorders Medications Allergies *Any weight loss*

Particular 'red flag' symptoms have been identified that are commonly associated with abdomino-pelvic and systemic malignancy (Table 21.4). Early referral to secondary care is of paramount importance when the GP suspects a malignant urogenital disorder. Most gynaecology, urology and general surgery units in the UK offer a 'rapid access' service for assessing suspected malignancy. This ensures that women with suspected cancer are assessed and diagnosed within 2 weeks of the date of referral, in accordance with National Health Service (NHS) cancer diagnostic pathway target.

Specific conditions

Pelvic mass

The discovery of a pelvic mass in a postmenopausal woman is a 'red flag' finding (Table 21.4). The differential diagnoses include:

- Ovarian: epithelial ovarian cancer; benign ovarian cyst.
- Uterine: fibroid, carcinoma, pyometra, leiomyosarcoma.

Table 21.2 Gynaecological examination in elderly women

System	Characteristic
Higher brain CNS	Mini Mental State Examination (if cognition appears impaired)
	Any typical features of neurological disease (Parkinson's disease, stroke)
Cardiovascular system and respiratory system	Evidence of congestive cardiac failure
Breast	Breast lumps, nipple abnormalities
Abdominal	Abdominal masses: any midline aortic aneurysm
	Pelvic masses: location, consistency
	Inguinal and femoral hernias
	Hepatosplenomegaly
	Rectal examination: *detect constipation, rectal lesions and assess ability to correctly contract the pelvic muscles (useful when assessing urinary incontinence).*
Lymph nodes	Inguinal, axillary, supraclavicular
Perineum and External genitalia	Prolapse examination is difficult with Cuscoe's speculum: consider examination in left lateral Sim's position with a Sim's speculum to show cystoceles or rectoceles.
	A cough urinary stress test, with or without replacement of the cystocele, may indicate a crude measure of the benefit of possible surgical bladder neck elevation or cystocele repair.
	Consider examination in upright position to detect minor degrees of prolapse.
Pelvic speculum and bimanual pelvic examination	Urogenital atrophy
	Pelvic masses
Neurological: CNS and peripheral	Lower limb: examine peripheral nervous system (ankle, knee-deep tendon reflexes, sensation)
	Pelvic: sensation S2–4, anal wink, bulbocavernosus reflex, anal sphincter tone (see above)
Musculoskeletal	Vertebral tenderness, decreased back flexion
	Gait: ability to walk to toilet
	Manual dexterity: able to remove clothing in timely fashion
Urine dipstix	

- Gastrointestinal tract: diverticular abscess, colorectal cancer.
- Bladder: urinary retention, bladder cancer.
- Metastatic tumour.
- Retroperitoneal: sarcoma, lymphoma.

History and examination may help to suggest the underling diagnosis; however, it is imperative that referral to the relevant specialty is promptly made. The key investigation is pelvic ultrasound, which is often conducted on the same day in rapid access clinics.

Postmenopausal ovarian cyst and ovarian cancer

Ovarian cancer is the most common gynaecological cancer in the UK. The lifetime risk of developing ovarian cancer is 1.4%, which increases to a 5% risk if the woman has a first-degree relative with ovarian cancer. Each year in the UK, >6600 cases of ovarian cancer are diagnosed and ~4400

Table 21.3 Risk factors for gynaecological cancers

Uterine cancer	Age
	Obesity
	Endometrial hyperplasia
	Hypertension
	Diabetes
	Polycystic ovarian syndrome
	Hormone replacement therapy
	Tamoxifen use
	Hereditary non-polyposis colorectal cancer
Cervical cancer	Cervical intraepithelial neoplasia
	Human papilloma virus
	Smoking
Ovarian cancer	Family history of ovarian cancer
	BRCA1 or *BRCA2* gene
	Nulliparity
	Ovulation induction drugs
	Endometriosis
Vulval cancer	Lichen sclerosus
	Vulval intraepithelial neoplasia
	Paget disease
	Melanoma *in situ*

women die from the disease. Ovarian cancer accounts for ~6% of all female deaths from cancer. Survival is strongly associated with stage at diagnosis; 5 year survival is 90% for stage 1A/1B, 60–70% for stage 2, 15–35% for stage 3 and 5–14% for stage 4. In addition, older age at diagnosis means lower 5 year survival rate.

Unfortunately, most ovarian cancers are diagnosed late, at an advanced stage. Around 50% of cancers are identified to have progressed through convoluted referral pathways before being correctly diagnosed, i.e. not being directly referred to the gynaecology oncologist. This may be inherent to the insidious nature of the disease in terms of symptoms and signs being recognized late by both women and their GP. However, there is encouraging preliminary evidence suggesting that a symptom index (Table 21.4), coupled with historical risk factors (Table 21.3) and clinical signs (Table 21.2: pelvic mass, ascites), may help to distinguish people with cancer from healthy women

Table 21.4 'Red flag' symptoms and signs suggestive of malignancy

Postmenopausal bleeding
Pelvic or abdominal pain
Increased abdominal size or persistent bloating
Ascites
Haematuria
Difficulty eating and feeling full
Weight loss

The frequency, persistency, severity and new onset of these symptoms may help to distinguish cancer and non-cancer causes.

early in the disease process. The following symptoms are frequent in patients who go on to be diagnosed with ovarian cancer: pelvic and abdominal pain; increased abdominal size/persistent bloating; difficulty eating and feeling full. Furthermore, it appears that the frequency, persistency, severity and new onset of these symptoms may help to distinguish between ovarian cancer and non-cancer causes.

Ovarian cysts may occur in ~20% of postmenopausal women. The majority of cysts are asymptomatic and benign in origin. Ovarian cysts are often discovered incidentally following investigations carried out for other reasons (e.g. pelvic pain, postmenopausal bleeding), or may be identified as part of a pelvic mass investigation or specific ovarian screening study. Management is focused on determining whether the postmenopausal ovarian cyst is benign or has malignant potential. In the UK, it is recommended that postmenopausal ovarian cysts should be assessed using transvaginal sonography and serum CA125 measurement in secondary care. A 'risk of malignancy index' (RMI) may then be calculated (Table 21.5) and used to triage the woman as follows:

◆ *Low risk*. RMI <25; <3% risk of cancer. Management in a gynaecology unit. Simple cysts <5 cm in diameter with a serum CA125 level of <30 U/ml may be managed conservatively. Conservative management involves repeat ultrasound scans and serum CA125 measurement every 4 months for 1 year. If the cyst resolves or does not increase in size at one year, then the woman may be discharged. Laparoscopic oophorectomy may be offered if the cyst increases in size or the woman is concerned about the risk of malignancy.

◆ *Moderate risk*. RMI 25–250; ~20% risk of cancer. Management in a cancer unit. Laparoscopic oophorectomy is acceptable in selected cases.

◆ *High risk*. RMI >250: >75% risk of cancer. Management in a cancer centre. Full staging laparotomy procedure.

Menopause

The menopause may be symptomless or associated with three classes of symptoms:

1) Vasomotor: hot flushes, night sweats.

2) Urogenital atrophy: vaginal dryness, dyspareunia, recurrent urinary tract infections.

3) CNS-related: depression, agitation, insomnia, concentration (hormone replacement therapy (HRT) does not prevent or protect against a decline in cognitive function).

There continues to be controversy on the indications for, type, and route of delivery for, HRT given the recent publication of large multicentre studies that have showed adverse side-effect

Table 21.5 Calculating the risk of malignancy index (RMI)

RMI = $U \times M \times$ CA125
$U = 0$ (for ultrasound score of 0); $U = 1$ (for ultrasound score of 1); $U = 3$ (for ultrasound score of 2–5).
Ultrasound scans are scored 1 point for each of the following characteristics: multilocular cyst; evidence of solid areas; evidence of metastases; presence of ascites; bilateral lesions.
$M = 3$ for all postmenopausal women.
CA125 is serum CA125 measurement in U/ml.

Risk RMI	Risk of cancer (%)
Low: <25	<3%
Moderate: 25–250	20%
High: >250	75%

profiles with long-term usage. Current consensus is that risks and benefits of HRT use are individually assessed and discussed with the woman, and that HRT should be administered ideally on a short-duration basis (≤6 months) for those women with the following symptoms:

♦ Moderate-to-severe vasomotor symptoms that substantially impair quality of life.

♦ Urogenital symptoms (but HRT does not improve urinary incontinence). Consideration should be given to using a 2–3 week course of a topical vaginal oestrogen preparation to minimize systemic side-effects (this is the average duration of one oestrodiol medicated tube). The risk of inducing endometrial hyperplasia or cancer with such low doses of vaginal oestrogen is extremely low and has not been widely reported in published literature. At secondary care level, women with ring or shelf pessaries *in situ* might have longer courses of treatment, or even once-a-week indefinite treatments, to protect the vaginal epithelium from traumatization, as these women are likely to be under regular GP or secondary care follow-up. Alternatively, consideration could be given to using vaginal gels (such as Replens®, a vaginal bioadhesive moisturizer that substitutes for vaginal secretions) or lubricant gels such KY® jelly.

♦ Low libido (use tibolone or add in androgens; see 'Sexuality' below).

HRT increases the risk of venous thromboembolism, stroke, endometrial hyperplasia and endometrial cancer (both these latter risks are reduced by a concomitant progestogens), breast cancer, and ovarian cancer; there is an increased risk of coronary heart disease in women who start combined HRT >10 years after the menopause. HRT reduces the risk of osteoporosis and bowel cancer. Nonetheless, an overall summary of the literature suggests that the benefits of short-term HRT outweigh the risks in the majority of HRT users who are aged <60 years.

Importantly, there are specific first-line therapies for osteoporosis prevention and treatment (e.g. bisphosphonates, calcium) which do not include HRT. There is insufficient data on HRT usage in women aged >65 years, hence particular caution is recommended if HRT is being started, or its use extended, in women aged ≥60 years.

Urinary incontinence

Urinary incontinence (UI) (see also Chapter 18) in elderly women occurs due to progressive weakness in detrusor contractility, decreased detrusor distensibility, increasing unprovoked overactivity of the bladder, weakening of the urethral sphincter, and poor urinary tract support due to pelvic floor weakness. Importantly, UI is symptomatically categorized into *urge, stress* or *mixed* based on history-taking, and this discrimination process is considered sufficiently reliable to inform initial, non-invasive treatment decisions as detailed below. A 3 day bladder diary, recording input, output and UI or urge episodes, is particularly useful and recommended in the initial assessment of UI in both primary and secondary care settings.

Genital tract prolapse and UI frequently coexist, as they share common antecedent factors. Daily urinary incontinence is experienced by between 4% and 14% of older women. The lifetime risk of having surgery for UI and/or genital tract prolapse in those aged ≤80 years is ~10%.

Urinary incontinence may have non-gynaecological or gynaecological contributory factors and assessment should explore these domains. Identifying non-gynaecological and gynaecological factors helps to determine the most effective therapy.

Non-gynaecological UI factors

♦ *Mobility* (e.g. degenerative joint disease): unable to get to the bathroom in time to void. In frail elderly women whose immobility and function cannot be improved, the chance of restoring continence is very low.

♦ *Manual dexterity*: inability to undress in time to void, perhaps due to arthritis.

◆ *Environment and access to toilets*: no downstairs toilet.

◆ *Cognition*: dementia, neurological (e.g. stoke, Parkinson's disease, normal pressure hydrocephalus) and psychiatric disease (e.g. depression) may alter normal voiding urges or voiding behaviours.

◆ *Medical disorders*: diabetes can lead to polyuria and diabetic neuropathy may cause detrusor overactivity. Congestive cardiac failure, sleep apnoea, chronic constipation and chronic bronchitis may also lead to UI.

◆ *Medications*: angiotensin-converting enzyme inhibitors may cause a chronic cough and stress UI. Potent diuretics can cause sudden large urinary volume voiding. Calcium blockers, opiates, and anticholinergics can impair bladder emptying.

Gynaecological UI factors

◆ *Urinary tract infection (often repeated episodes)*. A urine dipstix and mid-stream specimen of urine are useful to exclude infection which may be contributory to UI, or microscopic haematuria which could indicate a urinary tract neoplastic disorder. A urine dipstick may also detect blood, glucose or protein, suggesting other potential conditions.

◆ *Genital tract prolapse*. Symptoms that may indicate prolapse, in addition to UI, include: increasing vaginal discomfort, vaginal pressure or dragging sensation, difficulty with defecation (perhaps needing to insert fingers in the vagina to replace posterior vaginal rectocele in order to defecate completely) and any vaginal swelling (particularly noticed after standing or physical exertion).

◆ *Stress UI*. A cough stress test may demonstrate stress UI in a woman with a full bladder (Table 21.2). Treatment options include pelvic floor physiotherapy, bladder neck support with a ring/shelf vaginal pessary, medical treatment (duloxetine—is more effective when used as an adjunct to pelvic floor exercises), peri-urethral bulking agents (e.g. bovine collagen for women with intrinsic sphincter deficiency) and surgery (such as tension-free vaginal tape, laparoscopic or open Burch colposuspension).

◆ *Urge UI (detrusor overactivity or overactive bladder syndrome)*. Urge UI is more prevalent than stress UI; ~40% of continent women aged >65 years show detrusor overactivity on urodynamic testing. First-line treatment option is bladder retraining (gradually increasing the interval when urge is experienced and learning urge suppression techniques) for cognitive-intact persons, and prompted voiding for those who are cognitively impaired. Pelvic floor physiotherapy is also advised but has a less effective role in treating urge UI compared with stress UI. Antimuscarinic drugs are considered a second-line treatment and act to reduce involuntary detrusor contractions and increase bladder capacity. Several proprietary brands exist such as modified release oxybutynin (which is also available as a transdermal patch) and tolterodine. However, all predispose to adverse side-effects (Table 21.6). Antimuscarinics should be initiated at a low dose, then increased slowly to achieve efficacy without causing excessive side-effects. Women with urge UI that is refractory to conservative treatments may be offered sacral nerve stimulation or injection of botulinum toxin A (Botox) directly into the bladder detrusor.

◆ *Mixed UI*. Initial treatment is often directed at the predominant urge or stress UI component, but could also be combined (e.g. commence bladder retraining and pelvic floor physiotherapy concurrently). Alternatively, urodynamic investigations may be conducted to help determine the optimum surgical or non-surgical management.

◆ *Continuous UI*. This symptom is suggestive of a bladder fistula. Any history of gynaecological surgery, pelvic malignancy or vaginal delivery complicated by perineal trauma may lead to the development of a vesico-vaginal fistula.

Table 21.6 Drugs used to treat detrusor overactivity (antimuscarinic side-effects)

Examples of drug	Oxybutynin Tolterodine Solifenacin
Systemic side-effects	CNS stimulation, such as restlessness, disorientation, hallucination Dry mouth, dry eyes Blurred vision Constipation Reduced sweating, leading to heat sensations and fainting in hot environments
Contraindications	Bladder tract outflow obstruction Angle-closure glaucoma Myasthenia gravis Significant bladder outflow obstruction or urinary retention Severe ulcerative colitis, toxic megacolon, and in gastrointestinal obstruction or intestinal atony

- *Nocturia*. This is defined as the need to void more than once during sleeping hours. The prevalence of the condition increases with age, such that 90% of women experience nocturia at age 80 years. Nocturia in premenopausal women is often characteristic of detrusor overactivity, but in older women nocturia may also arise due the development of other conditions (such as polyuria, pedal oedema and primary sleep disorders).

- *Overflow UI*. Describes frequent small urinary leakage caused by a bladder that will not completely empty. Causes include neurological disorders, impaired detrusor contractility, and simultaneous detrusor hyperactivity with impaired contractility. Treatment options include intermittent self-catheterization, double voiding or long-term catheterization and use of antimuscarinics if detrusor hyperactivity is present.

UI: specialized investigations

- *Post-void residual (PVR) urine volume*. An elevated PVR volume may indicate either bladder outlet obstruction or impaired detrusor contractility; distinguishing these components requires formal urodynamic studies. Bedside portable ultrasound devices are in widespread use to measure PVR volumes, and should be performed prior to urodynamic studies. There is no agreed consensus or a normal limit; however, a PVR volume of 150 ml suggests the need for daily clean intermittent self-catheterization, whereas a residual of 400–500 ml indicates the need for ≥2 weeks of continuous indwelling catheterization followed by clean intermittent self-catheterization.

- *Urodynamic studies*. Urodynamic testing is not necessary prior to commencing conservative medical or pelvic floor physiotherapy measures. There is no evidence that routine urodynamic testing improves outcome. Secondary care specialists vary in their selection criteria, although urodynamics may be useful in the following situations:

  a. Pelvic floor physiotherapy or trial of medical therapy (Duloxetine or antimuscarinics) has failed.

  b. There has been previous surgery for stress incontinence or anterior compartment prolapse.

  c. There are symptoms suggestive of voiding dysfunction.

  d. Prior to any surgical continence procedure or vaginal pelvic floor repair, particularly if urge UI present as this could potentially worsen after surgery.

e. Uncertainty in clinical diagnosis (e.g. mixed symptomology: urge, nocturia, stress incontinence).

f. Existing complicating co-morbidity (e.g. neurological disease).

Generic UI treatment strategies

Management needs to recognize the inter-relationship between gynaecological and non-gynaecological factors (e.g. co-morbidities, motor impairment, cognitive decline) to ensure that treatment is individualized and effective. Generic strategies, in addition to the specific measures detailed earlier, should also be considered in the management plan, and include:

- Treat any urinary tract infection.
- Reducing polypharmacy.
- Lifestyle changes (e.g. weight loss if body mass index >30 kg/m^2).
- Help to limit effect of any cognitive decline, such as scheduled toileting, bedside commodes, large simple signs on the bathroom door, and simple protective garments that do not involve complex straps.
- Using pads together with prophylactic protection of the perineum with a barrier agent.
- Controlling daily fluid intake (<21) and reducing daily caffeine.
- Supervised pelvic floor physiotherapy, for at least 3 months' duration, for stress, urge and mixed UI women. Elderly women often have weak pelvic floor function which predisposes to both stress UI and uninhibited bladder contractions characteristic of urge UI. Both rapid (3 s) and sustained (5–10 s) contractions should be practiced several times daily. Checking the contraction strength at each visit reinforces its importance. Biofeedback and/or electrical stimulation should be recommended if the patient is unable to learn pelvic floor muscle contractions with physiotherapy support. Repeated pelvic floor contractions can suppress detrusor contraction and may be used by the woman as an urge suppression technique.

Consideration should be given to ensure that the intervention will optimize the patient's quality of life. With this in mind, it may therefore be inappropriate to refer women for incontinence assessment who have end-stage terminal illness or severe cognitive impairment or physical immobility. Palliative treatment by intermittent self-catheterization, incontinence pads and specialist female undergarments may be advisable for older women in such circumstances (see Chapter 19).

Postmenopausal bleeding

Around 10% of women aged >50 years experience an episode of postmenopausal bleeding. In the vast majority, the cause is due to benign atrophic changes of the genital tract (Table 21.7). However, in all cases, postmenopausal bleeding indicates urgent clinical assessment and secondary care referral, as the symptom must be considered a potential presentation of endometrial carcinoma until proven otherwise.

Assessment in primary care should include a relevant history which may identify risk factors for genital tract cancer (Table 21.3 and 21.4), systemic clinical examination and pelvic examination (particularly inspection of lower genital tract and cervix and bimanual pelvic examination).

For most women, assessment in secondary care involves history taking, clinical abdominal and pelvic examination, obtaining a cervical smear if a clinically suspicious cervical lesion is identified, and conducting a transvaginal pelvic ultrasound. A sonographically determined endometrial thickness, measured in the mid-fundus sagittal plane of the uterus, that is ≤4 mm in width, is considered unlikely to yield any underlying uterine pathology (that is either benign or malignant)

Table 21.7 Causes of postmenopausal bleed (PMB)

Cause	Prevalence in women presenting with PMB
Atrophic uterus or cervix or vagina	50–60%
Submucous fibroids	10–15%
Endometrial polyps	15%
Endometrial hyperplasia	15%
Endometrial cancer	2–5%
Cervical polyp	2%
Other genital tract cancers (cancer of vulva, vagina, cervix, Fallopian tube or ovary)	<1%

with excellent sensitivity, specificity and positive predictive value. However, an endometrial thickness >4 mm warrants, at a minimum, histological analysis of the endometrium (e.g. outpatient endometrial Pipelle biopsy) and further investigation of the uterine cavity (either hysteroscopy or saline infusion sonography).

Transvaginal pelvic sonography and hysteroscopy/endometrial biopsy in combination are considered the gold standard investigation for postmenopausal bleeding, as the combination accurately diagnoses both intra- and extrauterine (e.g. uterine fibroid, ovarian cyst) pathology.

Genital tract prolapse

Pelvic organ prolapse is often associated with urinary and bowel dysfunction. Genital tract prolapse may involve vaginal walls anteriorly (cystocele, urethrocele), posteriorly (rectocele, enterocele), cervix (first-, second- and third-degree descent) and vaginal vault post hysterectomy.

Although rare, management should ensure that there is no underlying abdominal or pelvic mass (particularly cancer) predisposing to the genital tract prolapse. Hence, it is important to obtain a comprehensive systemic history and perform an abdominal pelvic examination, including bimanual pelvic examination. Any suspicion of a pelvic mass representing malignancy can be reliably excluded by conducting a transabdominal and transvaginal pelvic ultrasound.

Management for prolapse depends on the location and severity of prolapse, association with any urinary incontinence, impairment in quality of life, whether she is sexually active or not, and co-morbidities (particularly fitness for surgery). Principles normally adopted include:

- *Expectant management.*
- *Pelvic floor physiotherapy* (discussed earlier in the chapter).
- *Insertion of vaginal ring or shelf pessaries.* These devices are highly effective, provide immediate symptomatic relief and avoid exposure to the potential risks of anaesthesia and surgery. It is important that the correct device (usually ring) is selected, and fitted correctly; the final fitting size may require a degree of trial and error. The pessary creates a supporting platform between the pubic symphysis and the coccyx, thus elevating the intervening redundant vaginal epithelium. Sexual activity is not obstructed by the vaginal pessary.
- *Surgical correction.* Anterior and posterior vaginal wall repairs plicate the levator ani complex over the bladder and rectal fascia, respectively, and can be performed in combination with vaginal hysterectomy if indicated. Newer techniques, involving vagina mesh insertion at the time of pelvic floor repair, are currently under evaluation. Vaginal vault prolapse can be corrected through a vaginal (vault sacrospinous fixation) or laparoscopic (sacrocolpoplexy) approach.

Vulval disorders

Vulval disorders tend to present as vulval bleeding, pruritus, pain and ulceration. In general, it is reasonable to commence a short trial of treatment to 'treat, watch and wait' as a method of management. However, if symptoms persist, referral should be made on a non-urgent basis to a general gynaecologist or specialist multidisciplinary vulval clinic. If vulval cancer is suspected then the woman should be *urgently referred* to the local gynaecological cancer rapid access clinic and be reviewed by a gynaecological oncologist.

Specific conditions to consider include:

- *Vulval and perineal dermatitis.* This is caused by longstanding urine or bowel incontinence and characterized by diffuse erythema, skin breakdown and excoriations. Ideal treatments are personal hygiene advice, hydrophobic protective perineal barrier creams and exposure of the skin to air drying.

- *Folliculitis.* Well-demarcated raised pustules, which, if allowed to progress, develop into labial and perineal abscesses. Treatment options include topical antibacterial cream (e.g. mupirocin ointment), oral antibiotics (e.g. flucloxacillin) and incision, and drainage.

- *Lichen sclerosus.* A chronic labial skin disorder characterized by pruritus, hypopigmented labial skin edges and fusion of the anterior and posterior vaginal fourchette. Although it is usually clinically suspected, *all women* should have their diagnosis confirmed by vulval biopsy; this can be performed under local anaesthetic. Management is usually long term with initial topical high potency steroid treatment (e.g. clobetasol propionate (Dermovate®)) thinly applied to the area of labial itching no more than twice daily for 4 weeks. The treatment is then gradually tapered down to a maintenance to moderate (e.g. clobetasone butyrate (Eumovate®)) or mild potency (hydrocortisone) steroid once remission is achieved. Once discharged to primary care, any worsening of vulval ulceration or new ulceration warrants urgent referral back to the appropriate specialist as this could indicate onset of vulval carcinoma. Long-term follow-up is required for women diagnosed with lichen sclerosis, as a small proportion (2–5%) may develop vulval cancer over the long term.

- *Vulval carcinoma.* Vulval cancer is a rare disease and, on average, a GP will only see a new case once every 7 years. Any elderly woman who presents with an unexplained vulval lump or suspicious ulceration warrants urgent referral to a general gynaecologist or gynaecology oncologist. Vulval cancer presents as a bleeding ulcerating lesion. Initial management is referral for urgent biopsy to obtain a histological diagnosis.

- *Vulval melanoma.* Vulval melanoma is a very rare disease, and may present as a newly pigmented mole, rapidly increasing mole, with irregular edges and bleeding. Initial management is referral for urgent biopsy to obtain a histological diagnosis.

Sexuality

Until recently, there has been little awareness and understanding of the sexual needs of older women. Women express an interest in sexual intimacy well into their eighties and beyond. Furthermore, sexuality impacts favourably on general health, quality of life and relationships.

In practice, women rarely directly volunteer problems with sexual function. Furthermore, the decision to enquire about such activity is often perceived as embarrassing.

Atrophic vaginitis and vaginal dryness are a common cause for dyspareunia that can be relatively easy to treat through vaginal instillation of aqueous lubricating gels prior to intercourse.

Licensed treatments for diminished libido (now termed as hypoactive sexual desire disorder) in elderly women include tibolone (continuous combined oral hormone replacement therapy) or testosterone (transdermal patches (Intrinsa®)). Tibolone combines oestrogenic and progestogenic activity with weak androgenic activity; it is given continuously, without cyclical progestogens.

Primary preventive strategies (screening)

1) *Cervical cancer screening.* The NHS cervical cancer screening programme offers cervical smear testing (liquid based cytology) every 3 years (if aged 25–49 years) or every 5 years (if aged 50–64 years). Women aged ≥65 years who have had three consecutive negative results are taken out of the call–recall system, as the risk of developing cervical cancer thereafter is virtually non-existent. However, cervical smears may still be appropriate if the woman has had a history of treatment for cervical dysplasia. Similarly, women who have undergone hysterectomy for cervical dysplasia, carcinoma *in situ*, or endometrial cancer, would require vaginal vault smears to continue on a yearly basis, as there remains a 10% risk of vaginal cuff recurrence.

2) *Breast mammography and breast self-examination.* The NHS Breast Screening Programme offers breast screening every 3 years for all women aged between 50 and 70 years. Women aged >70 years can have screening mammograms on request.

3) *Annual gynaecological pelvic ultrasound or pelvic examination.* The rationale for an annual gynaecological examination (pelvic or ultrasound) would be to detect cancer (mainly vulval, ovarian and uterine types) at an early stage and intervene before the cancer has significantly spread. However, there is no evidence to show that routine population-wide annual gynaecological examination or pelvic ultrasound improves cancer detection and survival. A 10 year study of screening for ovarian cancer (UKCTOCS) is currently underway. The purpose of this study is to determine whether transvaginal ultrasound or serum CA125 testing will detect ovarian cancer at an early stage when treatment is more effective and therefore reduce the number of deaths due to the disease.

4) *Genetic screening.* Women with first-degree family histories of breast or ovarian cancer extending to two or more relatives may be referred to a clinical geneticist for genetic screening. Identification of defective *BRCA1* or *BRCA2* genes has an estimated lifetime risk of developing ovarian cancer of ~50%.

Conclusion: key learning points

- Be vigilant for an underlying abdomino-pelvic malignancy when asked to review—look out for 'red flag' symptoms and signs.

- Ensure that assessment and treatment are individualized; in particular, consider co-morbidities and her functional level (the extent of any physical or cognitive dysfunction).

- Postmenopausal bleeding must be considered as uterine cancer until proven otherwise, and requires urgent assessment and rapid gynaecological referral.

- The benefits of short-term HRT outweigh the risks in the majority of women wishing treatment for their menopausal symptoms who are aged <60 years.

- Pelvic floor physiotherapy is beneficial in restoring urinary continence in women with stress, urge, or mixed urinary incontinence conditions.

- Transvaginal sonography combined with hysteroscopy and endometrial biopsy is considered the gold standard investigation for postmenopausal bleeding.

- All women with possible lichen sclerosus should have this confirmed by vulval biopsy.

Further reading

Clark TJ, Barton PM, Coomarasamy A, Gupta JK, Khan KS. Investigating postmenopausal bleeding for endometrial cancer: cost-effectiveness of initial diagnostic strategies. *Br J Obstet Gynaecol* 2006;113: 502–510.

Eve Appeal/Ovacome. *Ovarian Cancer UK Consensus Statement*. Available at: http://www.ovacome.org.uk/Resources/OvarianCancerUKConsensusStatement/consensus_statement.pdf

Davey DA. Hormone replacement therapy: time to move on?. *J Br Menopause Soc* 2006;12:75–80.

Moroney JW, Zahn CM. Common gynecologic problems in geriatric-aged women. *Clin Obstet Gynecol* 2007;50:687–708.

National Collaborating Centre for Women's and Children's Health. *Urinary Incontinence. The Management of Urinary Incontinence in Women*. NICE Clinical Guideline 40. London: National Institute for Health and Clinical Excellence; 2006.

Pitkin J, Rees MC, Gray S, *et al*. Managing the menopause: BMS Council Consensus statement on HRT. *J Br Menopause Soc* 2004;10:33–36.

Royal College of Obstetricians and Gynaecologists. *Ovarian Cysts in Postmenopausal Women*. RCOG Green Top Guideline No. 34. London: RCOG Press; 2003.

Royal College of Obstetricians and Gynaecologists. *Management of Vulval Cancer*. Working Party Report. London: RCOG; 2006.

Chapter 22

Psychiatry

David Anderson and Jim George

Introduction

The ageing population around the world is now recognized as one of the greatest challenges facing all health economies. The absolute numbers of older people with mental illness will increase proportionately but because the oldest old are increasing at the greatest rate the demand for health and social care will be disproportionately greater. The prevalence of mental disorder in the community is shown in Table 22.1. Lesser degrees of psychological distress will affect a similar number.

When there are high concentrations of people with physical illness, disability and social adversity the prevalence of mental illness rises. This is most obvious with depression. In contrast to younger adults the older population is characterized by multi-morbidity, requiring more knowledge and understanding of the interaction between physical and mental health. Older people tend to have a different set of psychosocial needs, obviating the requirement for a strong bio-psycho-social approach.

A close personal working relationship with mental health services for older people will enable primary care physicians to manage patients more successfully, often with advice and shared care. These services are based on a multidisciplinary team model that involves different disciplines at different times determined by the needs of the patient. They have a strong community focus, attempting to provide all services to patients' homes wherever possible. Psychiatrists, community mental health nurses, social workers, occupational therapists and psychologists form the core.

Dementia and depression are the most common conditions, and for primary care new cases of these will occur with a frequency of nine and 24 per 1000 population aged >65 years per year respectively.[1,2] The increasing numbers and emphasis on early diagnosis means that primary care will need to develop capacity and skills to detect and treat more mental illness in old age.

A study of elderly primary care attenders in Greater Manchester found that 26.1% had a diagnosable mental disorder (9.6% organic, 16.5% depression) and an additional 33.9% displayed psychological distress (mostly anxiety, phobic and undifferentiated depressive symptoms).[3] Despite high levels of psychological distress, detection of mental health problems by the primary care team was low and decision to treat or refer those cases detected was rare.

Only one-third of older people with depression discuss it with their general practitioner (GP) and less than half of these receive treatment. Nearly half of older people who commit suicide visit their GP in the preceding month.[4] The highest rate of suicide is among older people, who are the only age group in the UK where suicide rates have not declined. Less than half of people with dementia have a formal diagnosis and only 30% of GPs feel they have sufficient knowledge and skills to diagnose and manage dementia.[5]

The principles of assessment are those of medicine in general, namely a comprehensive history (including third parties), mental state examination, medical investigation, diagnosis and treatment plan. A large number of instruments are available for screening and diagnosis but nothing can replace the skills of history-taking and examination and engagement with patients and carers. Indeed, immediate engagement will form the basis of the doctor–patient relationship that will provide the foundation of successful treatment and outcome.

Table 22.1 Community prevalence of diagnosable mental disorders in individuals aged >65 years (%)

Dementia	5
Depression	10–15
Delirium	1–2
Neurotic disorders	2–5
Alcohol misuse	2–4
Total	20–30

Assessment and diagnostic instruments

Well in excess of 100 instruments to detect, rate and diagnose cognitive impairment, dementia, depression and mental distress have been described and extensively reviewed.[6,7] They can provide useful information, but do not provide clinical solutions and do not replace a comprehensive medical and psychiatric assessment. There is no evidence to support the use of routine screening for dementia or depression in primary care at this time.

If used, GPs should become familiar with only a few instruments and understand their values and limitations. All tests are influenced by a number of factors that can give spurious results and those designed for younger people may need to be interpreted differently with older people, particularly those with multiple morbidity, frailty and sensory impairments.

Typically, shorter cognitive tests such as the Mini Mental State Examination (MMSE)[8] do not test frontal/executive function, and this means that some dementias may be missed. Longer tests have a small additional benefit in sensitivity and specificity and have a role in defining patterns of cognitive loss, and to rate disease severity.

The six-item screener (SIS) is an example of a short test which can be used as part of an initial general practice consultation. It takes only 2 min to perform and consists of three orientation questions (day, month, year) and a three-item recall task derived from the MMSE (Box 22.1). A score of ≤3 suggests cognitive impairment.

The MMSE is a 30-point assessment test which takes ~10 min to perform. It has been adopted by the National Institute for Health and Clinical Excellence (NICE) guidelines for the evaluation of dementia. Scores of ≤25 for patients who have had a secondary school education suggest significant cognitive impairment. Though not designed to rate severity, the NICE guideline and clinical trials usually consider a score of 18–26 mild, 12–17 moderate and <12 severe dementia once the diagnosis is made.[9] The score is affected by a number of variables other than cognitive impairment, including educational attainment, sensory deficits and physical illness.

A more comprehensive test, which also tests for executive function and is an extension of the MMSE, is the Addenbrooke cognitive examination (ACE) which takes ~20 min to complete.

Box 22.1 Six-item screener (SIS)

1.	Day.
2.	Month.
3.	Year.
4–6.	Three-item recall after 2 min, e.g. apple, table, piano.

Total score: 6.

The Geriatric Depression Scale (GDS) is probably the most widely used screen for depression validated in older people.[10] The full version consists of 30 questions with yes/no answers taking 5–10 min to complete. It can be self-administered and comes in short versions of 15, 10 and 4 items. With the full version a threshold of 11/30 gives good sensitivity and specificity, and with the 15-item version a threshold of 4/15. It is not suitable for assessing depression in dementia. The Cornell Scale for Depression in Dementia takes 20 min with a carer and 10 min with the patient rating symptoms and signs.[11] Very short scales such as GDS-4 perform acceptably well.[12]

Commonly used scales for depression such as the Hamilton Depression Rating Scale may not be suitable for elderly people. The GDS deliberately avoids somatic symptoms which can artificially inflate depression ratings if people have certain significant physical disorders.

GPs should be able to use a simple screening test, such as the SIS and GDS, and be aware of their limitations and at least be familiar with the MMSE and ACE, which may be used by specialist services as part of a comprehensive assessment.

Dementia, delirium and cognitive impairment

As we age our intellectual function becomes less efficient and people often notice a decline in mental agility and memory. When this is accompanied by some demonstrable mild impairment of cognitive performance, the term mild cognitive impairment (MCI) is used. Although it may not signify a disease process, complaints of this sort should not be ignored. At least 10% of people with MCI convert to a diagnosis of dementia per year, suggesting that for some it is the very early stage of dementia and, while there are no certain ways of identifying these individuals, they perform worse on simple cognitive tests at the outset than those who do not progress.[13] At this stage, alternative causes should be considered, for example depression, prescribed medication, alcohol, or physical illness.

Of people referred to a memory clinic, 30% do not have a diagnosable disorder.[14] They should be honestly reassured and reviewed for the changes of dementia.

Dementia

Dementia is a clinical syndrome of progressive intellectual decline that is usually irreversible and occurs in the absence of clouded consciousness. Clouded consciousness is a sign of delirium. If a person with dementia develops clouded consciousness (states of drowsiness), or their condition rapidly deteriorates, then superimposed delirium should be suspected and an acute physical illness sought. This situation is not unusual, as dementia is a major risk factor for the development of delirium which is a common presentation of acute physical illness in people with dementia.

Increasing age is the strongest risk factor for dementia, with prevalence increasing quite rapidly beyond age 65 years (Table 22.2). Only 2.2% present when aged <65 years (young onset) and, even among the oldest old, the majority do not have dementia, implying that this is not normal ageing. People from Black and ethnic minority groups are prone to develop dementia younger (6.1% young onset) and have a higher risk for vascular dementia.

Dementia costs public services more than cancer, heart disease and stroke combined. The current cost in the UK is £17 billion per annum, with a third of that borne by informal carers, and predicted to rise three-fold by 2050.[15]

The management of dementia is like that of any long-term condition and it is helpful to have a structured approach (Table 22.3). It is a terminal condition and models of palliative care can be a helpful framework.

Early diagnosis and intervention are important. They give an opportunity for patients and carers to receive essential information and plan for their future, while patients are able to make their wishes known and make provisions for a time when they may have impaired decision-making

Table 22.2 Prevalence of dementia by age

Age (years)	Female (%)	Male (%)	Total (%)
65–69	1.0	1.5	1.3
70–74	2.4	3.1	2.9
75–79	6.5	5.1	5.9
80–84	13.3	10.2	12.2
85–89	22.2	16.7	20.3
90–94	29.6	27.5	28.6
≥95	34.4	30.0	32.5

Source: Alzheimer´s Society (2007).

capacity, for example financial management, wills, advance directives. Early intervention produces long-term gains by reducing cost of care at later stages.

Success depends on engaging carers positively from the first contact, understanding the person's circumstances and their life story, a good initial assessment, reliable diagnosis with a focused approach to problems, and ensuring easy access to services as they become necessary.

Necessarily, the assessment must be holistic, taking account of carers' needs and patients' conditions. It is useful to explore three domains: (i) cognitive; (ii) functional; (iii) behavioural. As dementia progresses, it is the functional and behavioural that will usually cause most difficulty and distress for patients and carers. In the early stages, cognitive problems dominate. Function includes activities of daily living (washing, dressing, toileting, feeding) and instrumental activities of daily living (complex tasks like finance, shopping, cooking). The more complex tasks will usually cause problems first.

Step 1: syndrome diagnosis

Recognition of the syndrome dementia depends on a history of progressive cognitive decline, i.e. it is cognitive, becoming worse and interfering with normal function. By the time patients present

Table 22.3 Structured approach to managing dementia

Syndrome diagnosis	History MSE Life story Engage patient/carer	Progressive intellectual loss Full consciousness
Pathological diagnosis	Investigations Course Features	Irreversible v treatable
Problem list	Treat reversible illness Risk assessment	Root analysis
Problem solving	Primary loss/dependence BPSD/analysis Carers/carer breakdown Co-morbid health	Compensatory services Focussed intervention Anticipate/supports Optimal treatment
Monitor	Identify individual	What to do

to a doctor, the history is usually of ~12 months' duration. Ideally, the history should come from a third party informant, and such a history from someone who knows the person well is a reliable indicator of dementia even when measured cognitive impairment is mild.

A mental state examination, concentrating on cognitive function, is performed to confirm impairment and give an idea of the severity.

Step 2: pathological diagnosis

Dementia always has an underlying organic pathology and >95% will be due to an irreversible neurodegenerative disorder. In a small number it can be caused by a potentially treatable condition (Box 22.2).

In most cases the neurodegenerative cause can only be confirmed by postmortem examination but, in life, the course of the dementia and associated medical features allow a reliable probable diagnosis for most, and this is important for the patient, carer and management. In 35% of cases postmortem shows two or more neurodegenerative diseases, usually combinations of Alzheimer, cerebrovascular and Lewy body pathologies, and these are more difficult to recognize.

Alzheimer's disease (AD) is responsible for 60% of all dementia. Insidious in onset, people often cannot pin-point the time of onset. It starts with short-term memory problems; risk factors include a positive family history, vascular risk factors, Down syndrome and depression. Three causative gene abnormalities are now identified with autosomal dominant inheritance but accounting for <5% of all cases. These are referred to as familial AD. Neurological signs only occur very late in the disease.

Vascular (VD), either pure or mixed, is responsible for 5%. Several subtypes exist though the most common is multi-infarct. It may date precisely from events such as stroke or transient cerebral ischaemia and typically follows a stepwise deterioration. Location, frequency and size of lesions can make presentation and course unpredictable. Neurological signs may occur early. An exception is small vessel vascular disease, for example that accompanying diabetes mellitus. Individuals with type II diabetes—which often develops insidiously, like AD—are 1.6 times more likely to develop dementia (both AD and VD). Typically vascular risk factors are present and the risk is much higher in those of African-Caribbean descent.

Lewy body disease is responsible for ~10% of all dementia cases. Classical dementia with Lewy bodies (DLB) is a triad: (i) fluctuating cognitive impairment; (ii) visual hallucination; (iii) parkinsonism. The diagnosis is more difficult when the complete triad is not present. Several symptoms that support the diagnosis are described, including rapid eye movement (REM) sleep disorder and unexplained falls.[16]

Box 22.2 Treatable causes of dementia

- Depression
- Severe anaemia
- Organ failure: cardiorespiratory, renal, hepatic
- Endocrine: hypothyroid
- Chronic infection: tuberculosis, syphilis
- Tumours: cerebral, primary, metastatic
- Subdural haematoma
- Normal pressure hydrocephalus

If a patient with Parkinson's disease of >12 months' duration develops dementia this is, by convention, called Parkinson's disease dementia (PDD), and up to 80% of people with PD develop dementia over an 8 year period.[17] If dementia occurs with <12 months' duration it is called DLB. The prevailing view is that these conditions are part of a spectrum of Lewy body disease and the clinical symptoms relate to the distribution of Lewy bodies in the brain.

Frontotemporal dementia (FTD) used to be called Pick disease. Whereas most of the common dementias present with short-term memory impairment, this is an exception. The presentation is with frontal lobe syndrome (decline of personal and social standards, personality change, poor judgement and insight, urinary incontinence) with or without progressive problems of language.

The early cognitive changes in the more common dementias involve memory and orientation but this is not invariable. It is not the case in FTD and may not be so in PDD or DLB. In the Lewy body diseases the most common early features are related to poor concentration, attention and dysexecutive symptoms. The dysexecutive syndrome is the inability to translate an intention or plan into productive self-serving activity needing to initiate, sustain, switch and stop sequences of complex behaviour in an orderly and integrated manner. It is rather like the difficulty with movement experienced by people with PD. This description will only come from the history, and routinely used instruments, such as the MMSE, will not reveal these problems.

Other, less common conditions typically have characteristic neurological signs or family history, e.g. PD, Huntington disease, Creutzfeldt–Jakob disease.

Routine investigations are essential for all cases of suspected dementia and NICE now extends this to include neuroimaging (Box 22.3). These investigations are primarily to exclude treatable conditions; however, in the hands of skilled neuroradiologists, neuroimaging can now provide more diagnostic information. Nevertheless, neuroimaging alone will rarely give the pathological diagnosis unless considered in the context of the clinical features.

Clinical situations which require more urgent investigation include:

◆ Short histories (<6 months).

◆ Atypical presentations.

◆ Early unexplained peripheral neurological signs.

Box 22.3 Investigation of suspected dementia[a]

1. Routine haematology.
2. Biochemistry (electrolytes, calcium, glucose, renal and liver function).
3. Thyroid function tests.
4. Serum vitamin B_{12} and folate.

Neuroimaging

MRI or CT (MRI preferred).

(HMPAO) SPECT (differentiate Alzheimer's disease, vascular dementia, frontotemporal dementia, if diagnosis in doubt).

(FP-CIT) SPECT (assist diagnosis dementia with Lewy bodies if in doubt).

[a] Source: National Institute for Health and Clinical Excellence.[9]

MRI, magnetic resonance imaging; CT, computed tomography; HMPAO, ^{99m}Tc-hexamethyl propyleneamine oxime; SPECT, single photon emission computed tomography; FP-CIT, fluoropropyl-carbomethoxy-iodophenyl-tropan.

Step 3: identify problem list and problem-solving

Patients and carers usually consult a doctor because problems are beginning, though with increasing public awareness they are seeking advice much earlier when still independent, wanting diagnosis and treatment. All people want information, and providing the diagnosis in a way which the patient and carers can understand should be routine. One advantage of early diagnosis is the opportunity to involve patients in a fully informed way and allow discussion of prognosis, anticipated difficulties and life planning. Diagnosis is usually reassuring for patients. It is the unknown that creates fear.

General advice:

- Maintain mental stimulation (conversation, social interaction, keeping abreast of news, word games, crosswords, bingo).
- Sensible physical exercise.
- Good healthy diet.
- Optimal treatment of medical conditions and reduce vascular risk.
- Healthy lifestyle advice on smoking and alcohol use.

There is no evidence that over-the-counter remedies such as vitamin supplements or herbal remedies are useful.

Supplementary advice:

- Despite difficulties, people should be encouraged to live as full and rewarding a life as possible.
- Inevitably, cognitive problems create frustration and sometimes conflict with carers, though staying calm and avoiding arguments will facilitate cognitive performance.
- People should be encouraged to be active, independent and work things out for themselves, with carers stepping in only when it is clear that the patient is struggling to manage.
- *Aide-mèmoires*, such as keeping a diary, calendar, watch, and keeping all important things in one place (keys, bills, pension book) will help orientation and recall.
- Familiar surroundings and routines using long-term memory reduces risk of mistakes. Long-term memory is more resistant to damage.
- A sense of humour helps everyone.

Each patient's situation is unique and so will the problem list be, but they will usually fall into certain categories. Understanding the origin of the difficulty is the key to finding the most appropriate intervention.

Primary problems

Primary problems are the direct consequences of lost cognitive abilities. Therefore, short-term memory impairment leads to losing things, forgetting appointments, medication or to switch off the gas; dyspraxia: inability to dress; agnosia: difficulty recognizing simple objects; calculation: difficulty managing money, etc. These problems lead to increasing dependence on other people to perform daily tasks.

The response usually requires mobilizing domiciliary services and shared care with informal carers.

Because the consequence of short-term memory impairment is the inability to learn new information, established routine and familiar surroundings that rely on intact long-term memory are helpful. This helps the person stay oriented and reduces the chance of mistakes that create risk.

Part of this process involves evaluating and minimizing risk. Occupational therapists can be particularly helpful in this process.

Secondary problems

Secondary problems are the behavioural and psychological symptoms of dementia (BPSD). These are more complex and require an analysis of root cause. There may be multiple aetiological factors, therefore do not assume it is all just due to brain failure. Ninety-five per cent of people will develop these problems at some point in their dementia, becoming more common as the condition progresses. Though they often resolve spontaneously they are frequently replaced by a different set of symptoms.[18]

Psychiatric symptoms can be approached in the same way as they would be in a person without dementia. For example, depression might be related to loneliness, boredom, pain, separation, and loss, etc. Treatment could include antidepressants, social intervention or analgesia. Often, particularly in more severe stages, depression is expressed in atypical ways such as recent irritability or aggression, restlessness, social withdrawal, resistance to care, non-compliance, food refusal and insomnia.

Behavioural symptoms require a good description of what actually takes place. Words like 'aggression' or 'wandering' are used loosely to mean many different things. Verbal abuse in someone who has always been abusive is different to indiscriminate violence. People in care homes who are only physically aggressive during personal care usually do not understand what is happening to them and need more skilful carers, not drugs. But people who are violent because they believe they are being poisoned or are visually hallucinating may need an antipsychotic drug. Sudden behavioural change may indicate delirium secondary to an acute physical illness.

Knowing patients' life stories is not an academic exercise, for it may well explain their behaviour later in the disease when familiar patterns become pervasive. It will give opportunities to prevent problems and improve quality of life when their pre-morbid personality, likes, dislikes and routines are appreciated and can form the basis of personalized care plans.

The problem may not be the patient, but rather the care environment. If carers are not equipped to meet the needs of a patient, the response may need to be training or a change of care environment rather than doing something to the patient to make them compliant with an unsuitable situation.

Persistent behaviour problems are a major determinant of moving to 24 h care.

Tertiary problems

Tertiary problems are those of the carers, and these may be the critical problem. Carers are the mainstay of all management. Engagement with them and understanding their aims at the outset will prove critical. Fifty per cent of carers become depressed and this will affect their ability to care effectively. Their problems may arise from other aspects of their lives, their ability to adjust to the distress of dementia, competing demands on their time through work and their own families. Surveys of carers find that the majority, at some time, have felt under such stress that they become frustrated by the person with dementia and lose their temper. The resultant verbal or physical abuse creates guilt, adds to their own distress and may lead to more serious abuse.

The result of unrelieved carer stress is carer breakdown, and this will usually herald a move into 24 h care. Unsupported, isolated carers and those who have a poor pre-morbid relationship with the patient are likely to break with care more quickly.

The prevention of carer breakdown will be facilitated by their close involvement in the care plan, recognizing their aims and limitations early, and by access to good support systems. Carer groups, Alzheimer's Society, day care, respite care, flexible and reliable care which is easy to access are important.

A useful shorthand approach to the problems of dementia is given by the 4 Ds: Describe (the problem), Decode (the real problem), Devise (a treatment plan) and Determine (if it works).

Contributing causes that need to be Decoded are cognitive impairment, psychiatric symptoms/syndromes, physical/medical problems, environmental factors and carer approach. The Determine emphasizes the need to be specific about the aims of an intervention with clear and measurable goals to evaluate response.

Step 4: physical health

Optimal control of all physical health problems is essential, including sensory deficits, bowel function, dentition, foot care. Any of these may become the cause of BPSD either directly or by precipitating a delirium, and may only become apparent by a sudden deterioration of behaviour or function. Good physical health care will provide the best protection for failing cognitive reserves and reduce the likelihood of complicating disability.

Step 5: monitoring

By definition, dementia is progressive and inevitably changing. Someone will need to perform a monitoring function because the problem list may change and need to be reviewed. Many people can provide this function, for example, doctor, district nurse, health visitor, social worker or informed formal or informal carer. It needs to be clear who does this and what they should do if needs change.

People's circumstances, not just their dementia, may change: new physical illness or disability, loss of carer or carer's health, change of domicile or change in carer's circumstances. All may impact on the problem list.

Drug treatments

It is important to consider the prescription of psychoactive medications to people with dementia. Organic brain disease reduces tolerance with greater susceptibility to adverse effects, particularly sedation and balance. Anticholinergic drugs have the potential to impair cognitive function and should be avoided. Antipsychotic drugs may cause parkinsonism, sedation and falls and reduce life expectancy in dementia.

Cognitive enhancers

In the UK the acetylcholinesterase inhibitors donepezil, rivastigmine and galantamine are licensed for mild and moderate AD. Rivastigmine is also licensed for PDD. NICE recommends they only be used for moderate AD based on cost-effectiveness, though they can also be used for the treatment of psychotic symptoms in DLB if these do not respond to other approaches or atypical antipsychotic drugs.[9]

There is no evidence that they differ in effect in clinical situations even though they have slightly different pharmacological properties. They are generally well tolerated and the most common adverse effects are gastrointestinal. There are contraindications, notably cardiac conduction defects, asthma and peptic ulceration.

They are initiated by specialist services but can be monitored under shared care arrangements between primary and secondary care. Response should be reviewed every 6 months.

BPSD

No other psychoactive drugs are licensed specifically for use in dementia but the indications for psychotropic drugs are essentially the indications in people without dementia. If a person with dementia is sufficiently depressed, antidepressants should be prescribed, but those with high anticholinergic properties should be avoided. Psychosocial interventions are appropriate for milder depression.[9]

Antipsychotic drugs are indicated for the treatment of psychotic symptoms, such as hallucinations, delusions and severe agitation or aggression. There is evidence that these drugs are overprescribed and not reviewed, particularly in care homes.[19] The rule is: only prescribe for these specific problems; when severe and distressing; only when non-pharmacological approaches are ineffective or unsuitable; review benefit and consider drug withdrawal if symptoms are controlled for 3 months because some will spontaneously resolve in that time. Atypical antipsychotics are preferred because of safety profile and traditional antipsychotics avoided, but none should be prescribed casually.

If distressing psychotic or behavioural symptoms in DLB fail to respond then cholinesterase inhibitors can eliminate psychotic symptoms in 50% of cases.[20]

People with dementia are more sensitive to the adverse effects of psychotropic drugs, which should only be necessary in very small doses. Caution is recommended with the use of olanzapine and risperidone because of the small increased risk (2–3% absolute risk) of cerebral ischaemia, though it is not clear whether this is specific to them or to a class effect of atypical or all antipsychotic drugs. The best available evidence of effectiveness for psychosis and severe agitation is for olanzapine and risperidone. There should be particular caution in DLB and PDD because of the neuroleptic sensitivity syndrome (sedation, rigidity, postural instability, falls, confusion, mortality increased two- to three-fold). In all of these cases the risk:benefit ratio needs to be considered carefully and discussed with patients and carers.

Other

Insomnia can be a difficult problem for patient and carer, and simple sedatives for short-term use can be used. Dependence, particularly in moderate and severe stages, does not have quite the same importance as usual. Benzodiazepines impair cognitive function to a small degree, though of uncertain clinical significance, and this is related more to duration of use than to dose.[21]

The evidence base for the effectiveness of psychotropic drugs in FTD is particularly poor but serotonin reuptake inhibitors can be helpful. Trazodone, a predominantly serotonin reuptake inhibitor, is quite sedative and can be effective as night sedation and for agitated behaviour.

If this range of approaches is unhelpful then specialist advice should be sought.

Driving and dementia

Unfortunately, there are no validated assessment tools with standardized thresholds currently available for clinicians to assess fitness to drive.[22] The Driver and Vehicle Licensing Agency (DVLA) stresses the importance of a holistic clinical assessment of the ability to drive.

It is recognized that the course of a dementia can be variable but patients with dementia must inform the DVLA of their diagnosis, and the issue of a licence may be subject to an annual review. GPs may need to give a medical report and patients with very poor short-term memory, disorientation and lack of insight or judgement are almost certainly not able to drive. A formal driving assessment may be necessary in borderline cases.[23] In extreme cases, where the general public may be put at risk, then it may be necessary for the doctor to discuss with relatives or carers removal of the vehicle and to inform the DVLA directly of concerns.

It is the patient's responsibility to inform the DVLA (similarly their insurer, otherwise their insurance will be invalid) but the doctor should also advise a relative as the patient may forget this information. If a patient refuses to do so, or there is no relative, then it may be necessary for the doctor to inform the DVLA; if there is genuine concern about safety of the public, this professional obligation would not be considered a breach of confidentiality.

Stopping driving in a patient with dementia should never be undertaken lightly as it has many negative consequences, limiting access to family, friends and services.[23] The risk of an accident seems to be acceptably low for up to 3 years after the onset of dementia.[23]

Delirium

Delirium (acute confusional state) is present in ~20% of older patients admitted to hospital and also 1–2% of older people in the community.[24] Delirium is often unrecognized in older people and has a high morbidity and mortality. National guidelines have been produced in order to improve its detection and management in both hospital and community settings.[25]

The key to successful management is early detection and treatment of the underlying physical cause.

The cardinal features of delirium are recent onset of cognitive impairment with fluctuating awareness, impaired attention and disorganized thinking (Box 22.4). Patients with delirium often have pre-existing dementia (acute on chronic confusion) and dementia is a recognized risk factor for delirium. Patients with delirium may present with visual hallucinations or paranoid delusions and sometimes it is the first presentation of pre-existing dementia. Delirium is due to an underlying medical cause, e.g. drugs, drug or alcohol withdrawal, infection, metabolic or electrolyte disturbance. Commonly with older people there may be multiple contributing causes, e.g. a recent medication change in an elderly man with a chest infection, constipation and urinary retention and vascular dementia.

Delirium has three clinical forms:

- Hyperactive: the older person is restless, agitated and wandering.
- Hypoactive: the patient appears drowsy and apathetic (sometimes mistaken for depression).
- Mixed hyperactive/hypoactive.

Risk factors for delirium include increasing age, dementia, severe illness, dehydration, renal impairment, visual impairment and polypharmacy. It is important for GPs to recognize delirium in its early stages (especially the hypoactive type which has a higher mortality) and treat the underlying cause, or causes, promptly as this may prevent social care breakdown and admission to hospital. A few simple blood tests, e.g. full blood count, urea and electrolytes, C-reactive protein, calcium and liver function tests—combined with a physical examination and a drug history—will identify most causes of delirium. In addition, mid-stream specimens of urine may be useful in identifying an underlying urinary tract infection, but only if this is clinically suspected, because asymptomatic bacteriuria is common in frail older people and can often be an incidental finding. Similarly, a chest X-ray in selected cases may help to diagnose heart failure or chest infection.

Common drug causes of delirium are listed in Box 22.5. Drugs with potent anticholinergic properties are particularly implicated. Alcohol withdrawal is a common cause and needs specific treatment in hospital with benzodiazepines and intravenous thiamine replacement. In other

Box 22.4 Clinical features of delirium in older people

- Recent onset of confusion or increased confusion.
- Fluctuation of symptoms.
- Cognitive impairment.
- Impairment of attention/concentration, e.g. difficulty counting backwards from 20 to 1.
- May have reduced conscious level, visual hallucinations, paranoid delusions, disturbance of sleep/wake cycle.
- An underlying physical cause, e.g. drugs, drug or alcohol withdrawal, infection or metabolic/ electrolyte disturbance.

Box 22.5 Common drugs which can cause delirium in older people

- ◆ Analgesics: especially tramadol, codeine and morphine.
- ◆ Sedatives: especially benzodiazepines and benzodiazepine withdrawal.
- ◆ Antidepressants: especially tricyclic antidepressants.
- ◆ Steroids.
- ◆ Anticholinergic drugs: especially oxybutinin.
- ◆ Cardiac drugs: especially digoxin (check level).
- ◆ Anti-parkinsonian drugs: especially dopamine agonists (reduce or stop if possible).

forms of delirium, sedation should be avoided as far as possible as it may worsen outcomes and lead to complications, such as falls and pressure sores. However, for patients who put themselves, or others, at risk because of severe delusions, hallucinations or agitation, then small doses of haloperidol (0.5–1.0 mg) may be needed, but only in the short term. An alternative for patients with parkinsonism is lorazepam at a similar dose.

GPs can help to prevent delirium in older people by avoiding drugs that cause delirium and by ensuring that older people have prompt treatment for chest and urinary tract infections; also by taking steps to avoid dehydration in vulnerable older people, especially in nursing and residential homes.

Depression and mood disorder

Depression is the most common mental health problem in older people and an excellent review is provided by Alexopoulos.[26] Older people with depression have an increased mortality rate (3-fold in males, 2-fold in females). It is considered an independent risk factor for cardiovascular disease with effect equivalent to that for smoking and diabetes.[27] Untreated and unresolved depression are associated with the greatest risk.[28]

It is the commonest cause of suicide and self-harm. Older people who self-harm should always be taken seriously as most will have a mental disorder and the risk of subsequent suicide is significant. Older people expressing suicidal ideas are more likely to commit suicide than younger people and use more violent methods, especially males. Age is a major risk factor for suicide.

A 20 year follow-up of older people presenting with self-harm found that 75% involved high suicidal intent and only 15.3% were under psychiatric treatment; 23.7% had a history of self-harm and 41.3% had previous psychiatric treatment. They commonly had co-existing physical illness (46.1%), social isolation (33.5%), relationship problems with family or partner (29.4%, 25.9% respectively) and bereavement or loss (16.7%). In the subsequent 20 years, death by suicide and open verdict were 49 and 33 times, respectively, more frequent than expected by population death rates.[29]

The defining symptoms are the same for all adults. It is much more common in people with physical illness and disability (Table 22.4). Older people with physical handicap are five times more likely to suffer depression. The health burden of depression is substantial and incrementally worsens health in combination with long-term conditions, producing the greatest decrement in health when compared to angina, arthritis, asthma or diabetes mellitus.[30]

Table 22.4 Prevalence of depression with co-morbidity (%)

Care homes	16–44
General hospital	29
Primary care attenders	30
Dementia	25
Neurological disorders	24
Parkinson's disease	50
Huntington disease	40
Stroke acute	25
Stroke at 12 months	16
Stroke at 36 months	30
Myocardial infarction	
Acute and at 12 months	15–30
Coronary heart disease	
Major depression	20
Minor depression	27
Cancer	20
COPD clinic	42

COPD, chronic obstructive pulmonary disease.

In some physical conditions it is the major predictor of quality of life and outcome. The apathy and hopelessness of depression may lead to non-compliance with treatment of physical illness, failed attendance at appointments, serious neglect and a variety of poor outcomes (Box 22.6)

Depression in older people often has more serious consequences than younger adults. In severe depression and advanced old age, cognitive impairment may be prominent and lead to a false diagnosis of dementia (depressive pseudodementia). Despite some variations in the way depression presents in older people, the core features are the same and may be elicited with simple questions. It is worth considering in some less obvious clinical scenarios (Box 22.7).

The main risk factors are being female, previous depression, family history of depression, bereavement, other loss events, physical illness, disability and handicap and psychosocial adversity. Protective factors include being married, having a confidante, good physical health and religious faith.

It is also now recognized that some people develop depression in association with vascular brain disease. This was discovered with the advent of magnetic resonance imaging and led to the concept of vascular depression.[31] This association was found to respond less well to conventional antidepressants and have a poorer prognosis. It seems likely that vascular brain disease acts as just another aetiological risk factor, particularly when there is evidence of large lesions in the anterior frontal and basal ganglia areas.[32]

Assessment

The core features are elicited from a mental state examination. This should also gauge the severity of the disorder. All patients with depression should be asked about suicidal thoughts and this evaluated in terms of risk of self-harm. Most people with depression have had fleeting thoughts

Box 22.6 Consequences of depression

◆ Increased mortality.

◆ Increased death by suicide and open verdict.

◆ Increased health burden.

◆ Poorer outcome of depression.

◆ Poorer outcome of physical health.

◆ Worse quality of life.

◆ More medical investigations.

◆ More prescribed treatment.

◆ Worse independent function.

◆ Worse health care compliance.

◆ Predicts readmission to general hospital.

◆ Greater health and social care cost.

of this sort, and as the severity increases they become more prominent. An older person with suicidal thoughts needs prompt specialist assessment.

The examination should determine how prominent suicidal thinking has become and whether there have been any plans on method or intention. Contrary to common concerns, patients are usually relieved to be able to discuss these thoughts which typically worry them and sometimes invoke guilt. Thoughts of hopelessness, guilt and being a burden should raise concern.

Psychomotor disturbance with either marked retardation or agitation is a sign of more severe depression.

Rare, but most serious, is the presence of psychotic symptoms. These are usually described as mood congruent, i.e. consistent with the negative and morbid thought processes of a depressed

Box 22.7 Scenarios in which to consider depression

◆ Cognitive impairment.

◆ Non-compliance.

◆ Failure to attend appointments.

◆ Frequent attendance.

◆ Unexplained deterioration of physical health.

◆ Increased alcohol use.

◆ Increased use of analgesics, hypnotics, tranquillizers.

◆ Increased isolation.

◆ Anorexia, weight loss, insomnia.

◆ Self-harm.

◆ Medically unexplained symptoms.

person. Occasionally they are not, and this can confuse diagnosis. Mood-congruent delusions commonly involve guilt (having done bad things, needing punishment, being wicked or bad, undeserving) or are hypochondriacal (having terminal or infectious diseases that could infect others); examples may include a belief in being poisoned, or people trying to kill them or their family. Hallucinations are less common and usually auditory (threatening, accusatory voices saying that they are bad), olfactory (smelling their disease or rotting), gustatory or somatic.

Typically, depressed people are preoccupied with their deficiencies and are self-critical. When more severe they can be importuning and plead for help. Preoccupation with physical symptoms is not uncommon. A useful clue to the presence of depression is that the company of a depressed person usually makes one feel sad.

With a good history and thoughtful mental state examination the presence of depression is not difficult to detect but it is important to be sure that there is no physical health problem to explain symptoms, particularly when somatic symptoms are prominent. Knowledge of medical history supplemented by simple blood count, biochemical profile and thyroid function as a baseline are usually sufficient.

Finally, social aspects of depression, either aetiological or part of a treatment plan, must be considered. This may involve loneliness, isolation, care needs, consequences of physical ill health or disability. Alcohol misuse may develop as a secondary problem.

Treatment

Evidence indicates that, even when recognized, depression in older people is undertreated. This may be related to the misconception that depression in later life is a normal reaction or has poor prognosis, and to the old-fashioned dichotomy of endogenous versus reactive depression, implying that antidepressants were only indicated when depression was endogenous, and that reactive depression is 'just life'. This dichotomy is obsolete as it is now recognized that depression often follows life events and that antidepressants relieve symptoms regardless of antecedents.

On the contrary, treating early and vigorously should be the rule because long duration of symptoms and incomplete recovery are poor prognostic factors for the longer term.

If depression is mild, the preferred approach is psychological, involving problem-solving or cognitive behaviour therapy (CBT). When moderate this may be combined with or replaced by antidepressants. The best results with most sustained effects come from the combination. The more severe the depression the more antidepressant and physical treatments will dominate acute treatment. The evidence shows that older people are as likely to respond to all modalities of treatment as younger adults.[26]

Severe depression and psychotic depression require urgent attention and should be considered psychiatric emergencies. There should be no delay in involving mental health services. Psychotically depressed older people will almost always need admission to hospital.

First-choice antidepressants are selective serotonin reuptake inhibitors (SSRIs) or mirtazapine. The latter is more sedative and, paradoxically, with the lower dose. Of the SSRI group, some pharmacological differences may influence choice. Sertraline and citalopram have least interaction with other drugs; escitalopram is purported to have a faster onset; fluoxetine has a longer active half-life that may be an advantage with erratic compliance; and paroxetine has been most implicated in inducing withdrawal states possibly because of its shorter half-life. Mirtazapine is least likely to interfere with sexual function.

All are relatively safe in overdose. Hyponatraemia is particularly common with SSRIs and this is more likely with older people, especially those taking diuretics—it has been reported in up to 25%, though at symptomatic levels in about half that number. It is worth checking sodium levels a week or two after initiation and also to consider hyponatraemia in people who fail to progress, as the symptoms can be similar to those of depression (e.g. lethargy, anorexia).

It is always worth considering an antidepressant that has been effective if the patient has suffered depression before.

About 60% of people will respond to monotherapy and the response in older people is comparable to younger adults. Traditional wisdom is that response may take 2–3–weeks or more with older people. However, there is some evidence that effects are much quicker in those who go on to make the best recovery.[33]

When patients fail to respond to monotherapy there are a number of strategies available, though the first requirement is to check compliance, as non-compliance is common. First, change to an antidepressant of another class, e.g. swap SSRI to mirtazapine or vice versa. There is no rationale or evidence that changing within class is worthwhile unless there are problems with tolerance.

Treatment resistance

Treatment resistance is taken to mean a failure to respond to treatment with two antidepressants in therapeutic dosage after 6 weeks. The choice of strategy will depend on the severity, previous response and medical factors. Electroconvulsive therapy (ECT) is most effective for psychotic and severe depression. NICE recommends it be used for life-saving situations (psychotic or severe associated with refusal of food and fluids or serious suicide risk) or when all other treatments have failed.

The best evidence is for the addition of lithium salts to an antidepressant (lithium augmentation) and this can produce a quick response. Plasma levels of lithium need careful monitoring and its excretion is entirely dependent on renal clearance. Older people often have impaired renal function, obviating careful dose adjustment, maintenance and monitoring.

Thereafter, the evidence base is poor but considerations include monoamine oxidase inhibitors, anticonvulsants (usually as an alternative to lithium), addition of atypical antipsychotics or various combinations of antidepressants used for monotherapy. More exotic combinations have been advocated but are relevant to very few patients.

Although tricyclic antidepressants are less used now because of their side-effect profile, they remain valuable in treatment resistance. There is some evidence that they may be more effective than new-generation antidepressants for severe depression.

Before embarking on complex drug regimens it is always important to review diagnosis, previous treatments and factors that might be impairing response. Complex treatment should only be managed by specialist services.

Co-morbidity

Depression occurring with co-morbidity is the norm with older people. The choice of antidepressant will be influenced by its effects on these conditions and interaction with other medication. There is no evidence that a particular co-morbidity is best treated with a particular approach but there are developing indicators that depression with particular co-morbidities may differ by causal mechanism and need different approaches. For instance, the best evidence for safety and effectiveness after myocardial infarction or with angina is for sertraline,[34] particularly if depression is severe or recurrent, and SSRI treatment is associated with reduced risk of subsequent death or non-fatal myocardial infarction.[35] SSRIs may have benefits for recovering executive function after stroke;[36] depression with marked executive dysfunction may respond better to behavioural approaches than to antidepressants;[26] and pramipexole (a dopa agonist) has been shown to have antidepressant effects[9] and may be a consideration in Parkinson's disease depression as part of an overall treatment plan.

In general, treating depression with significant co-morbidity is more difficult, though still effective.[37]

Bipolar affective disorder and mania

Bipolar disorder is defined by the patient having suffered hypomania or mania at some time. Its recognition has implications for treatment, especially prophylaxis. Lithium salts or anticonvulsants are the prophylactic agents of choice. A subtype of bipolar disorder is rapid cycling, defined as experiencing four or more episodes per year, and they are commonly lithium resistant. For this group, anticonvulsants seem to be more effective and the emphasis is to concentrate on more effective prophylaxis, because changes in acute phase treatment carry the risk of increasing the cycle frequency. Psychological therapies are also helpful.

Little is known about mania developing for the first time in later life. Most of these patients have a history of depression, 50% having had at least three episodes of depression with the latent period between first depression and first mania usually being 15–20 years.[38] When mania occurs in the absence of a history of depression, thoughtful assessment is required as this can be associated with physical pathology, particularly intracranial.

Mania (or the milder form hypomania) can be very serious as patients become disinhibited, behave out of character, their judgement is poor and they can enter into personal and financial relationships that put themselves at great risk of exploitation. The evidence suggests that hallmark symptoms when beginning in later life are the same as those in younger adults, and consist of elated irritable mood, grandiosity, overactivity, increased speed of thought and activity, insomnia, pressure of speech, incessant talking and disorganized thinking including flight of ideas, where thoughts move quickly from one subject to another.[38]

The treatment of mania in later life follows the same principles as younger adults with drug regimens involving antipsychotics and mood stabilizers.

Maintenance treatment

Depression is a relapsing disorder, and as many as 90% without prophylaxis will relapse in 3 years but with continued treatment this rate is reduced by 50–60%.[39] Once a single episode of depression recovers it is crucial to continue treatment for ≥12 months and probably for 2 years from the point of recovery (not from the point of treatment).[40] The evidence clearly shows that continuing treatment at the dose necessary to bring about recovery is the most effective approach. The previous fashion of reducing to a lower maintenance dose is no longer accepted.

With a first episode after 12 months of sustained symptom-free recovery, the antidepressant can be withdrawn gradually. If symptoms recur, slow withdrawal prevents catastrophic decline and the full dose can be reinstituted. Attempted withdrawal is then postponed for 6 months. It is wise to initiate withdrawal when the patient's life and health are stable. If a stressful situation is present or anticipated it is better to postpone withdrawal.

Once treatment is withdrawn, people should be told to seek treatment immediately if, at any time in the future, they experience depressive symptoms. The earlier treatment is initiated the better the prognosis. An individual patient's episodes usually follow a recognizable pattern (the patient signature) and if made aware of this they can recognize subsequent episodes quickly. It is worth explaining these things—with the patient's agreement—to key people, like family members.

If patients have recurrent depression, the decision to withdraw treatment needs careful thought and discussion with the patient. If someone has two episodes of depression then it is recurrent and they are at risk of more. If two episodes are separated by many years, withdrawal may still be appropriate. If closer together, and where several episodes have occurred, long-term maintenance treatment is the best option. For those with three or more episodes, maintenance should be continued for ≥3 symptom-free years.[26]

Patients will have their own views about these decisions, and full discussion on the risks and benefits is essential.

Bereavement

Grief is a normal human experience. In the early period it has many of the features of depression and may be accompanied by perplexity, disbelief, guilt, self-reproach and pseudohallucinations (seeing, hearing, sensing the dead person but insight is retained). The bereaved may be preoccupied with the deceased person, but when morbid preoccupations extend beyond the lost person this usually indicates depression. Depression complicates ~12% of grief reactions.

Grieving is a very individual process and people are not helped by being told that there is a right and wrong way to behave. This can cause guilt. Moving through grief is a process of adjustment and is classified as an adjustment disorder. Whereas the emotional aspects attract most attention, there can be very practical consequences which are often overlooked. If one loses a partner of 50 years' duration, life changes overnight. A division of labour during these years may leave the survivor bereft of a range of skills and knowledge previously provided by the deceased. So an older man may have no domestic skills, an older woman no knowledge of their financial business.

Distinguishing grief from depression, especially in the early weeks and months, can be difficult. Features better explained by depression are severe biological symptoms, failing to function, preoccupations with guilt and self-reproach, suicidal thoughts and generalized morbid thoughts. Psychotic symptoms are not explained by grief. If depression is present it should be treated and, even though antidepressants do not change what has happened, relieving symptoms may enable a person to deal with their psychological difficulties and adjustment.

Those who fail to progress through bereavement, more likely with complicated deaths or highly interdependent relationships, may have an adjustment disorder requiring skilful psychological guidance.

Most people will manage their adjustment with the help and support of family and friends in an entirely normal manner. When this is not the case they need psychological and practical help.

Paranoid states

A paranoid state is characterized by a morbid distortion of beliefs. This is not the same as psychosis though this too is characterized by morbid beliefs and comprises an important part of the larger term. The content of these distortions may include persecution, grandiosity, hypochondriasis, jealousy and guilt.

This term could be applied to ~5% of older people in the community[41] with ~45% due to organic brain syndromes, 35% mood disorders and 20% other conditions including schizophrenia.[42] The incidence of psychotic symptoms increases with age beyond 60 years.[41] About 10% of those aged 70 years without dementia and 20% aged 85 years develop first-onset psychotic symptoms and the most common are visual hallucinations and persecutory delusions. Of these, 45% eventually acquire a diagnosis of dementia compared to 25% of those without.[43]

The nature and content of paranoid beliefs is rarely diagnostic in itself and it is a full appreciation of other symptoms, the onset, course and past history which leads to diagnosis. Consequently a good history, ideally involving third parties and thorough mental state examination, is crucial. Medical investigations are frequently important. In general the presence of visual hallucinations indicates an organic pathology.

Differential diagnosis of paranoid states (Box 22.8) requires a knowledge both of medicine and psychiatry.

Organic brain syndromes

Delirium (acute confusional state)

At least 50% of people with delirium will have paranoid thinking. Characteristic of delirium is the rapid onset, short history, and fluctuating course. The onset is usually days or a week or two.

Fluctuation can be marked with symptoms both appearing and receding throughout the day and changing. No other disturbance of mind shows such sudden onset and fluctuation. Visual hallucinations, cognitive impairment and clouded consciousness are common accompaniments.

Dementia

Paranoid thinking is common and usually understood as a consequence of cognitive impairment. These symptoms usually develop in the moderate and severe stages of dementia when it becomes more difficult to understand and remain in touch with the outside world and the inconsistencies with one's own thinking.

Forgetfulness leads to purses and money being mislaid and the conclusion that they have been stolen. Not recognizing people, or forgetting, leads to suspicion about people's intentions and thoughts of persecution that may result in hostility, forcefully ejecting them from the house or refusing access. These events are often forgotten and may, subsequently, be vehemently denied but when present tend to be the same ideas.

Some people confabulate to fill in their gaps in memory and may describe completely fictitious events or events of a previous period in their life which remains prominent in their consciousness.

Box 22.8 Differential diagnosis of paranoid states

Organic

- Delirium.
- Dementia.
- Hallucinatory disorders.

Mood

- Depression.
- Mania.

Non-organic, non-affective

- Schizophrenia.
- Delusional disorder.
- Schizoaffective disorder.

Other

- Paranoid personality disorder.
- Sensory impairment especially deafness.
- Abuse.

Visual hallucinations also occur and may explain people with dementia reporting strangers entering the home.

These problems are rare in early dementia and, when present, the chronic progressive course of intellectual decline should be evident. Demonstrable cognitive impairment is usually obvious. Beware the person with dementia who suddenly develops paranoid thinking, as that may indicate delirium. People with dementia are at greater risk of developing delirium even with minor physical illness.

The exception is DLB, where visual hallucinations and paranoid thinking can be a presenting feature and prominent symptoms of this sort are characteristic.

Because people with dementia may have a variety of carers and are vulnerable, a high degree of suspicion is needed not to dismiss all reports of suspicious events or accusation because it is easy for people to steal from, or exploit, people with dementia. This can be difficult to prove but any doubt should prompt a formal investigation.

Mood disorders

Depression

Morbid thinking is typically mood congruent and in keeping with the negative, self-critical sadness of depression. Feeling a burden, guilt, and hypochondriacal worry are common. These may be overvalued ideas, when the patient can recognize that they may have things out of proportion, but if depression is of psychotic degree these become delusions, i.e. fixed beliefs not amenable to reason.

Hallucinations occur in psychotic depression and are typically mood congruent. Auditory hallucinations tell them how bad and wicked they are, somatic hallucinations convince them of physical disease, olfactory hallucinations are the smell of their body decaying.

When morbid thinking is present, depression will be of at least moderate and usually severe degree. The biological symptoms of depression are usually pronounced (poor appetite, weight loss, insomnia, fatigue). A past history of depression, that may have had similar presentation, is a diagnostic clue.

Mania

People with mania (or the milder form hypomania) are typically grandiose. They are full of confidence in their own abilities and may portray themselves as more successful and talented than they are. Like depression, mania can be of psychotic degree when these ideas become fixed delusions.

Irritability and lability are common and people with mania can be very suspicious and accusatory.

Recognition is straightforward when the diagnosis of bipolar affective disorder is already established and, like depression, episodes usually follow a recognizable pattern for any individual. If a first episode occurs then a previous history of recurrent depression is common.

Other characteristic features of elation, overactivity, excessive energy, overfamiliarity, disinhibition, pressure of speech, flight of ideas and insomnia are likely to be evident.

Organic delusional and hallucinatory disorders

These are conditions where the mental disturbance is the direct result of an identifiable organic disorder. Myxoedema psychosis is an example. In this case psychosis arises exclusively from a severe hypothyroid state. These conditions are rare but most likely to be seen in older people. They can be indistinguishable from the more common 'functional' mental illnesses that they mimic. The resulting paranoid state can take any form.

By definition there has to be a temporal relationship so that the organic condition precedes the paranoid state. This diagnosis can only be established by clear demonstration of the organic condition and it is here that medical investigations are essential.

Some conditions where this diagnosis would be more often seen may include cerebral tumours, temporal lobe epilepsy, endocrine disorders and prescribed drugs. Up to 50% of people with PD develop psychotic symptoms, which can present at any point in the disease.[44]

A condition almost exclusively seen in older ages is the syndrome of complex visual hallucination eponymously named the Charles Bonnet syndrome. While not strictly an organic hallucinatory syndrome it is associated with ocular disease that restricts vision and vertebrobasilar insufficiency. It has the hallmarks of an organic disorder.

Patients experience complex visual hallucinations in the absence of any other disturbance of mental state. Typically hallucinated images do not talk and patients describe whole scenes in detail. Sometimes patients recognize that the images must be unreal, but are so overwhelmed by them that they lose that insight and become very distressed.

Charles Bonnet hallucinosis can be a harbinger of dementia and a significant proportion do develop dementia, usually of vascular or Lewy body type. A community study found that 64% of those with first-onset visual hallucinations after age 70 years went on to develop dementia.[43]

The immediate need is to establish the underlying condition and treat that. Sometimes, psychotropic drugs are needed until the medical condition is controlled. In the case of Charles Bonnet hallucinosis, atypical antipsychotics are used with varying success. Patients often have difficulty tolerating side-effects of sedation or imbalance.

Schizophrenia

There are two peaks in the incidence of schizophrenia during the life span, the largest in young people between teenage years and early thirties. The second, smaller peak is after age 60 years. Symptoms overlap in both age groups.

Schizophrenic symptoms are conventionally separated into positive (delusions, hallucinations, thought interference, passivity) and negative (apathy, social decline, self-neglect, lack of emotional response, disordered thinking). The range of positive symptoms seen in both age groups is similar but negative symptoms are less common and much less marked in late onset. Very-late-onset patients are more likely to experience visual hallucinations.

The late-onset disorder is more common in females (not the case with younger patients) and associated with hearing impairment. People with late-onset schizophrenia are more likely to have suspicious, solitary natures and to be socially withdrawn. A positive family history (often taken to imply genetic predisposition) is far less likely with late-onset disorder.

Atypical antipsychotic drugs are the mainstay for treating positive symptoms and response is usually good. Doses will usually be 10–25% of that used in younger adults. Lack of insight often creates problems of compliance and intramuscular depot preparations can be valuable. Older people are at higher risk of developing tardive dyskinesia and involuntary movement disorders produced by typical antipsychotics.

Psychological support and understanding will help people manage their condition. Attention is also needed to sensory impairment or social isolation if these are evident.

If patients have suffered schizophrenia from younger ages and grown old with the condition (referred to as 'graduates') their tolerance to antipsychotic drugs is like that of younger adults. Consequently, they will regularly be on much higher doses than those beginning treatment in later life. If this is needed to control symptoms and causes no adverse effects, treatment should not be altered. However, as people grow older, effects of these drugs on movement and mobility can occur and gradual, controlled dose reduction is often beneficial. If people are taking traditional antipsychotics they should be offered the opportunity to convert to an equivalent atypical.

There is little information about the value of clozapine (powerful atypical antipsychotic for treatment-resistant schizophrenia that requires routine haematological monitoring) in older people. Most experience indicates problems with adverse effects, especially severe salivation, urinary incontinence, and impaired mobility. Fortunately, most late-onset disorders show a good response to conventional treatment. Clozapine would only be considered by specialist services.

Schizoaffective disorder

This term is used when a patient meets the diagnostic criteria for schizophrenia and a mood disorder simultaneously. It is usually recurrent. In terms of symptoms, course and response to treatment, it lies somewhere between schizophrenia and mood disorders.

It usually involves a combination of approaches for mood disorder and schizophrenia. Drug treatments often involve antidepressants, antipsychotics and mood stabilizers.

Persistent delusional disorder

This condition typically develops in middle age or older. The defining feature is a fixed and persistent delusional belief. Otherwise, these people often function quite normally and, for this reason, the condition can be of several years' duration before coming to attention.

The content of the delusion varies but remains the same and unchanging in any individual. A striking example is delusional jealousy where the person has an unshakable belief of a particular person's (usually partner's) infidelity. This can be a dangerous condition as they may kill the person who constantly denies their accusations.

The delusion may be persecutory (certain people wanting to kill them), grandiose (special talent or wealth), hypochondriacal (an example is delusional parasitosis or Ekbom syndrome with the conviction that they are infested with parasites) or erotic (particular person (usually famous) loves them).

Paranoid personality disorder

These people are not ill in the strict sense of the word but their character can result in a very unhappy life. As they get older their life becomes more lonely, and adversity in later life that brings them into closer contact with people may be the trigger that brings them to attention.

They are suspicious, excessively sensitive to setbacks or rejection, bear grudges, self-referential with a pervasive tendency to see conspiracies to undermine them and distort experience to misconstrue people's behaviour to be antagonistic. They are usually self-important and attribute any failures in themselves to be brought about by others.

This is their nature and to establish this needs good evidence from others that this is the way they have been from adolescent or early adult life.

Inevitably, they have difficulty forming and sustaining relationships. When adversity befalls them they blame someone else.

This is difficult as patterns are entrenched when people reach later life. The approach is a sympathetic understanding of a person who may now be in a situation creating perceived conflict and without natural confidantes. Helping them to adjust has to be combined with limit-setting of their behaviour.

Others

Two situations are encountered, particularly with older people, that may seem to be paranoid disorders but are not.

Deafness can easily lead to misinterpretation of people's behaviour and isolation. Whereas most people respond to other people's disability by offering assistance, deaf people are often avoided purely because of the difficulty in communication and this avoidance is obvious to the deaf person. Without hearing people's words their behaviour can be misunderstood. Suspiciousness can develop.

To a lesser extent similar things may arise from blindness, though this sensory deficit tends to invoke greater assistance.

Older people can be vulnerable to exploitation because they often rely on other people and tend to be more trusting. Exploitation is not confined to strangers such as formal carers but might involve family. It is important not to disregard accusations they may make, but to investigate possible abuse.

Neurotic disorders

This is a disparate group of disorders, often considered to represent the milder end of the mental health spectrum, but they can be severe and very disabling. With the exception of agoraphobia they are much less common in older people than young adults. Partly for this reason, they have received little research attention and there are, at present, no treatments specific to older patients. Even from age 65 years their frequency continues to decline.

The major message is that these presentations for the first time in later life will frequently be symptomatic, i.e. secondary to another mental or physical disorder and a common way in which patients present in primary care. So, whereas neurotic symptoms are quite common in older people, primary neurotic disorders are not. The primary condition is likely to be depression, an organic brain disorder or physical illness. In this case, investigation and treatment of the primary disorder is the approach.

When they are the primary disorder there is usually evidence that the onset predated later life but that circumstances have caused them to present at this later stage. A large epidemiological study in the USA, the Epidemiological Catchment Area Study,[45] showed that 90% of all neurotic disorders occurred by the patients' early fifties. These syndromes can date from the time of another mental disorder, particularly incompletely recovered depression, when the core symptoms of depression resolve leaving a neurotic disability. Co-occurrence of neurotic disorders is quite common.

However, the occurrence of neurotic symptoms is more common. For example, in the studies conducted by Copeland et al.[46] they identify 'cases' when they are of degree to be diagnosable disorders and 'subcases' when they are below that diagnostic threshold, i.e. symptoms (Table 22.5). The strongest association is with depression, which is considered the primary condition; for example, 74% of older people who are cases of depression also have significant symptoms of anxiety.[46] These studies also compare the 1 month prevalence between London and New York using the same method and showing considerable consistency.

Table 22.5 Neurotic syndromes versus symptoms[a]

	London		New York	
	Cases	Subcases	Cases	Subcases
Generalized anxiety	1.1	17.2	0.7	16.0
Phobic disorder	0.0	1.8	0.0	1.4
OCD	0.6	9.3	0.0	0.7
Hypochondriasis	0.5	0.0	0.7	0.2

[a] Source: Copeland et al (1987).
OCD, obsessive-compulsive disorder.

What is also clear, and contrary to the situation with most mental disorders, is that an individual can suffer different neurotic syndromes at different times; although neurotic symptoms are commonly chronic their form is changeable.[47] Therefore at one time it is a phobic problem, at another an anxiety problem or even depression.

Perhaps the exception is obsessive-compulsive disorder (OCD), which tends to be the most discrete, though obsessive-compulsive symptoms are common in depression and far more common than primary OCD presenting in later life. OCD is also the only one which is not more common in females.

Generalized anxiety and panic disorder

Of those with generalized anxiety disorder, 97% have onset before the age of 65 years and panic disorder with onset after this age is particularly rare. In general, anxiety disorders are consistently more common in females and have been associated with lack of support network, lower education, extreme war experience and those with less sense of control over their world. It is usually triggered in susceptible individuals by stresses commonly involving losses and chronic physical illness.

Treatment is preferably with psychological therapies such as anxiety management or CBT. Antidepressants, particularly SSRIs, can sometimes be helpful.

It is important to be sure that symptoms of late-onset disorder are not arising from physical symptoms. For example, paroxysmal cardiac dysrythmia, hyperthyroidism, or hypoglycaemia can easily be mistaken for the somatic symptoms of anxiety disorders or panic.

The course tends to be chronic, with acute exacerbations at times of stress, though there is evidence that late-onset cases are less likely to remain cases than with younger people.

Obsessive-compulsive disorder

Seventy-five per cent of OCD has onset before age 30 years and <5% after age 40 years. Consequently, onset in later life is extremely rare. In this situation another primary condition should always be suspected. Most commonly the primary disorder is depression or an organic brain disorder. The latter may be a dementia, particularly frontotemporal, but also space-occupying lesions like cerebral tumours.

By definition, obsessive-compulsive symptoms are resisted and this creates mounting anxiety until the compulsion is performed. In the case of organic brain lesions this aspect is often absent.

Treatment of the primary disorder is either behavioural (response prevention), where the patient resists or is prevented from performing their rituals until their mounting anxiety abates, or with SSRI antidepressants. The former is the preferred approach where compulsive acts are involved, e.g. hand washing or checking, but this is less effective when the obsession only consists of compulsive thoughts. In the case of compulsive thoughts, drug treatment may give greater success.

OCD is not more common in either gender and less likely to be stress-induced than the anxiety-based disorders, but stress can induce exacerbations. Of all the neurotic syndromes it is most likely to have a constitutional basis and family history.

Somatoform disorder and medically unexplained symptoms

This includes somatization and hypochondriasis. The former refers to people with multiple physical symptoms who constantly seek investigation and the latter a preoccupation with the thought that they have a particular medical condition. This is associated with increased attendance in primary care and is a predictor of quality of life.[48]

If late onset, be very cautious before ascribing these diagnoses as most patients do have physical illness or disability even though attribution of all symptoms to the known disorders may be difficult. Symptoms should always be taken seriously and investigated to a reasonable degree.

In a prospective study of elderly primary care attenders, somatization was found in 5% and associated with depression, physical illness and low perceived social support.[49] It was commonly transient even though 13.6% of attenders had a somatizing attributional style which was quite stable. Frequent attenders were characterized by high rates of depression (28.3%), psychological distress associated with physical symptoms and perceived lack of social support (40%).

In people with physical illness where somatic symptoms are not easily understood or out of proportion to known physical disease, there should be a strong suspicion that these arise from a mood disorder and this should be treated. Both antidepressants and CBT have been shown to be effective[50] and a trial of treatment is usually justifiable. Methods to improve perceived social support are also likely to be helpful.

Once a treatable physical condition or underlying mood disorder can be reasonably excluded, the response is to reassure and support patients in their distress. Their symptoms should never be dismissed as insignificant or fictitious. Regardless of their origin they are experienced in reality. A reasonable approach is to explain that while they have real symptoms the medical profession is not, at this time, able to explain how they are caused but that the investigations completed have excluded all the conditions known to produce this range of symptoms.

Once this position is reached, no further investigations should be pursued. Doing so only conveys the doctor's doubts about the position which undermines the patient's confidence. The aim is to convey sincerity and commitment to do all possible to help them adjust to the symptoms they have. With more severe and disabled patients, more sophisticated psychological approaches involving re-attribution (being able to re-focus understanding of the origin of symptoms) can be helpful.

Hysteria (conversion) disorder

This refers to symptoms, physical or behavioural, which are thought to arise from subconscious conflict. This is a very dangerous diagnosis to make in older people and should be avoided. It will result in failing to diagnose serious physical disease or mental illness.

Phobia

Simple phobias are common to all people and may persist throughout life. Fear of heights, enclosed spaces, insects, etc. almost always starts in childhood and rarely requires treatment. The most common and disabling problem in later life is agoraphobia. In most this develops following illnesses such as heart attack, falls or depression that shake confidence, or a traumatic event like mugging or assault. It could also be a symptom of depression.

Agoraphobia can be profoundly disabling for an older person who lives alone and the ensuing isolation impairs quality of life and may lead to depression. Prevention following common precipitants by active rehabilitation is crucial. Once established, the treatment is behavioural by graded exposure, initially being accompanied, and setting targets of feared situations. When people become accustomed to one situation they move on to a more difficult target.

This is supplemented by psychological support and anxiety management, and occasionally by antidepressants or short-term anxiolytics. If depression is evident it should be treated and may be the primary problem.

Graded exposure is a labour-intensive process requiring consistency of approach, positive reinforcement and the ability to remain in situations and tolerate uncomfortable anxiety until it dissipates. The aim is to leave a situation only when this is achieved, so that the memory of the experience is not one of exiting in fear.

Alcohol misuse

In general, as we get older our alcohol consumption naturally declines. Establishing the frequency of harmful alcohol use in older people, as with all ages, is difficult as we know that self-disclosure of drinking habits is always an underestimate. It also depends on the criteria used to define levels of problem drinking. The suggested prevalence of misuse or dependence is 2–4% but less restrictive terms like excessive alcohol consumption identify 17% of men and 7% of women. Those most at risk are male, socially isolated, single, separated or divorced.[51]

We can confidently assert that alcohol misuse in older people is underdetected. There are many reasons, including underreporting, low levels of suspicion, assumptions that older people don't imbibe, greater acceptance (don't stop them having fun when life is so difficult) or not wishing to embarrass one's elders.

There are also difficulties in knowing what level of alcohol intake is safe for older people, as guidance (21 units for men, 14 units for women weekly) may not apply. Screening instruments, e.g. CAGE, MAST-G, AUDIT, may not apply in the same way to older people because of their different life circumstances. Older people may present in different ways with falls, cognitive impairment, or depression, or the alcohol use may be masked by physical or mental illness.

The complications of alcohol misuse apply as much to older people and can be complicated by co-morbid physical illness, disability and prescribed medication. It is more likely to be apparent in physical and social functioning than in the social, legal and occupational aspects evident with younger adults.

Alcohol is neurotoxic and traditionally discrete syndromes have been described, including Wernicke–Korsakoff (caused by thiamine deficiency) or alcohol-related dementia. It is now recognized that these overlap and the umbrella term 'alcohol-related brain damage' is acquiring popular use.

In practice there are two groups of older drinkers: first, those who have consumed heavily all their life who present rather like younger drinkers with physical problems or deteriorating social circumstances; second, 'symptomatic drinkers', who start to use, misuse or escalate their alcohol intake secondary to another problem. Commonly, the underlying problem is bereavement, loneliness, depression or chronic physical illness and disability.

Symptomatic drinkers are very important to recognize—if not, their primary problem will become more complicated and established patterns of drinking may continue after it has resolved. The priority is vigorous and early treatment of the underlying problem, combined with open

Box 22.9 Features of alcohol dependence

- ◆ Desire or compulsion to drink.
- ◆ Tolerance (increasing amounts needed to achieve desired effects).
- ◆ Physiological withdrawal symptoms.
- ◆ Loss of control.
- ◆ Primacy (preoccupation with alcohol).
- ◆ Persistent use despite knowing harmful effects.

Box 22.10 Twelve tips

- ◆ Diagnose dementia early and engage patient and carers.
- ◆ Establish aims of dementia management with patient and carers early.
- ◆ Make the first contact a winner, it will set the scene for therapeutic alliance.
- ◆ Recognize carers as the foundation to success.
- ◆ Consider delirium for any sudden change in an older person's function or behaviour.
- ◆ Seek and treat depression early.
- ◆ Look out for the atypical presentation of depression.
- ◆ Suicidal thoughts are always serious—refer to specialist services early.
- ◆ Neurotic symptoms are usually a sign of something else.
- ◆ Spot the symptomatic drinker and the depressed bereaved.
- ◆ Information helps patients and carers manage their health problems.
- ◆ Form a close liaison with the local secondary care mental health provider.

discussion about the seriousness of developing a drink problem. In contrast to life-long heavy drinkers, symptomatic drinkers are usually eager to control drinking and often feel guilty about it.

For all people, education about safe drinking is important and this may not be as familiar to older people. Drinkers are likely to neglect diet, and supplementation, particularly thiamine, may be necessary. Thiamine deficiency can be severe and a daily dose of 300 mg over several months may be necessary to replace depleted reserves. Introduction of carer support might improve the home circumstance and introduce a watchful eye on consumption.

Engagement with a health care professional is the foundation on which to build a plan to disrupt harmful drinking patterns. Avoiding situations where drinking is likely, avoiding alcohol in the home and finding alternatives and distractions can be helpful.

For those with alcohol dependence (Box 22.9), specialist services should be involved. Admission for detoxification is a likely requirement and older people are prone to greater severity and duration of withdrawal symptoms, compounded by medical co-morbidity.

For those who do not engage, prolonged contact, support and long-term thiamine replacement may, eventually, bring dividends.

Conclusion

The mental health problems of older people are common, interesting and rewarding to treat. Often simple interventions produce gratifying results and substantially improve quality of life. Primary care equipped to respond to this challenge will be an essential part of the solution to the increasing demand of an ageing population.

References

1. Ferri CP, Prince M, Brayne C, *et al*. Global prevalence of dementia: a Delphi consensus study. *Lancet* 2005;366(9503):2112–7.
2. Copeland JR, Davidson IA, Dewey ME, *et al*. Alzheimer's disease, other dementias, depression and pseudodementia: prevalence, incidence and three-year outcome. *Br J Psychiat* 1992;161:230–9.

3. Watts SC, Bhutani GE, Stout IH, Ducker GM, Cleator PJ, McGarry J, Day M. Mental health in older adult recipients of primary care services: is depression the key issue? Identification, treatment and the general practitioner. *Int J Geriat Psychiat* 2002;17:427–37.

4. Age Concern. *UK Inquiry into Mental and Well-being in Later Life*. London: Age Concern; 2007.

5. National Audit Office. *Improving Services and Support for People with Dementia*. Report by the Comptroller and Auditor General. London: Stationery Office; 2007.

6. Burns A, Lawlor B, Craig S. *Assessment Scales in Old Age Psychiatry*. London: Informa Healthcare; 2004.

7. Woodford HJ, George J. Cognitive assessment in the elderly: a review of clinical methods. *Q J Med* 2007;100:469–84.

8. Folstein MF, Folstein SE, McHugh PR. "Mini-mental state". A practical method for grading the cognitive state of patients for the clinician. *J Psychiat Res* 1975;12:189–98.

9. National Institute for Health and Clinical Excellence. *Dementia: Supporting People with Dementia and their Carers in Health and Social Care*. London: NICE; 2006.

10. Yesavage JA, Brink TL, Rose TL, Lum O. Huang V, Adey M, Leirer O. Development and validation of a geriatric depression screening scale: a preliminary report. *J Psychiat Res* 1983;17:37–49.

11. Alexopoulos GS, Abrams RC, Young RC, Shamoian CA. Cornell Scale for Depression in Dementia. *Biol Psychiat* 1988;23:271–84.

12. Pomeroy IM, Clark CR, Philp I. The effectiveness of very short scales for depression screening in elderly medical patients. *Int J Geriat Psychiat* 2001;16:321–6.

13. Bruscoli M, Lovestone S. Is MCI just early dementia? A systematic review of conversion studies. *Int Psychogeriat* 2004;16:129–40.

14. Banerjee S, Willis R, Matthews D, Contell F, Chan J, Murray J. Improving the quality of care for mild to moderate dementia: an evaluation of the Croydon Memory Service Model. *Int J Geriat Psychiat* 2007;22:782–8.

15. Alzheimer's Society. *Dementia UK*. A report to the Alzheimer's Society on the prevalence and economic cost of dementia in the UK produced by Kings College London and London School of Economics. London: Alzheimer's Society; 2007.

16. McKeith IG, Dickson DW, Lowe J, *et al*. Diagnosis and management of dementia with Lewy bodies: third report of the DLB consortium. *Neurology* 2005;65:1863–72.

17. Aarsland D, Andersen K, Larsen JP, *et al*. Prevalence and characteristics of dementia in Parkinson disease: an 8-year prospective study. *Arch Neurol* 2003;60:387–92.

18. Ballard CG, Margallo-Lana M, Fossey J, *et al*. A 1-year follow-up of behavioural and psychological symptoms in dementia among people in care environments. *J Clin Psychiat* 2001;62:631–6.

19. All Party Parliamentary Group on Dementia. *Always a Last Resort. Inquiry into the Prescription of Antipsychotic Drugs to People with Dementia Living in Care Homes*. London: House of Lords and House of Commons; 2008.

20. McKeith I, Del Ser T, Spano P, *et al*. Efficacy of rivastigmine in dementia with Lewy bodies: a randomized, double blind, placebo controlled international study. *Lancet* 2000;356(9247):2031–6.

21. Bierman EJ, Comijs HC, Gundy CM, Sonnenberg C, Jonker C, Beekman AT. The effect of chronic benzodiazepine use on cognitive functioning in older persons: good, bad or indifferent?. *Int J Geriat Psychiat* 2007;22:1194–200.

22. Molnar FJ, Patel A, Marshall SC, Man-Son-Hing M, Wilson KG. Clinical utility of office-based cognitive predictors of fitness to drive in persons with dementia. A systematic review. *J Am Geriatr Soc* 2006;54:1809–24.

23. Breen DA, Breen DP, Moore JW, Breen PA, O' Neil D. Driving and dementia. *Br Med J* 2007;334(7608):1365–9.

24. Royal College of Psychiatrists. *Who Cares Wins. Improving the Outcome for Older people Admitted to the General Hospital: Guidelines for the Development of Liaison Mental Health Services for Older People*. London: Royal College of Psychiatrists; 2005.

25. Royal College of Physicians. *Concise Guidance of Good Practice, Number 6. The Prevention, Diagnosis and Management of Delirium in Older People. National Guidelines.* London: Royal College of Physicians; 2006.

26. Alexopoulos GS. Depression in the elderly. *Lancet* 2005;365(9475):1961–70.

27. Van der Kooy K, Van Hout H, Marwijk H, Marten H, Stehouwer C, Beekman A. Depression and the risk for cardiovascular disease: systematic review and meta-analysis. *Int J Geriat Psychiat* 2007;22:613–26.

28. Ryan J, Carriere I, Ritchie K, *et al.* Late life depression and mortality: influence of gender and antidepressant use. *Br J Psychiat* 2008;192:12–18.

29. Hawton K, Harriss L. Deliberate self-harm in people aged 60 years and over: characteristics and outcome of a 20 year cohort. *Int J Geriat Psychiat* 2006;21:572–81.

30. Moussavi S, Chatterji S, Verdes E, Tandon A, Patel V, Ustun B. Depression, chronic diseases, and decrements in health: results from the World Health Surveys. *Lancet* 2007;370(9590):851–8.

31. Alexopoulos GS, Meyers BS, Young RC, Campbell S, Silversweig D, Charlson M. 'Vascular depression' hypothesis. *Arch Gen Psychiat* 1997;54:915–22.

32. Baldwin RC. Is vascular depression a distinct sub-type of depressive disorder? A review of causal evidence. *Int J Geriat Psychiat* 2005;20:1–11.

33. Taylor MJ, Freemantle N, Geddes JR, Bhagwagar Z. Early onset of selective serotonin reuptake inhibitor antidepressant action: systematic review and meta-analysis. *Arch Gen Psychiat* 2006;63:1217–23.

34. Glassman AH, O' CM, Califf RM, J, *et al.* Sertraline treatment of major depression in patients with acute MI or unstable angina. *J Am Med Assoc* 2002;288:701–9.

35. Berkman LF, Blumenthal J, Burg M, *et al.* Effects of treating depression and low perceived social support on clinical events after myocardial infarction: the Enhancing Recovery in Coranary Heart Disease Patients (ENRICHD) Randomized Trial. *J Am Med Assoc* 2003;289:3106–16.

36. Narushima K, Paradiso S, Moser DJ, Jorge R, Robinson RG. Effect of antidepressant therapy on executive function after stroke. *Br J Psychiat* 2007;190:260–5.

37. Wilson K, Mottram P, Sivanranthan A, Nightingale A. Antidepressants versus placebo for the depressed elderly. *Cochrane Database Syst Rev* 2001;(2):CD000561

38. Broadhead J, Jacoby R. Mania in old age: a first prospective study. *Int J Geriat Psychiat* 1990;5;215–22.

39. Reynolds CF 3rd, Frank E, Perel JM, *et al.* Nortryptiline and interpersonal psychotherapy as maintenance therapies for recurrent major depression: a randomized controlled trial in patients older than 59 years. *J Am Med Assoc* 1999;281:39–45.

40. Old Age Depression Interest Group. How long should the elderly take antidepressants? A double-blind placebo controlled study of continuation/prophylaxis therapy with dothiepin. *Br J Psychiat* 1993;162:175–82.

41. Howard R, Rabins PV, Seeman MV, Jeste DV. Late-onset schizophrenia and very-late-onset schizophrenia-like psychosis: an international consensus. The International Late-Onset Schizophrenia Group. *Am J Psychiat* 2000;157:172–8.

42. Leuchter AF, Spar JE. The late onset psychoses. Clinical and diagnostic features. *J Nerv Ment Dis* 1985;173:488–94.

43. Ostling S, Pálsson SP, Skoog I. The incidence of first onset psychotic symptoms and paranoid ideation in a representative population sample followed from age 70–90 years. Relation to mortality and later development of dementia. *Int J Geriat Psychiat* 2007;22:520–28.

44. National Institute for Health and Clinical Excellence. *Parkinson's Disease: National Clinical Guidelines for Diagnosis and Management in Primary and Secondary Care.* London: Royal College of Physicians; 2006.

45. Regier DA, Boyd JH, Burke JD Jr, *et al.* One month prevalence of mental disorders in the United States. Based on five Epidemiologic Catchment Area Sites. *Arch Gen Psychiat* 1988;45:977–86.

46. Copeland JR, Gurland BJ, Dewey ME, Kelleher MJ, Smith AM, Davidson IA. Is there more dementia, depression and neurosis in New York? A comparative study of the elderly in New York and London using the computer diagnosis AGECAT. *Br J Psychiat* 1987;151;466–73.

47. Larkin BA, Copeland JR, Dewey ME, *et al.* The natural history of neurotic disorder in an elderly urban population. Findings from the Liverpool longitudinal study of continuing health in the community. *Br J Psychiat* 1992;160:681–6.

48. Sheehan B, Lall R, Bass C. Does somatization influence quality of life among older primary care attenders?. *Int J Geriat Psychiat* 2005;20:967–72.

49. Sheehan B, Bass C, Briggs R, Jacoby R. Somatization among older primary care attenders. *Psychol Med* 2003;3:867–77.

50. Drayer RA, Mulsant BH, Lenze EJ, *et al.* Somatic symptoms of depression in elderly patients with medical comorbidities. *Int J Geriat Psychiat* 2005;20:973–82.

51. O' Connell H, Chin AV, Cunningham C, Lawlor B. Alcohol use disorders in elderly people—redefining an age old problem. *Br Med J* 2003:327(7416):664–7.

Chapter 23

Ethical and legal issues

David Oliver

Introduction: why ethics and law matter so much in the care of older people

With the extension of the lifespan, most general practitioners (GPs) have become responsible for the care of increasing numbers of older people. Although many remain very independent, as they age they may increasingly suffer frailty, physical impairment, disability or dependency, sensory or cognitive impairment, an accumulation of long-term conditions often leading to hospitalization. Their interactions (positive or negative) with family members, informal carers or professional health and social care services may become more important and in some cases they may need to move to nursing or residential homes.[1,2] And with most people surviving beyond mid-life, most end-of-life care involves older people. All of these factors raise ethical and legal issues around consent, communication, capacity, autonomy and risk, personal finances and interactions with family members or health and social care.[4,5]

There is increasing evidence and awareness of ageist attitudes, both covert and overt,[6,7] which may lead to routine assumptions about older people and their abilities, and to actions or attitudes which would be considered unacceptable in younger patients. For instance, it may be assumed that they are unable to grasp or retain important information to make decisions affecting their own life, medical treatment or place of residence, or to take risks. They may fall victim to patronizing or condescending terminology or communication styles such as belittling 'elderspeak',[8] and to unfounded assumptions about the 'futility' of treatment or investigation simply on the grounds of age. Legitimate medical problems with treatable causes may be labelled 'social' or 'failure to cope'[9] in a way that would be unacceptable in the young. And although >50% of health and social care resource is spent on people aged >65 years, health systems are often not geared to the complex needs of older people with multiple problems or functional impairment, with such patients often being presented as a 'problem' for the system.[10] On the other hand, either through cognitive impairment or other factors such as fear, pain, anxiety or family pressure, the capacity of older people to make autonomous decisions about their own care may be compromised, raising issues for the practitioner around paternalism, advocacy and 'best interests', as well as balancing the previous known wishes of the older person and the views or wishes of their family members.[11]

Staff in primary care will often be called upon to deal with these complex issues, so this chapter aims to point them towards key underlying principles or practice frameworks and key points of law, which might guide them. Whereas the legal considerations might centre on the UK in this chapter, the underlying ethical principles are universal. There are many situations which might not have a 'ready-made' professional or legal rulebook or which are morally grey areas, therefore an understanding of these principles and how they are reflected in law is also important. So while the main focus of the chapter will be practical guidance for common scenarios which practitioners are likely to encounter, it is worth very briefly setting out some principles for practice.

A widespread approach to the teaching and study of applied healthcare ethics—initially set out by Beauchamp and Childress[12–14] and reinforced by others, e.g. Gillon[15,16]—has drawn together utilitarian schools of philosophy (focusing on maximizing benefits for the whole population) and deontological approaches (based on absolute rights of patients and the responsibilities of practitioners or organizations). Whilst it has attracted some criticism in philosophical circles, this is a useful and widespread approach to difficult decisions, which led to the setting out of the 'four principles' of health care ethics: (Box 23.1) namely *beneficence* (the duty to do good or maximize patients' welfare); *non-maleficence* (the duty to not to inflict harm or to take all reasonable steps to minimize harm); *respect for autonomy* and for *justice* (to do with fair allocation or resources—*distributive justice*—and to do with respecting *human rights* and avoiding discrimination). In order to turn these principles into rules for action in particular circumstances, it might be necessary to breach one of the four principles ('specification')[12–14] set out as 'balancing rules' for action (Box 23.2). Applying the rules in a given scenario often adds clarity to decision-making.

These principles are clearly reflected in professional codes of conduct, e.g. the General Medical Council,[17] which sets out professional duties of care, the need to obtain informed consent, to respect patients' rights, and to minimize harm (Box 23.3). They are also often reflected and codified in law (Box 23.4). Relevant law with regard to older people may be statutory (e.g. Mental

Box 23.1 The 'four principles' or 'prima facie moral norms' of healthcare ethics

1. Beneficence

- The obligation to provide benefits and balance benefits against risks.
- This is a positive duty to do good and means that health workers have a duty of care actively to promote and advocate the wellbeing of their patients.

2. Non-maleficence

- The obligation to avoid so far as possible the causation of harm.
- This is a negative principle, i.e. that workers have a duty to abstain from causing harm or at least to cause the least possible harm commensurate with achieving a good outcome.

3. Respect for personal autonomy

- The obligation to respect personhood and the decision-making capacities of autonomous persons.
- We should distinguish general respect for personhood from normative autonomy (i.e. the general right to make autonomous decisions) and from empirical autonomy (i.e. whether an individual has the capacity to make autonomous decisions at that time).

4. (Distributive) Justice

- Obligations of fairness in the distributions of benefits and risks (equity).
- Also has implications for equal rights to treatment or assessment.

[a] Source: Beauchamp and Childress.[12]

> ## Box 23.2 Balancing rules: necessary conditions for breaching one of the 'four principles' and specification for action in given circumstances[a]
>
> If one of the prima facie moral norms is to be overridden, then the following rules must be satisfied:
>
> - *Better reasons* can be offered to act on the overriding than infringed norm.
> - The moral objective justifying the infringement must have a *realistic prospect of achievement.*
> - The infringement is necessary in that *no morally preferable alternative* actions can be substituted.
> - The infringement selected must be the *least possible infringement* needed to achieve the primary goal.
> - The agent (i.e. doctor/nurse) must seek to *minimize any negative effects* of infringement.
> - Must *act impartially* in regard to all affected parties and not influenced by morally irrelevant information.
>
> [a] Source: Beauchamp and Childress.[13]

Health Act, Human Rights Act, Mental Capacity Act) or common (judge-made) law, e.g. around clinical or criminal negligence or various rulings on end-of-life withdrawal of food and fluids. However, even with statutes, these tend to be tested by rulings in the courts which form the basis for legal precedent. For those wishing to search for legal rulings there are databases (West Law, BAILI, Lexis Nexis)[18] which provide a similar role to medical databases. There are also a number of authoritative and frequently updated texts to which interested readers can refer.[19–21]

This chapter aims to provide practical guidance for the most common *predictable* scenarios likely to face primary care staff when dealing with older people.

A. Respecting the humanity and human rights of older people and providing adequate information and communication

Good primary care should always be patient-centred, holistic and mindful of the dignity and respect owed to the person. Older people should be afforded the same standard of care as younger patients,[22] with control over their own decisions, adequate information and communication, and freedom from discrimination on grounds of age or any other characteristic.

This includes a duty to respect the right of autonomous older people to take risks without being overruled by their family[23,24] and to be 'active participants in, rather than subjects of the care-providing process.'[25] Older people may easily become marginalized if they have hearing or memory problems, leading medical professionals to ignore them and deal directly with their relatives instead. Ingrained attitudes or assumptions towards older people may be potentially compounded by their higher prevalence of sensory deficit, communication difficulties and cognitive impairment. The doctor must strive to overcome these barriers, setting aside sufficient time for elderly patients and providing adequate information in an accessible form, without infantilizing or demeaning language.

Effective non-discriminatory communication with the elderly patient should include a duty to offer appropriate information relevant to the condition, i.e. evidence for the diagnosis and prognosis, including up-to-date treatment options, with the implications, drawbacks and side-effects

Box 23.3 Ways in which the 'four principles' are reflected in professional codes of conduct[a]

1. Respect for autonomy

- You must respect the patient as an individual (NMC).
- You must obtain consent before giving treatment or care (NMC).
- Respect patients' right to confidentiality (GMC).
- Listen to patients and respond to their concerns and preferences (GMC).
- Give patients the information they want or need in a way they can understand (GMC).
- Respect patients' right to reach decisions with you about their treatment and care (GMC).

2. Non-maleficence

- You must act to minimize the risk to your patients (NMC).
- Keep your professional knowledge and skills up to date (NMC).
- Recognize and work within the limits of your competence (NMC).
- Act without delay if you have good reason to believe that you or a colleague may be putting patients at risk (NMC).

3. Beneficence

- You have a duty of care to your patients, who are entitled to receive safe and competent care (NMC).
- Work with colleagues in the ways that best serve patients' interests (GMC).
- Protect and promote the health of patients and the public (GMC).
- Provide a good standard of practice and care (GMC).
- Keep your professional knowledge and skills up to date (GMC).

4. Justice

- You are personally accountable for ensuring that you promote and protect the interests and dignity of patients, irrespective of gender, ethnicity, age, etc. (NMC).
- Never discriminate unfairly against patients or colleagues (GMC).

[a] Sources: General Medical Council (GMC)[17] and Nursing and Midwifery Council (NMC).[47]

of treatment and main alternatives. In particular, it is essential that clear, unhurried and adequate explanations concerning the purpose and proper use of medication be given to older patients. Lack of understanding of their drug regimen may easily lead to non-compliance in older patients, whose treatment may already be compromised by co-morbidity and polypharmacy.[26,27]

A recent all-parliamentary enquiry into the human rights of older people in health and social care[28] set out potential ways in which their rights might be compromised. And although it concerned the treatment of younger adults with learning difficulties, the Bournewood Ruling at the

Box 23.4 Ways in which the law codifies the 'four principles' with potential relevance to older people

1. Non-maleficence

+ Criminal law on abuse, assault, manslaughter by gross (criminal) negligence.
+ Clinical negligence where a harm which was foreseeable and preventable has been caused by a breach in the duty of care.
+ Human right to prohibition of torture inhuman or degrading treatment (Article 3, ECHR).

2. Beneficence

+ Negligence law. The doctor has a duty of care to the patient (to provide safe competent care).

3. Respect for autonomy

+ Common law on consent to treatment and tort of battery if patient touched without consent.
+ Common law on mental capacity (to consent to treatment) and mental incapacity act.
+ Provisions 5, 8, and 9 of ECHR concerning liberty and security; respect for privacy and family life; freedom of thought conscience and religion.
+ UK Data Protection Act (1998).

4. Distributive justice

+ NICE guidelines.
+ Human right to freedom from discrimination (ECHR, Article 14).

ECHR, European Convention on Human Rights; NICE, National Institute for Health and Clinical Excellence.

European Human Rights court[29] also identified ways in which the human rights of dependent institutionalized adults could be jeopardized (in particular around restraints and restrictions), and set out rules for avoiding such a breach of human rights.

B. Consent, capacity to consent and the Mental Capacity Act (2005)

In medical care, the moral principle of respect for autonomy demands the patient's consent to treatment, based on his possession of adequate information and understanding of the treatment options.[30,31] Where an older person lacks autonomy due to mental incapacity or severe acute illness, the doctor may legitimately act on his behalf, i.e. without consent but motivated solely by the patient's welfare.[32,33] This is enshrined in common law, under which treatment without consent becomes the tort of battery,[34] but professionals acting in the patient's best interests out of necessity are protected.[20] Under common law, for consent or refusal to be valid, patients must have a general understanding of the decision to be made, the reason for it, and its likely consequences.

They must also be able to understand, retain, use, and weigh relevant information; be acting voluntarily and free from pressure; and be aware that they are free to give or refuse consent.

The Mental Capacity Act[35] has codified these tests, which should be applied to each decision at that time—as the level of capacity required for one decision may be higher than for another and capacity may fluctuate with time. The Act sets out five key principles:

1) A presumption of capacity unless proved otherwise.

2) The right of support for the patient in decision-making: all appropriate help should be given before any conclusion that a person cannot make his own decisions.

3) The individual retains the right to make what might be seen as eccentric or unwise decisions.

4) The aim of all action taken on behalf of a person without mental capacity should be that person's 'best interests'. Carers and relatives have the right to be consulted, and a person may also make a written statement of his wishes.

5) Where an intervention is applied in the best interests of a person without mental capacity, the intervention *least restrictive to basic rights and freedoms should be applied.*

The Mental Capacity Act also goes beyond common law in significant ways[36,37] with new concepts, services and a code of practice, e.g. making wilful neglect or ill treatment of people without capacity a criminal offence. It also introduced an independent mental capacity advocacy service and the concept of advance decisions. The role of several existing services, such as the Court of Protection, was expanded and new frameworks, such as lasting power of attorney and court deputies, established.

In addition, the Act also identifies factors to be considered when making a 'best interests' assessment (Figure 23.1). These include provision of practical help to assist the patient in decision-making; identifying factors that the patient would take into account if making his own decisions; reflecting his known wishes, values or statements made before capacity was lost; avoiding assumptions about best interests based on age, appearance, condition or behaviour; considering whether he or she is likely to regain capacity; and, where possible, consulting relevant others for their views.

C. Healthcare proxies, lasting powers of attorney and independent mental capacity advocates

The Mental Capacity Act[35] extended powers of attorney, previously used only for the management of assets, to health and welfare decisions for mentally impaired individuals. An older person facing possible future incapacity may nominate a relative, friend or other person to assume lasting powers of attorney on his behalf. Others may prefer their doctor to continue as decision-maker for them in the case of their acute medical illness or mental incapacity, acting under the 'necessity' principle.[20]

A valid lasting power of attorney must be a document written on a statutory form, signed voluntarily by both parties and specifying its nature and effect. Decisions then made by the attorney are as valid in law as those made by the 'donor' (i.e. patient) when competent, though its powers do not extend to refusal of life-sustaining treatment unless explicitly stated. Replacement attorneys may also be nominated.

The Act also requires the development of independent mental capacity advocates (IMCAs), adults who are empowered to make decisions for vulnerable, incapacitated and otherwise unsupported adults on matters such as serious medical treatment, long-term place of residence, care review or adult protection.

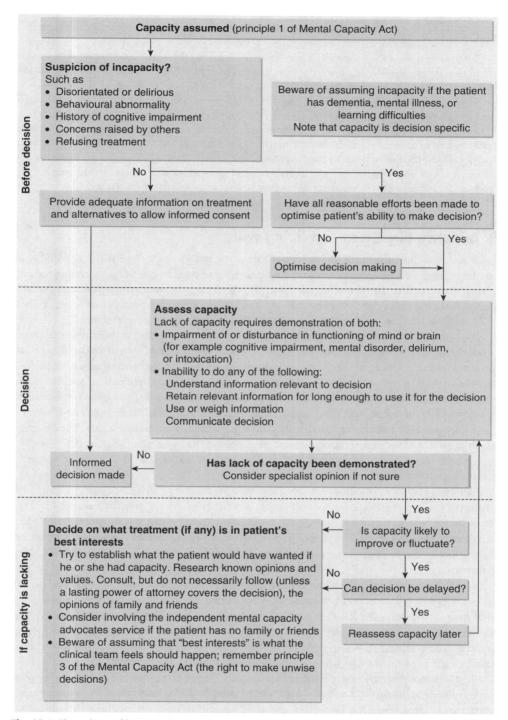

Fig. 23.1 Flow chart of how to decide whether or not a person aged ≥16 years has capacity. Redrawn with permission from Nicholson et al.[37] ©BMJ Publishing Group Ltd.

Case Example (illustrating issues in Sections B and C)

Mrs L is aged 85 years, with osteoporosis, hypertension, diabetes and chronic obstructive pulmonary disease related to smoking. She lives in a two-storey house heated with a log fire. Although she has suffered three admissions to hospital with falls and immobility in the past 6 months—one resulting in a hip fracture—and, according to her daughters, a number of other falls or 'near misses', she has always insisted on returning home and has only reluctantly accepted social services, making it clear that she is far from happy with the cost or the carers who visit, saying that 'they don't do anything when they come round.' She refuses to move her bed downstairs or to have a commode in the living room, and refuses Meals-on-Wheels. She continues to use the fire, even though once or twice her daughters have come round to find logs smouldering on the floor. She is increasingly unsteady on her feet but still refuses to use the walking aid provided by the hospital. Her daughters are increasingly concerned but she says she 'doesn't know what all the fuss is about.'

D. Advance directives and living wills

Older people facing impending loss of mental capacity may wish to exert control over their future care by making an *advance directive*, a written statement of their wishes to be enacted in the case of their serious illness or mental impairment. Directives do not necessarily cover every possible contingency, but are useful where the individual has strong views, predictable treatment options, or a condition likely to result in deterioration and a future of mental impairment.

When treating a patient who has made an advance directive, the doctor must make efforts to check the validity of the document. He should consider whether the current circumstances are those envisaged, whether the decision has been reviewed and updated and whether, since then, there have been new medical developments that could have affected the patient's wishes. On a personal level, he should check whether there is any evidence of a change of mind by the patient or behaviour inconsistent with the directive, such as appointing a healthcare proxy or attorney.

Advance refusal of treatment is also legally valid when certain conditions are met. The directive, which must not have been withdrawn, must have been made by an adult who, at the time of its drawing up was mentally competent but, by the time it was to be invoked, had lost decision-making capacity.

There are additional criteria for *refusing life-prolonging treatment*. Refusal of any recommended treatment can result in deterioration or death; nevertheless, where they intend specifically to refuse life-sustaining treatment, individuals must clearly indicate that it is to apply, even if life is at risk and death will result. The decision must be put in writing and duly signed and witnessed. If there is any doubt about the validity of the directive, referral can be made to the Court of Protection.

Advance requests or authorizations may also be made by individuals while still fully competent, and, although they are not legally binding, they are helpful in identifying how patients would like to be treated when capacity is lost. Where no advance discussion on such matters has taken place, the doctor must adhere to the principle of presumed best interests, in the light of his knowledge of the patient's wishes. However, doctors are not legally or morally bound to provide treatment with little chance or success or where the burdens will outweigh the benefits.

When advance directives have been drawn up, they can be carried by the person on a signed card or placed in the medical record. Ideally they should be drafted with the aid of health professionals and with sufficient information and clarification. In both verbal and written advance directives, clear, specific, unambiguous language should be used. If health professionals are asked to witness a directive, it might be assumed that they verified the patient's capacity at the time.

E. Paternalism, non-consensual treatment and 'best interests'

The principle of 'respect for autonomy' may legitimately be overridden under certain circumstances. When an older person is at risk of significant but preventable harm, the doctor has a duty of care to intervene, even if his action is against the wishes and without the consent of the individual. The action is considered justifiable if the doctor's intervention will prevent the harm, if the benefits to the patient outweigh the risks, and if the least restrictive alternative is used. Here the principle is that of 'paternalism', which must be invoked solely by consideration of the best interests of the person, and referring 'exclusively to [his] welfare, good, happiness, needs and interests and values.'[38] However, it is worth re-emphasizing that there is a difference between 'normative' autonomy (i.e. the general principle of patients' right to self-determination) and 'empirical' autonomy, i.e. whether the patient really does have the capacity to make an informed decision. This may be compromised not just by cognitive impairment but by factors such distress, fear, pain, disorientation, lack of information or misunderstandings, concern for or pressure from others. Thus we should not confuse respecting the humanity and dignity of older patients with respecting autonomy. This is why some authors distinguish 'weak' or 'soft' paternalism (i.e. acting on behalf of patients who lack autonomy) from 'hard paternalism' (where they possess it). The Bournewood Ruling[39] illustrated the risk of staff in institutions restricting the freedoms and choices of residents even in instances where they did possess sufficient autonomy, or excessively restricting those freedoms where they did not. This should be a powerful caution.

F. Testamentary capacity

GPs require a working knowledge of the law concerning testamentary capacity, as they may be asked by the family or solicitor of an elderly patient, for a variety of reasons, to assess the individual's capacity to make a valid will. The conditions for testamentary capacity are that the testator must understand the nature and effects of his making a will, the extent of the assets to be disposed of, the relative claims of potential beneficiaries and that he be free from significant mental disorder.[40]

There are a number of important, though time-consuming tasks here for the doctor: an excellent practical guide in this regard is to be found in Jacoby.[41] The patient should be assessed in the standard way for dementia, with, if necessary, a second opinion from a psychiatrist in geriatrics. The acting solicitor should be consulted on appropriate legal tests and the facts of the case, e.g. the extent of the estate, previous wills, and reasons for including or excluding potential beneficiaries. Patients' answers should be recorded verbatim. The 'golden rule' for the doctor is that he witness the making of the will himself.

G. Driving and the law

When questions arise concerning an older person's capacity to drive safely, relatives may seek the opinion of the family doctor and ask him to advise the individual to stop driving. Older drivers, fearing the loss of mobility, may be very resistant to surrendering their licences voluntarily, despite their increasing frailty, visual or cognitive impairment or physical disability.

Legally, age itself is no bar to holding a valid driving licence, but all licence holders must be considered fit to drive, as defined by the Driver and Vehicle Licensing Agency (DVLA).[42] Driving licences are normally valid until the age of 70 years and may be renewed by a self-declaration to the DVLA that no medical disability is present. Thereafter they are renewable for 3 year periods, subject to satisfactory completion of medical questions on the application form.

Disabilities which restrict or impose conditions on the holding of a valid licence are categorized in the Road Traffic Act (1988).[43] A *prescribed* disability is one which constitutes a legal bar to holding a licence, e.g. epilepsy. A *relevant* disability is any medical condition likely to render the person a source of danger while driving, e.g. a visual field defect. A *prospective* disability is any medical condition which, because of its progressive or intermittent nature, may in time develop into a *prescribed* or *relevant* one, e.g. insulin-treated diabetes. Persons with such disabilities may normally only hold a driving licence subject to medical review in 1, 2 or 3 years. Specific medical standards are set out for fitness to drive in epilepsy, syncope, stroke, post-head injury, cardiac arrhythmias, diabetes, visual and psychiatric disorders, alcohol or drug abuse, cardiorespiratory disease and carcinoma.

In the case of dementia in its early stages, appropriate skills and judgement may be retained and a driving licence can be issued, if supported by appropriate medical reports. A systematic review of the evidence on road safety and driving in dementia[44] concluded that accidents are infrequent during the first 3 years of the disease.

However, notification of the DVLA of all new cases of Alzheimer's disease is mandatory. On diagnosis, an immediate decision on the patient's fitness to drive must be made and the DVLA duly notified. The doctor's duties in this regard are set out in General Medical Council guidelines.[45] These include convincing the patient that his medical condition may impair his ability to drive, and advising him to stop driving. Where he continues to drive against advice, a second opinion may be suggested, the next-of-kin informed and the relevant medical information disclosed to the medical adviser of the DVLA, notifying the patient of this action.

H. Confidentiality, privacy and information-sharing

Doctors have been charged with a duty of confidentiality towards patients since the beginnings of organized medicine, from the Hippocratic oath to successive rulings of medical professional bodies, the General Medical Council and the British Medical Association in the UK, and the wider framework of the European Commission on Human Rights.

At the present time, the greater part of medical consultations take place in public settings— hospitals, clinics and nursing or care homes. Patients interact with large numbers of different people, not only medical professionals but ancillary, social care and administrative staff, and patient information, easily accessible in written or electronic form, is routinely transmitted between individuals, departments and organizations.

There is, however, a professional duty of confidentiality in dealing with all patient-related information which identifies or contains details about patients of whatever age or condition. Where patient information is required for teaching, planning or research purposes, it must be anonymized, and clinical and administrative information reported separately. Without this proviso, it cannot be divulged without the express permission of the patient, unless required by law or overriding public interest.

Professionals also have a duty to keep electronically stored or written information protected and secure. The Data Protection Act (1998)[46] requires that organizations must process information on patients fairly and lawfully, in a manner which meets legal standards for confidentiality, and that information shared between organizations should be only the minimum necessary and retained for only as long as it is needed. Further, patients must be made aware of what information is being processed about them. The National Health Service (NHS) care-record guarantee sets out rules governing information held electronically by NHS case records, including patients' access to their own records and control over access by others, while the General Medical Council[17] and Nursing and Midwifery Council[47] set out duties around confidentiality, privacy and data-sharing.

All patients have the right to object to the disclosure of personal information which has been provided in confidence. This includes disclosure to relatives when it is against the patient's wishes. However, when patients lack capacity, it is usual to assume that they would want those close to them informed, unless there is clear evidence to the contrary. Health professionals should always be able to justify the reason for their disclosure.

An aspect of confidentiality, physical privacy, is particularly critical in the case of elderly people, many of whom live out the last of their lives in public, in chronic hospitals, nursing and care homes. Vulnerable older people may feel keenly the loss of privacy implicit in mixed-sex wards, shared bathing and toileting facilities and confidential disclosures made within earshot, if behind curtains.[28] Despite the introduction of national minimum standards[48] for privacy and dignity in social care, these have not yet been reached in a number of care homes.[7]

Case Example (illustrating issues in Section H)

Mrs J is aged 87 years and has been widowed for several years. Though increasingly frail, she is still lucid and takes an active interest in literature and current affairs. She has decided views about her own health care—in particular, taking as little medication as possible and remaining in her own home 'till the end'. She is becoming more unsteady and her eyesight is failing. Over the past 12 months, she has been admitted twice to hospital—once with a fall and a fracture of the humerus and once with a urinary tract infection causing transient confusion and immobility. For all this, she is realistic about the risks, knowing that she might fall again, and says that she will accept help at home if you feel she really needs it. She has one daughter who lives in Canada and has complained vociferously to you and the hospital that 'No one has told me anything. I would like to know what's going on.' However, Mrs J is quite adamant that she does not want information about her medical history shared and that she will choose what to tell her daughter. She is particularly worried that her daughter might put pressure on her to go into a home.

I. End-of-life care, autonomy and communication

With better treatments for medical conditions in mid-life and more people surviving to old age, an increasing proportion of end-of-life care concerns older people. However, with insufficient provision of palliative and hospice care, all primary care health workers will find themselves caring for older patients with end-stage illness—either in their own homes or in long-term care settings.[49] It is therefore important for skills and training in general practice in end-of-life care to be improved, for staff be aware of the guidelines and available resources, and for them to understand the associated ethical and legal issues.

A key issue is that of care planning and open communication around end-of-life care. Although there is some variability[50] in the amount of information older people wish to receive on prognosis and treatment, virtually all older people do wish to know their diagnosis. The World Health Organization[51] has highlighted how older cancer patients generally 'want more information, want to be involved in decision-making, and experience better psychological adjustment if palliative care and good communication are part of their care from the time of diagnosis.' Despite some relatives' requests that information be withheld from older cancer sufferers, 88% of patients, aged from 65 to 94 years, wanted to know more.[52] Other conditions, such as heart disease, appear to stimulate less open communication from health professionals, and in this respect the general management of such conditions compares unfavourably, in terms of information and support, with that available to cancer patients.[52] Patients need to know what to expect in the period leading up to their death. For many people, loss of control is one of their main fears. Consciously giving patients the opportunity to take control of whatever aspects of their care can be controlled may have a positive psychological effect. They may need to take practical steps to put their affairs in order, ensure that a will is up to date, sort out finances, or seek reconciliation with relatives.

Help the Aged[53] found that, compared with younger terminally ill patients, older people not only have fewer opportunities to discuss the options available to them at the end of life but also are more likely to have both multiple health problems and financial difficulties, are less likely to receive specialist care, less likely to die in the place they would prefer, and less likely to have social support networks.

Many older people are particularly worried about the circumstances in which they are likely to die. They fear dying alone or being found only after they have been dead for some time. Most people want to be at home with people around them at the end. For some, it is particularly crucial to have present some specific relative, such as the eldest son. Primary health care teams and other care providers need to have a general awareness of the cultural customs of the population they look after, but in every case they need to check what are the individual's wishes.

The ability of attending medical professionals to recognize the key signs of when patients are approaching their last days or hours is important for the planning of a 'good death'. At this stage, members of the care team need to communicate well with each other and with the patient. It is important to avoid mixed messages which lead to poor patient management. Once dying is diagnosed, patient care needs to refocus. Relatives and patients themselves may initially want to collude with a pretence that death is not approaching, but often feel aggrieved and unprepared when the truth emerges. It is better for health professionals to explore patients' wishes sensitively, with the aim of encouraging them to recognize the reality of their situation.

Age Concern[54] has also set out principles, described below, which should form the basis of the care of terminally ill patients, as reflecting the wishes of perhaps the majority of people at the last stage of their lives. Aware of when death is coming and what can be expected, the individual should be afforded dignity and privacy, and as far as possible retain control of what happens—control of pain relief and symptoms, and control and choice over where death takes place and in the presence of whom. The dying person should have access to information and expertise of whatever kind is necessary—hospice care in any location, not only in hospital, and to any desired spiritual or emotional support. Opportunities should be offered for the individual to realize any last wishes, e.g. to issue advance directives in the knowledge that they will be respected, and to carry out any desired last actions. Finally, the dying person should have time to say goodbye, and be able to let go and not to have life prolonged pointlessly (see Chapter 25).

Case Example (illustrating issues in Sections I and J)

Mr C is a Chinese gentleman, whose English is good and who has lived in the UK for many years. He has recently moved to the area to live with his extended family and is now on your list. He has recently been losing weight rapidly and suffering widespread bony pain and new onset of leg weakness. You suspect disseminated prostate cancer with spinal secondaries and refer him to the hospital for urgent investigation. His son and daughter-in-law contact you to 'make sure' you or the hospital 'don't tell him' the results of any tests or what you are suspecting but 'speak to them first'. Later, when your suspicions are confirmed in a letter from the hospital, he not only requests full and frank information but also makes it clear that he does not want any additional treatment—including radiotherapy. His family put pressure on you and him to do 'everything possible' to 'fight' the condition and, although he has made it clear he is not hungry, also ask that you 'give him something to make him eat.'

J. Withdrawing and withholding treatment, nutrition, hydration and resuscitation

Decisions around the provision, non-commencement or withdrawal of life-prolonging treatment may be contentious and difficult for health professionals, patients, their families and in the public consciousness. A number of interventions such as resuscitation or dialysis might prolong life but not prevent death or modify the prognosis of the underlying condition. Treatments which might provide therapeutic benefit are not automatically used. Decisions are weighed using factors such as patients' wishes, the invasiveness/burden and likely success of the treatment, its side-effects, limits of efficacy and the resources available.[3]

Professionals are not morally or legally obliged to provide therapeutically futile treatment. But decisions to stop treatment should incorporate sensitive discussion with the patient and family ensuring that all understand the reasons for the decision and its implications. Such decisions should be based where possible on reliable data and not on assumptions about patients' wishes or their ability to gain benefit, even at an advanced age.

Oral nutrition and hydration

Where nutrition and hydration are provided by 'ordinary means' (e.g. hand-feeding or drinking from a cup or straw) this forms part of *basic care* and should not be withdrawn, though they should not be forced upon patients who resist or express a clear refusal or who are at risk of adverse events such as choking or aspiration. Where nutritional needs cannot be met meet by 'conventional' means, consideration should be given to whether artificial nutrition and/or hydration should be provided.[55]

Many older patients with a disability who require assistance with feeding can still safely swallow: this forms part of basic care. But when patients are terminally ill, they often no longer want nutrition and/or hydration, which may even worsen discomfort and suffering.[56] Good practice must, however, include good oral care to avoid the discomfort of a dry mouth.

Artificial nutrition and hydration

Whereas treatment may, in some circumstances, be withheld or withdrawn, appropriate basic care should always be provided unless actively resisted by the patient. Where patients lack the capacity to express preferences, procedures that are essential to keep the patient comfortable should be provided. If in doubt, we should presume in favour of providing relief from symptoms and distress and enhancing the patient's dignity. For the terminally ill, it is not usually appropriate to provide invasive treatment but the individual circumstances must be considered. The insertion of a feeding tube is legally classed as *medical treatment* rather than basic care, so that decisions not to insert a feeding tube, or not to reinsert it if it becomes dislodged, are legitimate medical decisions after assessment of the individual circumstances of the case, whereas a decision to stop providing hydration is not.

Artificial hydration and nutrition should be assessed separately. For example, with some terminally ill patients, subcutaneous or intravenous fluids may avoid dehydration, decrease pressure-sore risk and aid comfort, but the provision of nutrition artificially would be too invasive to be in a patient's best interests. With other patients, it is appropriate for both nutrition and hydration to be provided, withheld or withdrawn.

Cardiopulmonary resuscitation

In the discussions organized by Help the Aged,[53] some older people's experience of caring for their relatives led them to decide that they themselves would not want cardiopulmonary resuscitation (CPR) to be attempted on them. CPR should never be attempted on people who have clearly refused it in advance. But we cannot assume that all older people feel the same way, even when they have multiple morbidities and a poor prognosis. It might be considered discriminatory to decide against CPR merely on the basis of disability rather than as a carefully considered and individualized decision made case by case.

Establishments caring for older people (even nursing homes, which may feel that they are ill-equipped to provide CPR) should have a clear policy about this, and it must be readily available to, and understood by, staff.[57,58] It may not always be a question of providing the full panoply of CPR technology, but rather ensuring that personnel are trained to provide basic CPR. Where older patients have existing conditions which make cardiac arrest likely, consideration should be given in advance to formulating a management plan. Such plans should be discussed with patients who have capacity, or those close to patients who lack capacity, including informing them when a decision is made to not undertake CPR because the patient would not survive the attempt. Any such decisions, and the reasons for them, should be recorded in the medical notes. Although some professionals find it difficult to discuss the subject with patients, they should do so when appropriate. It is not necessary to raise the issue if it is clear that CPR would not be successful or if the patient has reached the terminal stage of life. Dying patients should not be subjected to CPR as this would be futile and inappropriate.

Conclusion

As the population increasingly survives into old age, primary care will increasingly focus on older people, raising a host of ethical issues for primary care practitioners. Such issues are not 'small print' but a common feature of front-line practice. In such circumstances practitioners can often feel the lack of relevant practical guidance. And where the decision or dilemma is grey with no clear-cut answer, practitioners may feel hesitant. This chapter has outlined some of the principles required to deal with moral uncertainty, and has supplied more concrete advice for the kinds of scenarios that practitioners might commonly encounter.

References

1. Department of Health. *Making Decisions. A Guide for People Working in Health and Social Care.* London: DoH; 2008. Available at: http://www.dca.gov.uk/legal-policy/mental-capacity/mca-guide-for-professionals/pdf

2. Wanless D, on behalf of King's Fund. *Securing Good Care For Older People. Taking a Long Term View.* London: King's Fund; 2006. Available at: http://www.kingsfund.org.uk/publications/kings_fund_publications/securing_good

3. British Medical Association, Medical Ethics Committee. *Working Together for Older People.* London: BMJ Publishing (in press).

4. Eccles J. Ethical considerations in the care of older people. *Clin Med* 2003;3:416–8.

5. Rai G (ed.). *Medical Ethics and the Elderly.* Oxford: Radcliffe Publishing; 2005.

6. Department of Health. *A New Ambition for Old Age Next Steps in Implementing the National Service Framework for Older People.* London: DoH; 2006. Available at: http://www.dh.gov.uk/en/Publicationsandstatistics/Publications/PublicationsPolicyAndGuidance/DH_4133941

7. Healthcare Commission. *Caring for Dignity: A National Report on Dignity in Care for Older People While in Hospital.* London: Healthcare Commission; 2007.

8. Williams K, Kemper S, Hummett ML. Enhancing communication with older adults: overcoming elderspeak. *J Geront Nurs* 2004;30:17–25.

9. Oliver D. Acopia and social admission are not diagnoses. Why older people deserve better. *J R Soc Med* 2008;101:68–74.

10. Rockwood K. What would make a definition of frailty successful?. *Age Ageing* 2005;34:432–4.

11. Woolhead G, Calnan M, Dieppe P, Tadd W. Dignity in older age: what do older people in the United Kingdom think?. *Age Ageing* 2004;33:165–70.

12. Beauchamp TL, Childress JF. *Principles of Biomedical Ethics*, 5th edn. Oxford: Oxford University Press; 2001. p. 12–13.

13. *Op. cit.* p. 15–20.

14. *Op. cit.* p. 57–9.

15. Gillon R. Promoting the four principles remains of great importance in ordinary medicine. *J Med Ethics* 2003;29:267–8.

16. Gillon R. Medical ethics. Four core principles plus attention to scope. *Br Med J* 1994;309:184–6.

17. General Medical Council. *The Duties of a Doctor Registered with the General Medical Council.* London: GMC; 2006.

18. Westlaw UK. Online legal information service. Available at: http://www.westlaw.co.uk/

19. Brazier M. *Medicine, Patients and the Law,* 3rd edn. London: Penguin Books; 2003.

20. Mason JK, McCall-Smith RA, Laurie GT. *Law and Medical Ethics,* 6th edn. London: Lexis Nexis; 2002.

21. Montgomery J. *Healthcare Law,* 2nd edn. Oxford: Oxford University Press; 2003.

22. Help the Aged. *Listening to Older people: Opening the Door for Older People to Explore End-of-life Issues.* London: Help the Aged; 2006.

23. Counsel and Care. *The Right to Take Risks.* London: Counsel and Care; 1993.

24. Department of Health. *Independence, Choice and Risk: A Guide to Best Practice in Supported Decision-making.* London: DoH; 2007.

25. Department of Health. *The National Service Framework for Older People.* London: DoH; 2001. Available at: http://www.dh.gov.uk/en/Publicationsandstatistics/Publications/PublicationsPolicyAndGuidance/DH_4003066

26. British Medical Association. *Evidence Based Prescribing.* London: BMJ Publishing; 2007.

27. Milton JC, Jackson SHD. Inappropriate polypharmacy. Reducing the burden of multiple medication. *Clin Med* 2007;4:514–17.

28. House of Lords and House of Commons Joint Committee on Human Rights. *The Human Rights of Older People in Healthcare.* London: Office for Public Sector Information; 2007.

29. Department of Health. Listening Events. The top "dignity" issues people have said they wish to see addressed. London: Department of Health; 2006. Available at: http://www.cardiff.ac.uk/medicine/geriatric_medicine/international_research/dignity/index.htm

30. Hill T. *Autonomy and Self-Respect.* Cambridge: Cambridge University Press; 1991.

31. General Medical Council. Consent: *Doctors and Patients Making Decisions Together.* London: GMC; 2007. Available at: 18/07/08 on http://www.gmc-uk.org/guidance/ethical_guidance/consent_guidance/endnotes.asp

32. Alderson P, Goodey C. Theories of consent. *Br Med J* 1998;317:1313–15.

33. Childress JF. Paternalism in health care and health policy. In: Ashcroft RE, Dawson A, Draper A, McMillan JR (eds), *Principles of Healthcare Ethics,* 2nd edn. London: Wiley; 2007.

34. Brazier M. Patient autonomy and consent to treatment. The role of law. *Legal Stud* 1987;7:72–6.

35. Mental Capacity Act (2005). London: Office for Public Sector Information. Available at: http://www.dh.gov.uk/PublicationsAndStatistics/Bulletins/ChiefExecutiveBulletin/ChiefExecutiveBulletinArticle/fs/en?CONTENT_ID=4108436&chk=z0Ds8

36. Mukerhjee E, Foster R. The Mental Capacity Act 2007 and capacity assessments: a guide for the non-psychiatrist. *Clin Med* 2008;8:65–9.

37. Nicholson TRJ, Cutter W, Hotopf M. Assessing mental capacity: the Mental Capacity Act. *Br Med J* 2008;336:322–25.

38. Dworkin, G. Paternalism. *The Monist* 1972;1:64–84.

39. Department of Health. *Briefing Sheet. Mental Health Bill. Bournewood Safeguards.* London: DoH; 2006.

40. Banks v Goodfellow [1870] 5 LR QB 549.

41. Jacoby R, Steer P. How to assess capacity to make a will. *Br Med J* 2007;335:155–7.

42. Driver and Vehicle Licensing Agency (DVLA), Drivers Medical Group. *At a Glance, for Medical Practitioners. Guide to the Current Medical Standards of Fitness to Drive.* Swansea: DVLA; 2008. Available at: http://www.dvla.gov.uk/media/pdf/medical/aagv1.pdf

43. Road Traffic Act (1988) Section 2: London: Office for Public Sector Information. Available http://www.opsi.gov.uk/Acts/acts1988/ukpga_19880052_en_2

44. Breen DP, Breen DA, Moore JW, Breen P, O' D. Driving and dementia. *Br Med J* 2007;334:1365–9.

45. General Medical Council. *Revised Guidance on Medical Assessment of Fitness to Drive.* London: GMC; 2008.

46. Data Protection Act (1998). London: Office of Public Sector Information. Available at: http://www.opsi.gov.uk/Acts/Acts1998/ukpga_19980029_en_1

47. Nursing and Midwifery Council. *Professional Conduct; Standards for Conduct, Performance and Ethics.* London: NMC; 2006. Available at http://www.nmc-uk.org/aFramedisplay.aspx?documentID=201

48. Care Standards Act (2003). London: Office of Public Sector Information. Available at: http://www.opsi.gov.uk/acts/acts2000/en/ukpgaen_20000014_en_1

49. National Council for Palliative Care (2006) Introductory Guide to End-of-life Care in Care Homes. London: NCPC. Available at: http://ncpc.org.uk/download/publications/GuideToEoLC%20 CareHomes.pdf

50. Meredith C, Symonds P, Webster L, Lamont D, Pyper E, Gillis CR. Information needs of cancer patients in West Scotland: cross sectional survey of patients' views. *Br Med J* 1996;313:724–6.

51. WHO Europe. *Better Palliative Care for Older People.* Geneva: WHO; 2004. p. 16.

52. Ajaj A, Singh MP, Abdulla AJJ. Should elderly patients be told they have cancer? Questionnaire survey of older people. *Br Med J* 2001;323:1160.

53. Help the Aged. *Dying in Older Age: Reflections from an Older Person's Perspective.* London: Help the Aged; 2005.

54. Age Concern. Debate of the Health and Care Study Group. *The Future of Health and Care of Older People; the Best is Yet to Come.* London: Age Concern; 1999.

55. British Medical Association. *Withholding and Withdrawing Life-prolonging Treatment.* London: British Medical Association; 2006.

56. Baines MJ. Symptom management and palliative care. In: Evans JG, Williams TF, editors. *Oxford Textbook of Geriatric Medicine.* Oxford: OUP; 1992. p. 693–6.

57. NHS Executive. *Resuscitation Policy (HSC 2000/028).* London: Department of Health; September 2000.

58. Conroy SP, Luxton A, Dingwall R, Harwood RH, Gladman JF. Cardiopulmonary resuscitation in continuing care settings: time for a rethink?. *Br Med J* 2006;332:479–82.

Chapter 24

Vulnerable adults

Margot Gosney

Introduction

Granny-battering was described in the UK in 1975, although much of the research in this area had previously been performed outside the UK.[1] In 1988 a Social Services survey[2] found that 5% of elderly clients were being abused and a 1990 study suggested that 45% of carers openly admitted to some form of abuse in a study of patients admitted for respite services.[3] Although few of the patients in the latter study admitted to having been abused, there is clearly a discrepency in the data between the two groups of individuals.

The first prevalence study of elder abuse in Britain was published in the *British Medical Journal* in 1992.[4] During the initial days following their study, there was outrage and much dispute about the reliability of the data. Action on Elder Abuse (AEA) was established in 1993 with the prime aim of preventing the abuse of older people.

What is adult abuse?

Adult abuse may be defined as a single or repeated act or lack of appropriate actions, occurring within any relationship where there is an expectation of trust, which causes harm or distress to an older person. In March 2000, the Department of Health issued *No Secrets*, which was comparable to the Welsh guidance publication, *In Safe Hands*. In *No Secrets*, abuse was defined as 'A violation of an individual's human and civil rights by any other person or persons. It may be physical, verbal or psychological, it may be an act of neglect or an omission to act, or it may occur when a vulnerable person is persuaded to enter into a financial or sexual transaction, to which he or she has not consented, or cannot consent. Abuse can occur in any relationship and may result in significant harm to, or exploitation of, the person subjected to it.'[5]

How common is abuse?

In the UK Study of Abuse and Neglect of Older People, published in June 2007, the achieved samples were representative of the general UK population aged ≥66 years who were living in private households.[6,7] They found that 2.6% of individuals aged >66 years reported that they had experienced mistreatment involving a family member, close friend or care worker in the previous year. This would equate to a quarter of a million people living in private households in the UK who were neglected or abused on an annual basis. If the definition of mistreatment is broadened to include incidents involving neighbours and acquaintances, prevalence increases to 4%, i.e. 342 000 older people will be subject to some form of mistreatment on an annual basis.

There is very little evidence as to the prevalence of elder abuse in nursing and residential homes. It must be remembered that the majority of patients within these settings are often physically frail, with marked cognitive impairment. Thus, physical injuries may be poorly reported and, without input from health care professionals and family and friends, many older people may suffer abuse that is poorly recognized and therefore underreported. Coincidential falls, the use of bed restraints, and high levels of medication may compound abuse and make it difficult to detect and quantify.

What type of abuse occurs?

Physical abuse usually takes the form of slapping, shaking or inflicting physical damage. Sexual abuse includes any sexual act to which a person has not agreed, and financial abuse is the stealing of somebody's money, or denying them access to their money or possessions. Older individuals may also feel pressure in connection with wills, property, inheritance or financial transactions. The misuse or misappropriation of property, possessions or benefit as well as exploitation, are defined as financial abuse. More difficult to define is psychological abuse. Any threat of harm, abandonment, humiliation, intimidation or verbal abuse that results in psychological distress, is a form of abuse.

There is evidence that psychological abuse is probably the most common form of abuse experienced by older people, but that which is taken least seriously by health care professionals. It could be considered that leaving an elderly person in a revealing gown or nightdress, in the absence of underwear in a public environment, is the commonest form of psychological abuse seen within many healthcare settings. Shouting at an older person is often considered to be acceptable due to an older person's deafness. It is neither helpful nor appropriate and may cause fear and distress. Much psychological abuse results from ignorance of health care workers and those dealing with an elderly population. Unfortunately it may occur in the person's own home or in a care home setting as the result of poor training and supervision, but must not be tolerated. Neglect by ignoring people's medical or care needs is a further example of abuse and includes depriving people of their medication, particularly pain relief; leaving people without easy access to food or drink; and failure to deal with issues of continence. Discriminatory abuse includes racist, sexist or other comments based on a person's disability.

Who is mistreated?

Women are more likely to say that they have experienced mistreatment than men. Men aged ≥85 years are more likely to experience financial abuse than men in the younger age groups, and women aged ≥85 years are more likely to have been neglected.

Mistreatment varies with socio-economic position, with those who live in rented housing tending to have higher prevalence rates than those who are in owner-occupied accommodation. Mistreatment also varies by marital status, with almost 10% of those who are separated or divorced having experienced mistreatment, compared to 1.4% of those who are widowed. Those living alone are more likely to experience financial abuse than those who live with others.

Who are the perpetrators?

In the 2007 study, which excluded stranger abuse, 51% of the mistreatment involved a partner or a spouse, 49% another family member, 13% a care worker and 5% a close friend.[6] When abuse is interpersonal, i.e. physical, psychological or sexual, perpetrators were four times more likely to be male, although when financial abuse occurred, 56% of the perpetrators were male. The perpetrators who carry out financial abuse are more likely to be younger than those carrying out interpersonal abuse. Over half of all perpetrators were living in the respondent's household at the time of abuse (25% financial abuse perpetrators; 65% interpersonal abuse perpetrators).

It must be remembered that perpetrators could be any individuals who come into contact with older people. They can be health or social care professionals, volunteers, friends and neighbours or someone well known to the vulnerable adult.

Is abuse reported?

Within the 2007 UK study, 70% of older people said that they had reported the incident or sought help, although only in 30% of cases had this been from a health professional or social worker.[6] What this study fails to address is the abuse that occurs in residential or nursing care, or in those who are not able through cognitive decline or disability, to convey the abuse that has occurred. The Commission for Social Care Inspection (CSCI) found that in 20% of care services no-one interviewed could remember receiving or understanding information about what to do if they had concerns about abuse.[8] Although in 82% of care services everyone interviewed said that they could speak to a staff member or manager if they felt unsafe, in only two-thirds of services (61%) did all interviewees feel that any concerns raised would be acted upon.

Is elder abuse and mistreatment only a UK phenomenon?

Studies have been undertaken in the USA,[9] Canada,[10] The Netherlands[11] and Germany[12] and have found that prevalence ranged from 2.6% (USA, 1988), to 5.6% (Amsterdam, The Netherlands, 1994). The studies were methodologically different. In Amsterdam and Germany face-to face interviews were carried out in a similar way to the 1992 UK study, and in the USA and Canada respondents were contacted by telephone. All studies were community-based and therefore excluded individuals in nursing or residential care.

A systematic review of worldwide prevalence of elder abuse and neglect was undertaken by Cooper and colleagues and published in *Age and Ageing* in 2008.[13]

What training do healthcare professionals receive about elder abuse?

Training of individuals about elder abuse is patchy, although many hospitals and primary care organizations now insist that all individuals managing the care of older people, or involved in the care of such individuals, should have Level 1 Safeguarding Adults training. However, CSCI found that no council had a systematic approach to prevent the abuse of people who direct their own care, although councils were beginning to provide options for this group. In the CSCI study it was found that 81% of relevant council staff had received training about safeguarding during 2007 to 2008, but only 46% of the independent sector have had this training.[8]

Risk factors for abuse

In one of the earlier studies of abuse of patients in the community who were subsequently admitted for respite, two characteristics of carers were associated with abuse: poor long-term relationships and a history of alcohol abuse.[3]

There is evidence that any carer who has significant other dependants is more at risk of being an abuser than those who have no other dependants of any age. A history of mental ill health, substance misuse, violence or abuse, either as a victim or as a perpetrator, increases the chances that an individual will abuse an older adult. When any individual is dependent on a vulnerable adult for financial support or accommodation, abuse is more common, for example in the case of a son or daughter who is living with an elderly parent in the knowledge that if that elderly parent goes into a nursing home, (s)he will loose not only financial benefit, but also the benefit of living under the parent's roof. Under these circumstances, healthcare professionals must be vigilant to ensure that carers do not insist that a vulnerable adult remains in the community, when 24 h care in a nursing home may be more appropriate. Many carers are faced with the loss of one parent or indeed of a spouse or partner just prior to taking on the role of carer. These people are at increased risk of abusing, as are those living in poor or inadequate living conditions. Any individual who has suffered abuse, either in childhood, or in later life, is more at risk of being involved in elder abuse, if they have significant contact with a vulnerable adult.

Within the nursing and residential home settings, a number of factors have been identified as increasing the abuse of older adults. Poor management and communication between staff and managers, which may or may not result in low staffing levels and a high turnover of staff, are often associated with abuse. Lack of supervisional support of staff working in an authoritarian atmosphere may put residents at increased risk. Lack of training, particularly concerning privacy and dignity, as well as basic nursing care, may result in abuse as a definite activity, or in neglect due to staff 'knowing no better'. Any institution where there is poor recording of complaints and little contact with the outside world may result in abuse being undetected for long periods of time. It is known that one of the major identified forms of abuse that occurs in the nursing home setting is the overadministration of medication to ensure that older residents are compliant and quiet. This may result in a sleepy older person, who has poor oral fluid and food intake, which may in turn result in infections and a higher incidence of falls.

Reporting elder abuse

All employees have a duty to report any suspicions of abuse that they may have, and individual organizations should operate a whistleblowing policy that protects people who report their concerns. Most social services departments have a lead for safeguarding adults, who should be the first point of contact, when abuse is suspected. These individuals will work with others from the multi-agency to ensure that all reports are fully investigated, that strategy meetings are held and that individuals are safeguarded where abuse has occurred or the potential for abuse exists. The quickest way to find one's local safeguarding adults co-ordinator is to search the website of the local Social Services organizations and find a link entitled 'Safeguarding Adults', where emergency numbers are usually provided.

Who forms the multi-agency Safeguarding Board?

Social Services' departments lead all multi-agency investigations and are responsible for documentation, communication with other professionals, leading strategy meetings, and for the future support of the individual who may have been abused. They work very closely with the police, who will be involved, not only if criminal charges are to be brought, but also in the investigation of suspected abuse. The CSCI works closely with the Safeguarding Board and is responsible for inspections of nursing and residential homes within a particular geographical area (see Chapter 26). Health is represented usually by both primary and secondary care trusts and a close working relationship is essential to ensure that patients move from one environment to another in a seamless fashion, and that abuse that has occurred within the community can be reported in secondary care and vice versa. The private and voluntary organizations are usually well represented, particularly since many of them will have contact with older people who may be poorly known to both health and social care services. Organizations bringing together all nursing and residential homes in an area will provide insight into reporting mechanisms, and their involvement will also ensure that there is consistent training across all organizations.

Points to remember

1) Abuse of older individuals occurs in healthcare, social care and private individuals' homes.

2) Perpetrators may be well known to the vulnerable adult and placed in a position of trust by healthcare professionals.

3) Many older individuals find it difficult to bring up the topic of elder abuse and the healthcare professional is therefore responsible for picking up clues that may enable them to ask targeted questions.

4) Social Services take the lead for all safeguarding adult issues and can be contacted through local unitary authorities.

5) Strategy meetings are convened and all interested parties represented. Decisions made at strategy meetings must then be conveyed to the multi-agency partners, even if they were not present at the strategy meeting.

6) Features commonly seen in older adults, such as falls, poor nutrition and pressure sores, may be indicators of abuse and if the history provided to the general practioner is not in keeping with the injuries observed, a high level of suspicion should exist.

7) It is better to express concerns that are investigated and found to be entirely innocent, than to wait for another individual to report on your behalf.

8) When reporting suspected abuse within one's own organization, a whistleblowing policy protects the informant.

References

1. Baker AA. Granny battering. *Mod Geriat* 1975;5:20–4.

2. Tomlin S. *Abuse of Elderly People: An Unnecessary and Preventable Problem*. London: British Geriatrics Society; 1988.

3. Homer AC, Gilleard C. Abuse of elderly people by their carers. *Br Med J* 1990;301:1359–62.

4. Ogg J, Bennett G. Elder abuse in Britain. *Br Med J* 1992;305:998–9.

5. Department of Health. *No Secrets: Guidance on Developing and Implementing Multi-agency Policies and Procedures to Protect Vulnerable Adults from Abuse*. London: DoH; 2000. Available at: http://www.dh. gov.uk/en/Publicationsandstatistics/Publications/PublicationsPolicyAndGuidance/DH_4008486

6. O' M, Hills A, Doyle M, *et al. UK Study of Abuse and Neglect of Older People. Prevalence Survey Report*. London: National Centre for Social Research; 2007. Available at: http://www.natcen.ac.uk/natcen/ pages/publications/research_summaries/NC234_RF_OlderPeople_web2.pdf

7. Action on Elder Abuse. *Briefing Paper: The UK Study of Abuse and Neglect of Older People 2007*. London: AEA; 2007. Available at: http://www.elderabuse.org.uk/Prevalence/Briefingpaperprevalence. pdf

8. Commission for Social Care Inspection. *How Councils Have Assessed their Progress in Delivering Services to Adults Needing Social Care*. London: CSCI; 2008. Available at: http://www.csci.gov.uk/ pdf/1SAS%20Report.pdf

9. Pillemer K, Finkelhor D. The prevalence of elder abuse: a random sample survey. *Gerontologist* 1998;28:51–7.

10. Podnieks E. National Survey on Abuse of the Elderly in Canada. *J Elder Abuse Negl* 1992;4:5–58.

11. Comijs HC, Pot AM, Smit JH, Bouter LM, Jonker C. Elder abuse in the community: prevalence and consequences. *J Am Geriatr Soc* 1998;46:885–8.

12. Wetzels P, Greve W. The elderly as victims of intrafamilial violence—results of a criminologic dark field study. *Z Gerontol Geriatr* 1996;29:191–200.

13. Cooper C, Selwood A, Livingston G. The prevalence of elder abuse and neglect: a systematic review. *Age Ageing* 2008;37:151–160.

Further reading

Age Concern England. *On the Right Track? A Progress Report of the Human Rights of Older People in Health and Social Care*. London: Age Concern; 2008. Available at: http://www.ageconcern.org.uk/AgeConcern/ 9730BC71BEB14E8999B1493FA1AF21B1.asp

Commission for Social Care Inspection. *Safe and Sound? Checking the suitability of new care staff in regulated social care services.* Available at: http://www.csci.org.uk. This document highlights recruitment and vetting practices and gives an overview on the new vetting and barring scheme.

Department of Health. Safeguarding vulnerable adults—Independent Safeguarding Authority (ISA): next step in transition to new Vetting and Barring Scheme. Under the Safeguarding Vulnerable Groups Act 2006, Parliament established a statutory body to take the decisions on who should be barred—The Independent Safeguarding Authority (ISA). The existing barred lists, PoCA (Protection of Childrens Act) and POVA (The Protection of Vulnerable Adults), will be replaced in October 2009, by the ISA, two new barred lists. From winter 2008, the employer's will make referrals to the ISA. Available at: http://www.dh.gov.uk/en/SocialCare/Deliveringadultsocialcare/Vulnerableadults/DH_088153

House of Commons, Health Committee. *Elder Abuse.* Second Report of Session 2003–04. Volume 1. Available at: http://www.publications.parliament.uk/pa/cm200304/cmselect/cmhealth/111/111.pdf. This is a Department of Health document that defines elder abuse and the prevalence, as well as many of the settings and how to tackle elder abuse in the community).

House of Lords and House of Commons Joint Committee on Human Rights. *Human Rights of Older People in Healthcare.* 18th Report of Session 2006–07, 14 August 2007. Available at: http://www.publications.parliament.uk/pa/jt200607/jtselect/jtrights/156/15602.htm

McAlpine CH. Elder abuse and neglect. *Age Ageing* 2008;37:132–133.

The Mental Capacity Act 2005: a new criminal offence. Available at: http://www.dca.gov.uk/menincap/legis.htm On 1 April 2007 the Mental Capacity Act 2005 came into force across England and Wales. Under Section 44 it sets out the new criminal offence of ill treatment or wilful neglect. It applies if a person ('D'): has the care of a person ('P') who lacks, or whom ('D') reasonably believes to lack common, capacity; is the donee of an lasting power of attorney, or an existing enduring power of attorney, created by ('P'); or is a deputy appointed by the court for ('P'). Such individuals will be guilty of an offence, if they treat or wilfully neglect the person they have cared for, or to whom the lasting power of attorney or enduring power of attorney or deputy appointment relates.

Association of Directors of Social Services. *Safeguarding Adults. A National Framework of Standards for good practice and outcomes in adult protection work.* This document gives the eleven standards which cover: joint planning and capability; prevention of abuse and neglect; responding to abuse and neglect; access and involvement. It has a useful bibliography, as well as a number of useful websites, pertinent not only to older individuals, but also to those caring for people with learning difficulties, who may be at risk of abuse, for women and children experiencing domestic violence and organizations concerned with working environments. London: ADSS. Available at: http://www.adass.org.uk/images/stories/publications/guidance/safeguarding.pdf

Chapter 25

Palliative care

Louise Robinson and Alexa Clark

Definition and philosophy of palliative care

Palliative care is 'the active total care of patients whose disease is not responsive to curative treatment. Control of pain, of other symptoms, and of psychological, social and spiritual problems is paramount. The goal of palliative care is achievement of the best quality of life for patients and their families'.[1]

Current NHS policy: palliative care provision and care of older people

The National Health Service (NHS) End of Life Programme[2] highlights the importance of palliative care for all those with a life-limiting illness. It emphasizes the need for equality of care wherever the person lives and dies, whether at home, in a care home, in hospital or in a hospice, and that 'the care of all dying patients must improve to the level of the best'. It promotes the use of three specific End of Life tools: palliative care standards, advance care planning, and a care pathway for the dying. These promote good communication and proactive planning.

Palliative care has been offered to patients with cancer for many years, and services developed in line with the NHS Cancer Plan,[3] NICE guidance for improving supportive and palliative care for adults with cancer,[4] and the Cancer Reform Strategy.[5] The importance of palliative care for non-cancer patients is also highlighted in the various Department of Health National Service Frameworks: Coronary Heart Disease (2000), Renal Services (2004), Long Term (Neurological) Conditions (2005) and the National Dementia Strategy (2009).

Specialist palliative care teams, in hospices, hospital and the community, now commonly care for those with non-cancer diagnoses including coronary heart disease, chronic lung disease, renal failure, multiple sclerosis, motor neurone disease, dementia, Parkinson's disease, as well as those with cancer. The guidance provided in this section is applicable to all older people with palliative care needs.

Provision of palliative and end of life care

Care in the community: role of the GP and primary care team

Standard 2 of the National Service Framework for Older People[6] highlights the importance of patient-centred care for older people through provision of information, choice, integrated and co-ordinated care, and support for their carers. In end of life care, the general practitioner (GP) and the primary care team are well placed to facilitate all of these, particularly as the GP is likely to have been involved from the beginning of the diagnosis of an incurable illness. The patient's wishes are central to the care provided by the community; however, the level of care provided by their family and friends cannot be assumed or estimated. A common difficulty in the provision of palliative care to older people is that their main carer, usually their spouse, will also have chronic health problems, as illustrated in the example of Mr S (Case Scenario). Both the patient's and the carers' needs require assessment in order to determine the most appropriate package of care.

In order to provide co-ordinated care in the community, effective teamwork is essential, with team members having a mutual understanding of each others' roles and responsibilities (see Figure 25.1). In the example of Mr S and his wife, the GP would traditionally discuss the diagnosis and prognosis of the disease, act as gate-keeper to secondary and community care services, provide information on practical, emotional and financial assistance and anticipate care requirements. Meanwhile, the community nurse would provide general hands-on nursing care, organize aids and equipment, provide emotional support and co-ordinate and access other services. Both would liaise closely with palliative care services, especially specialist palliative care nurses (often termed 'Macmillan nurses' in recognition of the charity that supports their role), in order to access specialist advice and hospice-based services, such as day care and respite care. In some areas a 24 hour (h) community nursing service is available; a night-sitting service may also be accessed, sometimes provided by Marie Curie nurses. The Case Scenario below provides an example of how such collaboration works in practice.

Case Scenario   Co-ordinated care in the community

Mr S, an insulin-dependent diabetic man aged 78 years, has for many years been the main carer for his wife, who has advanced Parkinson's disease. Following an emergency admission, he underwent a colectomy for bowel cancer. After surgery, the disease is confirmed as having spread into local lymph nodes and the peritoneum. He is fully informed of the diagnosis and offered chemotherapy; however, the consultant feels this will only be a palliative measure. On his return home, the community nurse attends to provide wound care; she also organizes a social services referral to discuss temporary home care support for both Mr S and his wife and an occupational therapy assessment. During a visit from his GP, the diagnosis and prognosis of the illness are revisited and the pros and cons of undergoing chemotherapy discussed. Mr S decides to forego this as he feels it will not greatly alter his prognosis and may affect his ability to continue to care for his wife. The GP refers Mr S to the palliative care team for support and to the local hospice, as both Mr S and his wife wish to attend for day care and complementary therapies. The GP also advises Mr S about the special attendance allowance (DS1500). The GP adds Mr S's name to the practice cancer and palliative care registers.

A new General Practice Contract was implemented in 2004 which defined core primary care services and optional enhanced services. It introduced a new concept: the provision of financial rewards linked to the achievement of clinical and non-clinical quality markers, through a Quality and Outcomes Framework (QOF) derived from evidence-based care.[7] The QOF for cancer requires general practices to maintain a register of all cancer patients and review their care within 6 months of diagnosis; the standard for palliative care stipulates the development and maintenance of a palliative care register and regular review of all listed patients. Patients eligible for the palliative care register are those whose death would not be unexpected within the next year.

Specialist palliative care services

Specialist palliative care services support and complement primary health care teams in providing palliative care to patients and carers. These services are for those with any life-limiting illness, not only cancer.

Community palliative care teams consist of a consultant and clinical nurse specialists in palliative care (Macmillan nurses); there may also be physiotherapists, occupational therapists and social workers working within the team. The team visit patients and families at home to assess and advise on physical symptoms (e.g. pain, nausea and vomiting, agitation), provide psychological support to patients and their relatives/carers, and address social and spiritual issues. They also

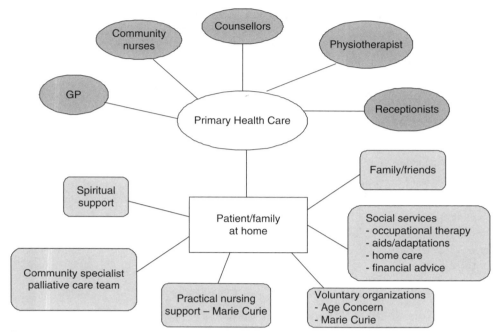

Fig. 25.1 Care in the community and effective teamwork.

provide telephone advice and support for health care professionals. Hospital palliative care teams work in a similar way but are based within hospitals.

Hospices provide specialist inpatient care for symptom control (physical, psychological, spiritual), end of life care and sometimes respite care. Services vary but most also provide day hospice facilities, day treatment service, e.g. for blood transfusion, complementary therapies, specialist lymphoedema services, and medical outpatients.

Management of common problems in older people towards the end of life

Many elderly patients are prescribed multiple drugs, which may cause side-effects independently or in combination. It is important to be aware if the patient has any renal or liver decompensation as this will affect the metabolism and excretion of some drugs (see Chapter 4). Regular medication review is essential; any non-effective medication should be discontinued and the number of drugs should be kept to a minimum. Patients' compliance, and their ability to swallow, will obviously affect whether the drug is actually ingested. Transdermal patches, where appropriate, help to ensure patient compliance.

Non-drug measures should be considered where possible, for example: Could a patient's pain be improved by a different mattress or seat rather than analgesia? Could anxiety be helped by relaxation techniques rather than benzodiazepines? It is important to include all members of the multidisciplinary team in assessment and treatment.

Pain management

A detailed pain assessment must be undertaken to identify different sites and types of pain present. In patients with advanced cancer, one-third are known to suffer from three or more types of pain.

The pain may be caused by the primary diagnosis (e.g. cancer, ischaemic heart disease), may be secondary to treatment (e.g. constipation, neuropathy), may be caused by general debility (e.g. pressure ulceration) or may be due to an associated co-morbidity (e.g. arthritis). Different pains may need a combination of analgesics to alleviate them. The pain may be caused by stimulation of the nerve endings (nociceptive pain) or caused by nerve dysfunction, e.g. due to compression or injury (neuropathic pain).

Nociceptive pain

This should be treated by following the World Health Organization three-step analgesic ladder:

- Step 1 analgesics: non-opioids, e.g. paracetamol.
- Step 2 analgesics: weak opioids, e.g. codeine, tramadol.
- Step 3 analgesics: strong opioids, e.g. morphine, diamorphine, oxycodone, buprenorphine, fentanyl.

Adjuvant analgesics (see subsequent sections) can also be given in addition to each of the above steps. Table 25.1 lists strong opioids commonly used in older people, together with instructions for their use.

Key points about opioids

One-third of opioid-naive patients experience nausea for 7–10 days on commencing morphine, or other opioids, which should respond to haloperidol 1.5–3 mg once daily. Strong opioids will cause constipation; regular laxatives should be prescribed to prevent this.

Hesitant patients should be reassured that patients rarely develop tolerance or addiction to strong opioids when they are used as analgesics.

When titrating oral or injectable opioids against pain, increase the 24 h dose by about one-third each time, e.g. increase from 60 mg twice daily to 80 mg twice daily to 110 mg twice daily. The prn (*pro re nata*: 'as needed') dose of oral or injectable opioids is one-sixth of total 24 h dose, and should be increased in proportion when regular dose is increased. The Case Scenario below illustrates how to use a stepwise approach to opioids.

Case Scenario   Titration of opioids and anticipation of opioid side-effects

Mrs P, who is aged 71 years with metastatic lung cancer, complains of a dull pain in her right chest, at the site of her cancer. It is eased partially by co-codamol, but she struggles to take the number of tablets. The GP decides to commence her on morphine and laxatives to prevent constipation. In addition, she is started on anti-emetics. He prescribes morphine immediate release (IR) solution 2.5 mg 4-hourly (total dose 30 mg). This helps the pain but does not ease it completely; he therefore increases the dose to 5 mg 4-hourly. The pain is better controlled on this dose, so he converts her to morphine sulphate modified release (MR) tablets 15 mg twice daily, with 5 mg IR solution prn hourly (i.e. one-sixth of total daily dose) for breakthrough pain.

One month later, her pain worsens but responds to morphine IR solution. The GP increases her morphine sulphate slow release (SR) tablets by one-third to 20 mg twice daily, and 4 weeks later by a further one-third to 30 mg twice daily in response to continuing discomfort. He also increases her prn dose to 10 mg (one-sixth of total daily dose). Her pain becomes well controlled.

Three weeks later, she becomes drowsy and confused. On examination, she appears opioid toxic: pinpoint pupils, myoclonic jerks, mild respiratory depression. Blood biochemistry reveals mild renal impairment. Her morphine is stopped and she is started on oxycodone SR tablets 15 mg twice daily (see Table 25.1). She is prescribed oxycodone IR capsules 5 mg prn (i.e. one-sixth of total daily dose).

Table 25.1 Opioid analgesics

Drug	Available preparations	Indications	Comments and guidance on opioid conversion
Morphine: IR	Oral: solution, tablets	First-line strong opioid; given 4-hourly as short acting	If opioid naive, starting dose is 2.5–5 mg 4-hourly. Also for breakthrough pain when taking morphine MR: calculated dose, one-sixth of total 24 h MR dose, and can be given hourly.
Morphine: MR	Oral: tablets, granules to make liquid	Modified release preparation for opioid responsive pain	To convert from morphine IR, add up the total 24 h dose taken; divide by 2 to give 12-hourly dose. Remember to also pre-scribe morphine IR for breakthrough pain.
Diamorphine	Injection (subcutaneous)	Use if unable to take oral morphine, e.g. vomiting or end of life	To convert from oral morphine MR, divide the total daily dose by 3, and give subcutaneously over 24 h. PRN dose is calculated as one-sixth of 24 h dose (given hourly subcutaneously).
Oxycodone: IR, e.g. Oxynorm	Oral: solution, capsules	Use if side-effects with morphine, e.g. drowsy, confusion. Safer in renal impairment than morphine.	Use first line only if contraindications to morphine.Used for breakthrough pain when taking oxycodone MR: calculated dose is one-sixth of total 24 h MR dose, and can be given hourly.
Oxycodone: MR, e.g. Oxycontin	Oral: tablets	Use if side-effects with morphine, e.g. drowsy, confusion. Safer in renal impairment than morphine.	To convert to oxycodone, halve the 24 h morphine MR dose. Remember to also prescribe oral oxynorm for breakthrough pain.
Oxycodone: injection, e.g. Oxynorm	Subcutaneous	Use if unable to take oral oxycodone, e.g. vomiting or end of life	To convert from oral oxycodone MR, divide the total daily dose by 2, and give subcutaneously over 24 h. PRN dose is calculated as one-sixth of 24 h dose, and can be given hourly subcutaneously.
Buprenorphine	Transdermal: BuTrans (7 day patch);	Safer in renal impairment and causes less constipation than morphine	Useful for opioid naïve patients with mild chronic pain, those with poor compliance or who struggle to take oral medication, e.g. dementia. Not for acute short-term pain, or severe pain.
Fentanyl	Transdermal patches Injection (subcutaneous)	Safe in renal failure. Causes less constipation than morphine.	Patches used if relatively stable pain and patient already taking alternative opioid. Not for acute short term pain, severe pain needing rapid dose escalation, or opioid naive; Fentanyl injection is more appropriate in these circumstances.

IR, immediate release; MR, modified release.

Her condition initially improves, but 2 weeks later she deteriorates and is thought to be dying. She is unable to take oral medication, so she is converted to injectable oxycodone: oxynorm injection 15 mg over 24 h subcutaneously (i.e. half the 24 h oral oxycodone dose). The addition of sedating drugs and anti-emetics are discussed further in the Liverpool Care Pathway. She is also prescribed 2.5 mg oxynorm injection prn hourly (i.e. one-sixth of total daily dose). She remains comfortable and dies peacefully at home.

Neuropathic pain

Pain in an area of absent or enhanced sensation is neuropathic. This pain is often described as a shooting, stabbing or burning pain. It can be treated with a tricyclic antidepressant and/or an anticonvulsant. A short course of dexamethasone can also often be effective, if side-effects do not preclude its use.

Tricyclic antidepressant

- Amitriptyline 10 mg nocte ('at night'), increased as needed to 75 mg nocte. Common side-effects are confusion, drowsiness, cardiac arrhythmias, urinary retention. These may prevent its use or upward titration.

Anticonvulsant

- Sodium valproate, starting at 200 mg daily, increased slowly to maximum 1500 mg: this tends to be better tolerated than amitriptyline but side-effects include drowsiness, ataxia and tremor.
- Gabapentin: this can be titrated quicker than sodium valproate. However, although the pharmaceutical guidelines state an initial dose of 300 mg and daily titration, clinical practice recommends a smaller starting dose in older people (100 mg daily) and titration over weeks rather than days. Side-effects include drowsiness and dizziness.
- Pregabalin: at lower doses, this is more expensive than gabapentin. It is a twice daily regime (gabapentin is three times daily) and can be tried if there are side-effects with gabapentin. In older individuals, it should be commenced at a lower dose than manufacturer's guidelines, i.e. 25–50 mg twice daily and increased slowly. Side-effects include dizziness and drowsiness.

Adjuvant analgesics

These can be used in combination with opioids and neuropathic drugs.

- Paracetamol.
- Non-steroidal anti-inflammatory drugs (NSAIDs) are useful for inflammatory pain but must be used with caution in the elderly population because of their many side-effects, especially gastritis and renal failure.
- Benzodiazepines and/or baclofen are effective in treating muscle spasm.
- Hyoscine butylbromide is effective for colic; it is poorly absorbed orally.
- Bisphosphonates (intravenous or oral) are effective in treating bone pain.
- Corticosteroids can help reduce inflammation and therefore ease pain, e.g. neuropathic, hepatomegaly; however, their likely effectiveness must be balanced against the risk of side-effects, and only short courses should be prescribed.

Nausea and vomiting

A detailed assessment needs to be made as the choice of anti-emetic depends on likely cause. If the oral route is not effective, the anti-emetic should be given subcutaneously via a syringe driver for a few days to ensure absorption, before being prescribed by the oral route again. This temporary use of a syringe driver must be explained clearly to the patient and relatives to avoid unnecessary anxiety, because they may only be familiar with their use at the end of life. However, at the end of life when the patient is drowsy and struggling to take oral medication, any regular oral anti-emetic should be continued subcutaneously via a syringe driver.

Table 25.2 shows the drugs commonly used to treat nausea and vomiting in older people. One-third of patients have more than one cause of nausea and vomiting. If symptoms continue, add in or substitute a different anti-emetic listed in the table.

Second-line, levomepromazine, a broad-spectrum anti-emetic, can be used but commonly causes sedation (starting dose: 6–12.5 mg once daily orally or subcutaneously). Ondansetron is rarely used in palliative care, except for chemotherapy-induced nausea and vomiting.

Table 25.2 Drugs used to treat nausea and vomiting

Features	Likely cause	Drug	Comments
Large volume infrequent vomiting, without nausea but often gastric fullness just prior to vomiting. Can also have belching, hiccoughs, early satiety	Gastric stasis, local tumour, hepatomegaly, ascites, subacute bowel obstruction	Prokinetic, e.g.: metoclopramide 10–20 mg orally three times daily or 30–60 mg subcutaneously over 24 h; domperidone 10–20 mg orally three times daily or 30 mg rectally three times daily	Metoclopramide: usual first line unless contraindications. Domperidone does not cause extrapyramidal side-effects; but is not available in injectable form. If tumour or hepatomegaly is the cause, dexamethasone 8 mg daily for 5 days, then tailed off. If patient is PEG-fed, consider reducing the amount of feed, as the patient may no longer require the prescribed amount of feed as deterioration progresses.
Nausea, with or without small volume, frequent vomiting	Drugs, e.g. opioids. Toxins, e.g. infection. Biochemical, e.g. hypercalcaemia, renal failure	Dopamine antagonist, e.g. haloperidol 1.5–3 mg nocte orally or sub-cutaneously (in sensitive patients, 0.5 mg once daily may be enough)	If the cause of the nausea is reversible, haloperidol should be stopped when the causal factor is no longer present.
Nausea, with or without small volume frequent vomiting	None of the above, middle ear involve-ment, vertigo, raised intracranial pressure, bowel distension	Histamine antagonist/ anticholinergic, e.g. cyclizine 50 mg orally three times daily or 150 mg subcutaneously over 24 h	For vestibular disorders, hyoscine hydrobromide 150–300 μg sublingually 6-hourly, or via a post-auricular patch (Scopoderm) can be used.

PEG, percutaneous endoscopic gastrostomy.

Constipation

Constipation is commonly experienced by elderly people towards the end of life, exacerbated by poor appetite and fluid intake, immobility, and prescribed drugs, particularly opioids and antimuscarinics.

A wide variety of laxatives are available. Patients will often need a combination of stimulant (e.g. senna) and softener (e.g. docusate). Lactulose is also a softener but is disliked by many patients due to its sweet taste, and the tendency to cause abdominal bloating. Combination drugs are available (e.g. codanthramer, codanthrusate). They are expensive but mean fewer tablets for the patient. Movicol sachets are an alternative, but can also cause abdominal bloating, and some patients struggle to swallow the volume.

If constipation causes discomfort in the dying phase, abdominal colic should be treated with hyoscine butylbromide subcutaneously (20 mg prn 2-hourly or 60–120 mg via syringe driver over 24 h).

Dyspnoea

The cause of the breathlessness needs to be assessed, and treated if possible. However, the sensation of breathlessness can be partially relieved by a small dose of opioids given regularly, e.g. morphine IR solution 5–10 mg prn 4–6-hourly. If the patient is anxious or frightened, this is likely to exacerbate the breathlessness, and can be treated with lorazepam 0.5 mg sublingually prn hourly. Oxygen is beneficial if the patient is hypoxic.

Modification of the patient's activities of daily living will help to reduce dyspnoea. Strategically placed chairs around the house will provide resting stops; a commode or urinal bottle will prevent the exertion of reaching the toilet; a stair lift and wheelchair may similarly help. Cool air (from a fan or open window), and relaxation techniques may also be beneficial.

In the dying phase, opioids given subcutaneously (from diamorphine 2.5 mg prn hourly or 10 mg over 24 h via syringe driver) may help relieve the sensation of dyspnoea. Midazolam subcutaneously (from 2.5 mg prn hourly or 10 mg over 24 h via syringe driver) helps ease the distress.

Excessive secretions

These are often present in the last few days or hours. Many relatives are distressed by the noise and may be reassured with an explanation. If the patient appears distressed, hyoscine hydrobromide can be given subcutaneously (400 µg prn 2-hourly or 1200–2000 µg via syringe driver over 24 h), to prevent the production of further secretions. If the secretions continue to distress the patient, glycopyrronium subcutaneously (200 µg prn 4–6-hourly or 600–1200 µg over 24 h via syringe driver) may be added or used instead.

Some patients experience excessive secretions earlier in their illness, particularly those with some neurological conditions. These may be prevented by applying a hyoscine hydrobromide (Scopoderm) post-auricular patch on the skin. If this is not effective, glycopyrronium can be given orally.

Terminal agitation

This is commonly seen in the last few days or hours. The patient may appear distressed and unable to settle, although not in pain. This usually responds to midazolam given subcutaneously (2.5–5 mg prn hourly or 10–20 mg over 24 h via syringe driver). If the patient does not settle, higher doses may be needed or, as a second line, levomepromazine may need to be added.

Caring for the carers

Practical and emotional support

Caring for older people with incurable disease can be rewarding but also emotionally and physically exhausting, particularly as older carers may also experience physical morbidity. In the year before the death of a cancer patient, one-third to one-half of carers experience symptoms of anxiety and depression. Carers require:

♦ *Information*: about the patient's diagnosis and prognosis, future symptoms, services and resources available.

♦ *Practical support*: advice on nursing care and sources of respite care, including night-sitting services (usually provided by Marie Curie nurses).

♦ *Psychosocial support*: coping with anger, guilt, uncertainty and depression.

♦ *Discussion about their concerns and expectations*: particularly around preferred place of care and the dying process.

Individual counselling for family carers can be provided from a variety of professional sources including the GP, community nurse or Macmillan nurse or via referral for counselling.

Financial and legal help

This area is traditionally regarded as the responsibility of social workers, nevertheless GPs and community nurses should also be aware of the financial benefits to which their older patients with incurable illnesses are entitled. These include:

♦ Attendance Allowance to be claimed by patients aged >65 years. A fast track system is available for those patients with a prognosis of <6 months; in addition to the standard form to be completed by the patient, a further form, DS1500, is completed by a doctor.

♦ Invalid Care Allowance to be claimed by the carer, should they be spending >35 h a week caring. Macmillan Cancer Relief and other charities also provide grants to patients with terminal illness for specific purposes such as installation of a telephone.[8] Equipment grants are also available via social services.

Application forms for the above allowances can be obtained from Social Services departments.

Decision-making at the end of life

People with terminal illness, and their family carers, face difficult moral decisions as they approach the end of their lives. These are often termed 'ethical dilemmas' (see Chapter 23) and may be associated with issues around communication about the diagnosis and prognosis; hydration and feeding; withdrawal of medication; respite and support care; advance decisions and the conflicting views of families and professionals. A key role for GPs is to ensure that patients and their families are sufficiently knowledgeable to make an informed choice and to support them, practically and emotionally, in these challenging areas. Decisions to adopt a palliative care approach and stop potentially curative measures lead to uncertainty, tension and distress and require detailed consideration and discussion, particularly if a patient or their family's wishes are different from the views of the health professionals concerned.

Autonomy has become increasingly important, especially with the introduction of patient-centred care and the Mental Capacity Act (2005). One practical method for eliciting and documenting a person's views is through an advance decision and the process of advance care planning in general.

Advance care planning

Advance care planning is now part of the NHS End of Life Care Programme.[9] It is defined as a process of discussion between a patient and a professional carer and sometimes their families. Possible outcomes of discussions around advance care planning include:

- *Advance statement*: documentation of patients' preferences for their future health care.

- *Advance decision*: documentation of patients' informed consent to refuse specific treatment, should they develop irreversible cognitive impairment in the future.

- *Preferred priorities of care*: documentation of their views and preferences on where they wish to be cared for in the future.

- *Lasting power of attorney (LPA)*: this refers to two legal documents, authorized through a solicitor, allowing a person (the donor) to give another (the attorney) the responsibility to act on the donor's behalf in relation to (i) property and financial affairs and/or (ii) health and social care issues.

Advance decisions and LPA are legally binding; advance statements and preferred priorities of care documents are not. An LPA is a new formal power of attorney introduced through the implementation of the Mental Capacity Act (2005), which replaces enduring power of attorney (EPA), although the latter remains valid if executed before the Act. LPAs extend the areas of power of attorney to include health care and medical treatment in addition to property and financial issues covered by EPAs. Currently only a very small percentage of patients have made any form of advance care plan (see Chapter 23).

Dying at home

On average, GPs can anticipate around 20 patients on their list dying each year, of which about a quarter will be at home.[10] If a decision has been made for the patient to die at home, family carers should be given the opportunity to discuss their anxieties and concerns with the GP/community nurse. Emergencies notwithstanding, the mode of death of many terminally ill patients can be anticipated and distressing symptoms generally optimally managed.

Care pathways for use during the last few days of a patient's life have been developed and are recommended by the National Institute of Health and Clinical Excellence as a means of improving the quality of end of life care.[10,11] They provide health care professionals with standardized protocols on the management of key symptoms and promote proactive, rather than reactive, care. They also allow appropriately trained nurses to verify the patient's death and agree to the removal of the body by the undertaker.

Care after death

After the patient's death, the relatives will require information about necessary procedures such as the registration of the death and the need to contact a funeral undertaker. The death certificate will normally be issued by the GP who attended the patient during his last illness. In certain circumstances the death must be reported to the coroner; these include:

- Deceased was not seen by a doctor within 14 days before death.

- There is doubt about a natural cause of death with concerns about neglect or abuse.

- There is uncertainty about the cause of death.

- Death was due to an industrial disease or poisoning.

The responsibility for notifying the patient's death rests with the relative, or in the absence of a relative, the owner of the premises in which the death has taken place, such as in care homes.

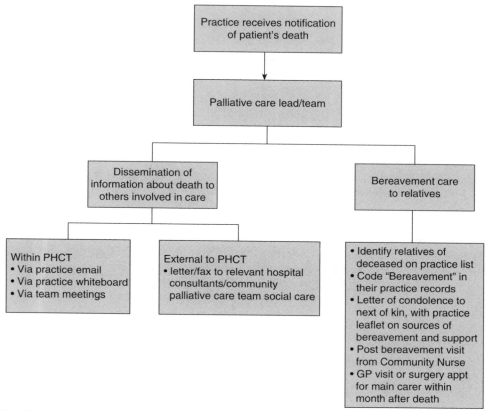

Fig. 25.2 Example of a bereavement care protocol for primary care. PHCT, primary health care trust.

The GP can advise the family that once they have registered the person's death and contacted a funeral director, the latter will provide all necessary support and advice regarding the burial or cremation. If the body is to be cremated, it must be seen by two doctors; first by the certifying doctor and then by a second independent medical practitioner who has been registered for a minimum of 5 years and who is not a partner or relative of the first doctor or of the deceased.

Although there is no legal obligation for GPs and their team to provide bereavement care to relatives of the deceased who are on their list, it is considered by many to be good practice. In addition, many primary care trusts now request a copy of the practice's bereavement care protocol (see Figure 25.2). This may include a bereavement visit to the deceased's spouse, providing advice on sources of bereavement support, and notifying other healthcare professionals who were involved in the care of the deceased. Organizations providing bereavement support include Cruse Bereavement Care (Cruse 2008) and Age Concern (Age Concern 2008).[12,13] See also Chapter 22 for further discussion of mental health consequences of bereavement.

References

1. World Health Organization. *Technical Report Series, 804.* Geneva: WHO; 1990.
2. Department of Health. *End of Life Care Strategy: Promoting high quality care for all adults at the end of life.* London, Department of Health, 2008. Available at: http://www.dh.gov.uk/en/publicationsandstatistics/publications/publicationspolicyandguidance/dh_086277

3. Department of Health. *The NHS Cancer Plan.* London: DoH; 2000.

4. National Institute of Health and Clinical Excellence. *Improving supportive and palliative care for adults with cancer.* London: NICE; 2005. Available at: http://www.nice.org.uk

5. Department of Health. *Cancer Reform Strategy.* London: DoH; 2007.

6. Department of Health. *National Service Framework for Older People.* London: DoH; 2001. Available at: http://www.dh.gov.uk/en/Publicationsandstatistics/Publications/PublicationsPolicyAndGuidance/DH_4003066

7. NHS Confederation. *Revisions to the GMS contract 2006/7.* 2006. Available at: http://www.nhsemployers.org/pay-conditions/primary-902.cfm

8. Macmillan Cancer Support. *Financial Help.* 2008. Available at: http://www.macmillan.org.uk/Get_Support/Financial_help/Financial_help.aspx

9. National Health Service—End of Life Care Programme. *Advance Care Planning: A Guide for Health and Social Care Staff.* NHS; 2007. Available at: http://www.endoflifecare.nhs.uk/eolc/acp/

10. Gold Standards Framework. *Palliative care and the GMS contract. Prognostic indicator guidance.* NHS; 2006. Available at: http://www.goldstandardsframework.nhs.uk/content/gp_contract/QOF_Introduction_Paper_1.pdf

11. Marie Curie Palliative Care Institute. *Liverpool Care Pathway.* MCPCI; 2005. Available at: http://www.mcpcil.org.uk/liverpool_care_pathway/view_the_lcp_and_associated_documentation

12. Cruse. *Cruse Bereavement Care.* 2008. Available at: http://www.crusebereavementcare.org.uk/

13. Age Concern. Age Concern website. 2008. Available at: http://www.ageconcern.org.uk/AgeConcern/info_guide_14.asp

Further reading

Regnard C, Hockley J. *A Guide to Symptom Relief in Palliative Care*, 5th edn. Oxford: Radcliffe Medical Press; 2004.

Twycross R, Wilcock A. *Palliative Care Formulary*, 3rd edn. 2007. Available at: http://www.palliativedrugs.com).

Chapter 26

Care home medicine

Clive Bowman and Emma Bowman

Introduction

In the UK, care homes have evolved from the ignominy of the Poor Laws through a period when they provided a more dignified refuge from poverty and inadequate housing for older people to their present principal role, providing a sanctuary for those with mental impairment and long-term care for people with complex needs. Recently, care homes are now providing a range of 'intermediate' care (subacute/convalescent/rehabilitative and end of life care) as hospitals focus on investigation, diagnosis and treatment and reduce their role as 'infirmaries'.

In the late 1980s and early 1990s many outdated and decrepit National Health Service (NHS) facilities providing long-term care were closed and in the absence of major capital investment their residents transferred to care homes. Patients became residents and a core of practitioners from the NHS followed their patients, becoming social care practitioners; this legacy has now largely been exhausted. Training, expertise and leadership for care home management is increasingly rooted within the care industry (and the use of the word industry is significant).

Care home provision is largely by small-to-medium size businesses with only some 20% of beds being managed by large corporate providers. Standards of care have been materially shaped through a combination of opportunity and constraints of commissioning, regulation, manpower and market forces. Diffidence characterizes the attitude of a wide array of professional bodies to care homes and it remains a regrettable truism that care home residents are defined more by their residence than clinical state.

There is a divide and lack of awareness and clarity between 'free at the point of delivery' NHS care and 'means-tested personal care' that continues to undermine long-term care. Generally, heavily dependent older people who previously would have been cared for in NHS wards are now classified as needing social care and their care means-tested. For individuals with the most complex needs and dependency, fully funded care may be commissioned by the NHS. Specified categories, for example, end of life care or specific contracted beds for intermediate care, may also be fully funded by the NHS. Long-term care residents not fully funded by the NHS are subjected to means testing for the hotel and personal care components of their needs and, for people with significant nursing needs, primary care trusts separately assess and provide supplemental payments to contribute to the cost of professional nursing. The financing of care home provision is principally dependent on fees predominantly from the public purse. These have to cover costs and enable adequate returns to justify the investment and considerable risks. The overall system is a patchwork of policies that are widely viewed as too complex, unfit and in need of modernization for the new ageing demography.

The scale of care home provision is seldom recognized. Viewed by some shapers of social care as an outdated provision, the NHS and its regulators have tended to regard them as being beyond its purview. In spite of this, some 80% of the social services' expenditure on care for older people is directed to care homes. Furthermore, for every NHS hospital bed (of all types) there are more than three care home beds and typically >10% of care home beds are commissioned by the NHS (divided equally between fully funded long-term and intermediate care). A reliable and sustainable care home sector is essential to enable social care and the NHS to function.

The overall length of stay in care homes has continued to decline and occupants now encompass a number of definable streams that include: dementia care, long-term care of a range of largely illness-driven disabilities, end of life care, intermediate care through to more traditional residential care and finally the care of younger people with acquired brain damage or inherited disorders such as Huntington disease. All of these have differing trajectories and outcomes but are typically lumped together. Care homes remain poorly defined regarding skill sets and capabilities with considerable overlaps. Care homes with nursing have a retinue of professional nurses; residential care will often not have professional nurses, though experienced social care workers are often very clinically able. Specialist dementia care residential homes should have a particular skill in positively managing generally physically able people suffering from dementia.

More than 60% of care home beds are occupied by people admitted principally because of a lack of mental capacity, largely as a consequence of dementia. Overall beds discharges and transfers exceed deaths, which in high dependency units may be of an order of 40 per 100 beds per annum—care homes provide more end of life care than hospices.

The general lack of research and development of medical practice and health service support to care homes means that this chapter relies largely on common sense, pragmatism and illustrative cases rather than strongly rooted evidence. A variety of issues are outlined with the purpose to both illustrate problems and also opportunities for progressive practice.

Communication and the relationships between primary care, hospital services and care homes

General practitioners (GPs) visiting care homes easily become frustrated by the apparent lack of responsiveness and unwieldy nature of 'getting things done'. There will always be a range of competencies but it is difficult for a typical care home of 50 beds with many visiting GPs, all with individual approaches to their work, to accommodate these. With patients resident in care homes frequently having to register with a new doctor, continuity of care remains a valued notion but is not the norm. Even a superbly run care home can produce poor outcomes through inadequate medical care, and exemplary medical care cannot overcome deficiencies in care provision. Clearly a sound working relationship between home and doctor is highly desirable.

At the time of writing there is no consistency in the arrangements that primary care trusts (PCTs) make for the medical and clinical support of care homes. A range of initiatives by PCTs have included inviting practices to tender for a contract to support care home residents, various visiting medical officer contracts (whose remuneration has been known to be based on the signature of the care home manager!), and having all calls from a care home directed to consultant nurses in the first instance. Some GPs have actively sought to avoid responsibility for care home residents, having them removed from their list. To encourage doctors to accept care home residents, retainer contracts have been used. Retainer contracts remain controversial and of unproven value for care homes or their residents. These contracts are typically devised in such a way as to not technically conflict or compete with GPs' General Medical Services responsibilities. They require a regular attendance to the home to be available to assist the home's management with a caveat that if no home business requires their attention then their visit may be used for seeing their NHS patients. This is a 'fudge' and given the increasing diversity and need for clinical support and team work, it is likely that either doctors will find new opportunities within PCTs to provide clinical officer support to contracted care homes or, alternatively, care providers awarded integrated health and care contracts may seek practices to develop clear contractual relationships. Either route is likely to improve the quality of clinical care provided compared with the present lack of a system.

Specialist support also lacks any consistency. Many geriatricians have 'retrenched' to acute hospitals, and consultant responsibility for, and experience of, long-term care is now patchy. Innovative appointments of community geriatricians have largely been of seasoned geriatricians used to working and decision-making without the panoply of hospital resources. Psychiatrists specializing in geriatrics have retained a greater community presence, and more recently district nurse support to residential homes has been overtaken by consultant nurses. The consultant nurse has yet to have a consistent structural role or professional standing, some being exemplary leading practitioners whereas others may lack depth of experience and be remote from peer and managerial support. The calibre of care home leadership can range from exceptional managers successfully leading a multi-million pound operation with a positively engaged stable team of nurses and support staff to those with worryingly weak managerial leadership and high staff turnover.

Communication and care

The admission of a resident to a care home is typically accompanied by fractured communication with adequate transfer information seldom being made available for care staff to provide a comprehensive care plan. Similarly, discharge notes may merely cite diagnoses such as, 'chest infection and dementia', while accompanying medication alludes to a far more extensive set of illnesses. It is exceptional for useful information such as functional capacities or resuscitation status to be communicated, indeed the very assessment of need that justifies care is often unavailable. These failings are often compounded by a long lag phase for full records to catch up with the new receiving doctor unfamiliar with the patient's past medical history. Frustrated GPs may gripe to the care home, energy that may be more usefully directed to the discharging hospital and the medical director of their PCT, who collectively could set local standards.

Care homes themselves often communicate poorly with GPs and particularly emergency out-of-hours' services. Home staff may have concerns regarding the deterioration of a patient's functioning and behaviour, ringing an out of hours' service with a request for a review. Made poorly, this can trigger inappropriate responses, for example compare and contrast:

> A. 'Mrs X is displaying challenging behaviour. She's attacked several staff members and pushed another resident to the floor—can you help urgently?'

> B. 'Mrs X has been resident with us on account of her dementia for 3 months; suddenly she has changed and become aggressive. This is not at all how she behaves and we think she may have an illness that has precipitated a delirium—could you review her urgently?'

Referral A has a strong probability of the receiving doctor becoming irritated about the failure of care home staff to cope and a possible prescription of sedation; referral B should trigger a much more inquisitive response.

For doctors confronted by uncommunicative residents and inadequate clinical information in care notes, the safety default may often be to refer a patient to hospital as an emergency. Such admissions can be clinically futile and may be averted by a simple statement from the GP with whom the patient is registered, for example:

> Mr A is in the final stages of a dementing illness. This is understood and accepted by his family and the care staff who agree with my assessment that distressing symptoms should be treated palliatively, and

that if at all possible he should be managed *in situ* in the care home. There is a collective agreement that Mr A should not be subject to resuscitation.

Such a simple statement properly signed and dated clearly informs decision-making for an emergency doctor. The reverse is also true; for example, if a patient transferred following a fracture fails to thrive in the care home, it is important that an attending doctor understands that recovery is anticipated and that, unless a clear and irredeemable clinical event has occurred to change that status, admission to hospital is necessary. In this instance a helpful statement in the care home records may read:

Mr B, usually entirely independent in all respects, fell while gardening and fractured his hip. Following an uncomplicated hip replacement and good initial postoperative course he was transferred for convalescent rehabilitation prior to return home.

A key issue in long-term care is the recognition, diagnosis and communication of the transition from living with a condition and its disabilities to entering a period of 'dying'. In cancer management there has been a great deal of progress in end of life care and greater clarity about the goals of treatments, transitions and palliation. Similar progress has been made in some chronic conditions such as respiratory diseases and renal failure, where measurable indices can bring helpful definition. In older people with neurological disease and various co-morbidities, these transitions can be missed or presumed—rightly or wrongly. Until such time that more sophisticated guidance is available it is incumbent for attending GPs to stand back and take a 360 degree look at an individual's status. For example, weight loss, repeated infections, increasing somnolence, all in the presence of good care and low probability of adverse drug reaction, may summatively indicate the transition. Understanding and communicating life status and transitions to care staff, family and friends is an important medical responsibility.

Regarding palliative care, although homes are often willing to extend their responsibilities they must maintain a 'joined up' approach to ensure that what the care home does is entirely agreed between doctor, district nurses and care staff. This approach is exemplified by the Liverpool Care Pathway, a validated shared care pathway for the last days of life that allows staff to act and treat in agreed ways with the patient's doctor. Unless care staff have clear guidance and there is a shared accountability, end of life care can be difficult (see Chapter 25).

The issue of resuscitation is difficult: in acute hospitals great trouble is taken to determine whether or not an older person with advanced frailty would seek to be resuscitated in the event of a cardio-respiratory arrest. Sadly, these decisions are seldom communicated on discharge and care homes are mandated to provide first aid but do not and cannot, through regulatory constraints, maintain full resuscitation resources. In consequence, in the absence of direction that an individual is not for resuscitation, emergency paramedics are summoned. In fact it is not unknown for what medically could be an anticipated death to be treated as suspicious, with police investigation yellow incident tape enlivening a homes' décor. Clearly, adequate and accurate communication can avoid this and instil a sense of dignity to both an individual's demise and respect for those around them (other residents and staff) (see Chapter 23).

Dementia

In spite of 'brain failure' and loss of mental capacity being the greatest risk to loss of independence and the principal reason for people to need long-term care home admission, it is disappointing how frequently clarity of diagnosis is missing. Good practice should be for receiving doctors to question and satisfy themselves that a firm diagnosis has been made and that potentially remediable conditions have been considered, as Case Example 26.1 demonstrates.

Case Example 26.1 Unscrutinized diagnosis

Miss X had been admitted to an acute orthopaedic ward having fallen in the street. She appeared confused and was seen by a junior doctor who prescribed antipsychotics in moderate dose for dementia; subsequently she was diagnosed by another junior doctor as having Parkinson's disease. Not having a fracture, she was expeditiously transferred to a nursing home where, during a 3 month period, she regained sufficient well-being to leave the care home all day (her property had been sold). She moved to residential care where 2 years later she was referred urgently after a further fall, followed by severe anxiety. Referred for specialist review for the first time, it became clear that her anxiety related to a fear of returning to the nursing home. Her intact mental capacity was confirmed by formal testing and her puzzle-solving ability. Both antipsychotic and antiparkinsonian medication were withdrawn and simple analgesia provided for her arthritis together with the provision of a walking frame. She remained well until death from an incidental illness some years later. In retrospect she had sustained a head injury at the time of her fall and concussion had been missed and an unscrutinized diagnosis and treatment by a junior doctor compounded by complicit acceptance by a receiving GP.

Dementia is generally progressive accompanied by a range of behavioural challenges that can lead to inappropriate long-term prescribing of antipsychotic medication. Care homes have been repeatedly criticized for sedating patients with dementia. Although care homes do not prescribe medication, some staff may overtly or inadvertently encourage doctors to prescribe. Importantly, more than half of antipsychotic prescriptions to care home residents are initiated prior to admission, either in NHS hospitals or in the community. In hospitals these drugs may be commenced to maintain the safety of the individual and those around them. In the community, prescription may be an attempt to extend a family's capacity to cope with extremely testing needs. Whatever the initial driver for the prescription, a well-run dementia care unit should be enthusiastic to see a reduction of medication use. There is a large and unwarranted variation in prescribing rates of antipsychotics with rates ranging from <5% to >40%; a positive clinical approach is to actively pursue a programme of medication reduction. The initiation of antipsychotic medication in care homes needs very careful reflection: Is the driver that the patient is displaying a delirium or is the home unable to meet an individual's needs? Is this a reflection of inadequate commissioning or simply inadequate care by inadequately trained staff?

The course of dementia means that a once good placement may need critical review, as the Case Example 26.2 illustrates.

Case Example 26.2 Reviewing a placement

An elderly widow was repeatedly found in a disoriented state wandering at night and after proper assessment a diagnosis of dementia confirmed. She was taken into the home of her caring son but this was not satisfactory, not least because of the disruption to family life of teenage children and their exam preparation. Retaining a good social functioning, this lady was placed in a residential home where she participated fully for some 8 months, after which she became increasingly withdrawn and lost weight. Review demonstrated a deterioration of her dementia and the simple fact that the good but not specialist residential home was unable now to meet her needs. She was transferred to a specialist dementia care home and, when reviewed, had regained weight and become fully engaged in the closely supervised activities and trips.

The prevalence of dementia over the forthcoming four decades in the UK is due to increase from 750 000 to ~1 500 000 at a time when the number of younger people (and likely care staff) are in decline. Any improvements in independent living, care and support in the community are unlikely to have a major impact on the implied increase in demand for residential care places.

There clearly is a pressing need for real strategic commitment to develop care and invest in this predictable demand (see Chapter 22).

Falls

A care home with no falls is either operating a no-risk approach to care or failing to record falls! The medical response to a fall in practice is generally a determination of injury and need for further action or not.

Falls are a symptom, a final common pathway, not a diagnosis. Referral and intensive investigation are only justified after a 'bedside' review. The GP has a unique opportunity to undertake this assessment, which almost certainly will take less time than writing a referral (see Chapter 13).

What were the circumstances of the fall? Was it poor footwear or poorly supervised ambulation? Was this a trip or was the individual pushed? What is the patient's usual mobility/stability status? Is the person's pulse acceptable and is blood pressure maintained in the upright position? Is an iatrogenic cause likely? If not too injured, watch the patient mobilize—this is often most revealing. Finally, is the care being purchased/supplied sufficient for the resident's needs?

A common presentation is that of serious fracture following a fall in late stage Alzheimer's disease. Although technically remediable, the stress, distress, limited potential health gain and high complication rate of an orthopaedic odyssey for some such patients should prompt careful consideration of whether a conservative palliative approach would be more appropriate, recognizing the fracture as a pre-terminal event. Such decision-making often needs careful discussion with care staff and family, fully informed by the patient's past medical history. Simply referring the patient to hospital will often lead to intervention with receiving teams not unreasonably taking a view that, as the patient has been referred, treatment is being sought.

Medication and chronic disease management

On average, care home residents are prescribed more than seven items. Whether individually or collectively these agents are helpful or harmful will vary from patient to patient, but generally speaking most patients are likely to be best served by critical review of their pharmaceutical burden. Specific targets might include:

- Antihypertensive treatment: nursing care homes can provide records of blood pressure and a significant number of patients taking antihypertensives will remain normotensive. As a practice point it is probably more useful to check standing blood pressure or, in the case of frailty, sitting. It is likely that this simple practice will lead to considerable withdrawal of hypotensives and can be accompanied with an instruction for the care home to monitor blood pressure with a request for reporting if reading exceeds a specified limit.

- Heart failure: diuretics are often more of a problem than acute deterioration of cardiovascular disease. Patients may present hugely congested, having multiple unresponsive chest infections (basically left ventricular failure) but more commonly dehydrated. For many patients with chronic disease, moderate weight loss and reduced activity may diminish the problems associated with heart failure and allow reduction of diuretic dosage.

- Treatments to control lipid profiles in the aged frail resident in care homes are beyond traditional evidence bases. We have identified that >20% of a sample of some 5000 care home residents continue to be treated with these agents. As these drugs interfere with metabolism and nutrition, and the original purpose may have been overtaken by events, there is potential for stopping them.

◆ In Parkinson's disease it is not uncommon for medication to become increasingly complex in an attempt to maintain sufficient mobility to live at home. Sometimes this preservation of mobility is at the expense of hallucination in an attempt to maintain physical independence; having been admitted to care it is likely that simplification of a regime will bring a clearer mind and a manageable increase in physical dependency. Certainly hugely demanding regimes are unlikely to be practicable and dosing schedules often can be rationalized.

Polypharmacy and complexity of dosing regimens impose a major risk to care home residents and a major challenge to care home medicine management. Often the rationale for various therapies has long been lost and critical medical review likely to be helpful.

Nutrition weight and hydration

Care homes should regularly weigh residents, and significant weight loss will often be reported to the patient's doctor. Medical inquiry should seek understanding of whether meals presented are being eaten, or whether adequate feeding help is being made available. Particularly common problems arise in patients with swallowing disorders arising from stroke or advanced Parkinson's disease. In both these settings, meal times may be significantly extended—there must be adequate care time to realistically ensure nutrition is maintained and sufficient skill to feed individuals with dignity and safety. Very often supplemental nutritional drinks are prescribed, but seldom are these indicated. Good homes can puree food and present it in an appetizing way rather than as a bowl of indeterminate sludge!

Malnutrition in care home residents is common, and though a concerning issue it should not be seen as synonymous with poor care. Cachexia may accompany a whole range of diseases including Alzheimer's disease as well as cancers and chronic cardio-respiratory disease. A positive diagnosis of cachexia is seldom made but should be considered and communicated. Malnourished residents are admitted to care homes from acute hospitals or sometimes present having failed to thrive in the community. These patients can often put on significant weight in care and need just as careful management as weight loss.

Particular problems arise with nasogastric tube feeding instigated in patients with very poor quality of life. Cases of severe stroke with significantly impaired consciousness, for which a good outcome is not expected, are typical. These cases may not need the resources of a district hospital, yet initiation of tube feeding may be followed by transfer to care home without a clear plan. Clearly, it is right and proper to maintain patient's hydration and nutrition until confidence regarding the prognosis is clear. It should be mandatory for full consideration of a long-term plan before the patient is transferred to care. A GP without extensive information and familiarity of the case is placed in an unacceptable position, and should seek full engagement of the consultant and multidisciplinary team regarding such cases.

Infection control and management

Care homes are fertile ground for uncomplicated, complicated, multi-resistant and exotic sporadic and epidemic infections and yet there is little routine surveillance or support compared with that made in acute hospitals. Care home regulations require good standards of hygiene. However, care homes are expected to receive cases infected with MRSA from hospitals and other resistant infections. Control of infection may be helped by the prevalence of single rooms and modern approaches to room cleaning, laundry management and food preparation, but undermined by poor antibiotic prescribing.

Poor antibiotic prescribing may include sequential broad-spectrum antibiotics for alleged chest infections that are probably heart failure and a lack of responsiveness to the onset of infection. A combination of slow referral and sluggish response to what may be an eminently treatable urinary/chest infection can lead to more extensive infection and a need for admission. Clear and speedy response is obviously desirable and usage of antibiotics in accordance with local guidance or best practice important. It is worth remembering to question whether a patient, particularly an unfamiliar one, has allergies.

A particularly common care home problem is scabies, and a useful clinical maxim is always to consider this when being asked to see a patient with rash or itch! (See Chapter 17.)

Conclusion

This chapter has focused on shortcomings and deficiencies in long-term care and sought to offer some understanding and description of opportunities for doctors in primary care to make a significant contribution to the health and wellbeing of the long-term care home resident. Issues relating to long-term care cannot simply be extrapolated to intermediate care. Although care homes are regularly (and sometimes deservedly) criticized, not unlike primary care, there are many more cards and notes of appreciation from families regarding the care provided than complaints and concerns!

Further reading

♦ Policy:

The King's Fund, Joseph Rowntree Foundation and the Royal Commission on Long-Term care have all produced extensive reports that are all available on the web.

♦ Understanding dementia:

Graham Stokes. *And Still the Music Plays: Stories of People with Dementia.* London: Hawker Publications; 2008.

♦ Long-term care failure:

Kane RL, West JC. *It Shouldn't Be This Way. The Failure of Long-Term Care.* Nashville: Vanderbilt Press; 2005. A personal account from America of the frustrations of navigating care, even as an expert.

Chapter 27

Rehabilitation and physical activity

Chris Turnbull and Steve Iliffe

Rehabilitation

Introduction

Older people commonly have complex disability comprising physical, psychological and social problems. In addition their functioning can easily deteriorate to a level where they are no longer able to undertake the essential basic activities of daily living. This inability to function independently often first becomes manifest following an acute illness or accident or sometimes following a social crisis. Many older people are dependent on their partner or other carers to enable them to manage in their own homes.

Rehabilitation is the process of learning to cope with a new lower functional level, or of improving function by physical therapy, by personal adaptation, or by adaptation to the environment.

In order to help patients with rehabilitation it is essential to have a full understanding of the nature of the disease processes, their personal psychological and social status, and also to understand their way of managing their life normally. Thus prior to effective rehabilitation and during rehabilitation it is necessary to carry out a full assessment. This will involve many members of a multidisciplinary team who are each skilled in different areas of assessment and therapy.

The doctor should make a comprehensive diagnosis and prognosis and should have a full understanding of the medication the patient is taking. Often by subtle adjustments to medication or by identifying an unsuspected diagnosis such as postural hypotension, non-tremulous Parkinson's disease or detection of joint contractures, the older person's functional level can be considerably improved.

It is useful to routinely undertake a comprehensive range of screening tests to detect problems that might otherwise go undetected. Thus a cognitive function test such as the Mini Mental State Examination (which tests for general cognitive dysfunction)[1] or the CLOX-1 (which tests for frontal executive dysfunction typical of Lewy body dementia)[2] and a depression test such as the Hospital Anxiety and Depression Scale[3] or the Geriatric Depression Scale[4] can be used to help detect occult depression which might benefit from treatment. In addition visual function can be tested by visual acuity testing, and visual field testing by the confrontation technique can detect visual problems which, when treated, might reduce the risk of recurrent falls. Physiotherapists will often use other tests such as the 'timed unsupported stand test', which detects impairment of strength and balance, and the timed 'Get up and Go test'[5] which also tests for walking and gait disorder such as frontal apraxia. Perceptual tests such as 'Albert's test' (crossing a series of lines drawn randomly on a page to detect visual neglect)[6] or drawing objects such as a flower or house, which can detect unsuspected parietal lobe dysfunction, are often done by occupational therapists who also assess the basic and sometimes extended activities of daily living.

Other professionals commonly involved in the assessment process are:

- Carers themselves who describe what a person can actually do for themselves.
- Community nurses who assess wound care, diabetes control, continence, stoma and catheter care, and bowel problems.
- Dieticians who assess dietary intake and requirements.
- Psychologists who assess the psychological profile.
- Speech therapists who assess speech and swallowing problems.

Rehabilitation in community settings

Community settings may include the patient's own home, a nursing or residential home or even a relative's or friend's home. If the patient is at home the advantage is that skills can be practised in the setting where the patient will be using them and that the environment is familiar and (it is hoped) secure for them as well. However, 'own homes' may be a problem in that providing 24 h care can be difficult and the design of the home may not be suitable, e.g. a patient needs a bed and toilet closely accessible on one floor but there are stairs. Homes may require significant adaptation to enable a patient to cope in the home environment. It may not be possible to get some equipment into the home, e.g. a hoist for transfers or parallel bars for practising balance and walking. Where many members of a multidisciplinary team have to travel individually to the patient's own home, travel costs can be high. In addition, having a weekly meeting to discuss cases will usually require a room in another setting. However, many patients are managed at home with the intervention of one discipline, commonly physiotherapy, when the problem is more restricted in nature. Some areas have developed generic therapist posts where one individual has physiotherapy, occupational therapy and other skills.

Nursing and residential homes have the advantage of a more home-like environment as compared to a standard hospital ward and have more privacy. Often there are communal rooms which provide the benefits of socialization and there is the incentive of getting to the dining area for meals which can be a very effective motivator for independent mobility. Care can be provided 24 h a day, though in a residential home this may not include nursing care, so frequent nursing observations such as standing and lying blood pressures, blood glucose monitoring, and pulse oximetry are more difficult to arrange. Therapists are often very positive about working in these sorts of environment as the type of patient is usually suitable for active treatment, but not very sick. Home carers are often very positive about the active process of rehabilitation as opposed to the usual passive approach of just providing care. Home carers can be taught many of the assessment methods and will undertake mental test scores, visual tests, basic continence assessment, inhaler technique assessment and assessment of patient understanding about medication use and likely concordance. In a care home it may not be possible to provide the whole range of equipment expected in hospital but, given a reasonable size room, equipment such as parallel bars, mirror, exercise ball, cycles, balance table and plinth can be provided (Colour plate 26). Equally an assessment kitchen is quite feasible to provide (Colour plate 27). It is perfectly possible to organize visiting specialist medical care to these environments and undertake blood testing, electrocardiogram and basic lung function testing. It is often possible to undertake more complex medical tests such as computed tomography (CT), ultrasound, etc., but this will usually involve a visit to the hospital. However, if patients require frequent and urgent medical review, blood transfusions, high flow oxygen (low flow oxygen can be provided; Colour plate 28), regular intravenous injections, or are extremely sick, they are better being hospitalized. Hospitalization carries the risks of hospital-acquired infection, hospital-related accidents and loss of privacy and the drive for independence.

Problems needing rehabilitation

In one residential intermediate care scheme, the proportion of cases with different main problems were:

- post-fracture/orthopaedic surgery 34%
- post stroke 23%
- chest problems (e.g. acute exacerbation of chronic obstructive pulmonary disease (COPD), recuperating from pneumonia) 15%
- depression/anxiety 15%
- arthritis 8%
- Parkinson's disease and others, including leg ulceration, etc. 5%.

It is important therefore to be familiar with the management of various fracture types and joint replacements and to have physiotherapists who know about neurological rehabilitation. Familiarity with falls assessment and rehabilitation is important, as this is a very frequent association with elderly patients receiving community rehabilitation. Many patients will attend fracture clinics for management of casts and splints which may include complex cases such as patients in a halo neck brace for unstable cervical spine fractures. It is important to know about preventive aspects of future care such as alternative treatment regimens for osteoporosis and cardiovascular risk management for patients with strokes or amputations, etc. The diagnoses of patients managed with rehabilitation at home are similar, though some areas have schemes dedicated to managing, for example, fractured femur, or early discharge following stroke, or with acute exacerbations of COPD. The evidence for effectiveness appears to favour specialist schemes (e.g. for stroke) though, from a cost-effectiveness point of view, a more generic scheme of at-home rehabilitation may be preferred.

The following Cases Examples A–C are typical of patients receiving rehabilitation in a community setting.

Case Example A

A female aged 74 years who lived alone with no nearby family was admitted after a short stay in hospital for insertion of a dynamic hip screw after a fractured hip. She suffered with depression, type 1 diabetes, spinal arthritis, and ischaemic heart disease. She was considering giving up her home and going into residential care. With leadership from the physiotherapist, the therapy assistant and care staff were able to get her independent in mobility and transfers within 4 weeks of care in a residential rehabilitation unit. She was re-educated to administer insulin herself. Soon she was able to climb stairs and went on a home visit, following which she was discharged with support of the home care re-enablement team.

Case Example B

A visually impaired man aged 80 years who lived alone was admitted to hospital after a fall resulting in loss of mobility. Brain CT showed lacunar cerebral infarctions. He was transferred to residential rehabilitation after a few days. After 5 weeks of rehabilitation with physiotherapy, occupational therapy and a home visit, he was able to return home with provision of hand rails in the house, various pieces of equipment for the visually impaired, and a care package.

Case Example C

A man aged 88 years living with his wife in a three-bedroomed terraced house had a stroke with left hemiplegia. He refused hospital admission. He was treated by the community therapy service with balance, walking, and personal activities of daily living skills training. He was provided with a hospital bed, commode, and a transfer turntable. He received twice weekly treatment for 6 weeks then weekly for a further 6 weeks. A stairlift was provided as he was unable to climb the stairs. No package of care was required.

Delivering rehabilitation

Rehabilitation has been provided in community settings in the UK for many years. Community physiotherapy services—sometimes working primarily in patients' own homes and sometimes in community hospitals and similar settings—and occupational therapy services at home have been provided by local authorities since 1974. Since the late 1990s integrated rehabilitation services have been provided in community settings, sometimes as a result of collaborative working between health and local authorities and sometimes following closure of geriatric day hospitals.

The national service framework for older people published by the Department of Health for England[7] formally established a new mode of rehabilitation in community settings called intermediate care. Intermediate care includes rehabilitation and is usually for up to 6 weeks. It can be based at home or in a care home (local authority, health authority or provided by the private sector) or in community hospital settings. There is some evidence for the effectiveness of this approach.[8–13]

Precise models of rehabilitation vary from area to area depending on existing local resources. Rehabilitation can be provided in a variety of different ways, some more traditional, e.g. day hospitals, community physiotherapy, and local authority occupational therapy, but also in community hospitals as well as the newer, more developed, community services arising out of intermediate care and other similar developments.

Collaboration by rehabilitationists

Some therapists work in relative isolation in community settings, receiving their referrals from members of the primary care team, usually general practitioners (GPs), and reporting back verbally or in writing to the rest of the primary care team suggesting, where appropriate, referral on to other therapists. In other areas the therapists work in a team, allocating out referrals as seems appropriate to the different expertise in that team, e.g. physiotherapist, occupational therapist, speech therapist, or nurse rehabilitationist. Well-developed teams will have multidisciplinary planning meetings, discussing management strategy for individual patients at case conferences. In some areas these teams are chaired by a doctor specializing in rehabilitation, either consultant or GP with special interest in older people or rehabilitation. Teams work best when sharing a common rehabilitation record rather than individual notes for different members of the team. Usually these records will be separate from the notes of the primary care team, and sometimes separate from hospital notes, but ideally they should provide written reports and letters describing progress and recommendations to others treating the patient.

Joint working with private and voluntary resources

In many areas the voluntary sector has developed where there are deficiencies in public sector services. Thus organizations such as Age Concern and the Alzheimer's Disease Society may provide day care or community support. In some cases these resources provide some limited rehabilitation or have ready access to other services by links with rehabilitation teams with a community base. In addition, with UK Government support, both local and health authorities have contracted out provision of day care or intermediate care to the private sector, often large nursing homes. Therapists working in these settings are usually employed by the health authority.

It is likely with the current UK emphasis on using private sector services that these sorts of arrangements will increase in number (see Chapter 29).

Setting up community-based rehabilitation services

This is largely a matter of experience combined with sensible use of existing resources. What is needed more than anything is an enthusiasm to get things working, knowledge of successful communication techniques and the ability to work in and develop a team. Resources are required, so a commitment from commissioners of services driven nowadays by targeted funding and a need to improve the effectiveness of joint working is essential. Administrative support will be needed for taking of referrals, liaison with the many agencies involved, and for typing letters and reports.

Managing functional impairment and disability

Many older people suffer with complex disability, with physical, psychological and social features. They may require special adaptations to maintain independence, such as provision of a raised toilet with a toilet frame. Chairs should be of the correct height with an appropriate angle (rake) on the seat and with arms to enable the person to push themselves up from sitting. A bed lever can be especially useful to help patients—particularly those with Parkinson's disease—get out of bed or turn over in bed. A rope ladder attached to the end of the bed can be helpful in getting people to a sitting position. Additional rails, particularly on stairs and in doorways, showers, or baths, can help patients get around safely.

Techniques of rehabilitation

The common problems among older people are orthopaedic and neurological, with some cardio-vascular and respiratory disorders. Pathology is multiple and patients are often taking complex medication regimens. It is essential that physiotherapists are familiar with the requirements of local orthopaedic surgeons with regards to weight-bearing status, management of plasters and splints, e.g. wicket splints (Colour plate 29) and Lancaster arm slings (Colour plate 30). Physiotherapists will need to be in regular communication with the relevant teams. It is also help-ful if physiotherapists are familiar with local strategies for managing stroke, such as the Bobath technique and proprioceptive neuromuscular facilitation. There is nothing worse than incurring the wrath of a hospital-based therapist who is in overall charge of stroke rehabilitation.

Access to appropriate equipment in a care home setting and to a variety of walking aids is appropriate. Many older people cannot manage to walk without their usual aid, e.g. a trolley (Colour plate 31) and some are used to furniture-walking or have made themselves dependent on a wheelchair. In general terms it is hard to get disabled people to change from equipment and techniques of coping that they are used to, so it is usually wise to stick with them. Some patients may require a special walking aid, such as an elbow gutter frame (Colour plate 32), because they are not allowed to weight-bear through their wrist because of a wrist fracture or severe arthritis. Some patients will have such severe problems with balance or general weakness that they require a platform or pulpit walking aid (Colour plate 33). Occasional patients with reasonable balance and wrist function but needing to reduce weight through the legs will be able to use elbow crutches. Axillary crutches are infrequently used except amongst a small number of amputees. Some patients with movement disorders, such as Parkinson's disease, require specific approaches to enable walking such as the use of music, metronomes or visual cues such as a series of yellow lines marked on the floor to enable them to practise stepping out. Heel toe walking will need to be encouraged to prevent Achilles tendon contractures. It is useful to have access to stairs or set of steps to enable quadriceps strengthening exercises and to establish that someone is strong and safe enough to manage stairs at home. A plinth is valuable to practise unsupported balance in sitting and also non-weight bearing exercises. A set of parallel bars is useful for patients with poor balance not quite ready to manage a zimmer frame and, with a mirror appropriately placed at the end, patients can appreciate faults in posture. Pulleys attached appropriately to weights can be used to develop strength in the upper limbs as required by amputees and wheelchair users.

Occupational therapists equally need to develop a range of skills and knowledge relevant to managing the types of problems that older people have. Tasks such as stretching sideways to improve balance and co-ordination and reordering skittles on a table of appropriate height can be used to counteract problems of visual neglect and to practise co-ordination skills. Many domestic skills need to be re-learned (or for some men learnt for the first time!) by patients who have acquired a new disability to which they must adapt, such as a stroke or upper limb weakness due to a ruptured supraspinatus tendon or a fixed joint following arthrodesis of a knee. Many of these tasks can be practised in a therapy kitchen or the patient's own kitchen. Sometimes special equipment such as a perching stool (Colour plate 34) is needed because of impaired functional balance or weakness such that prolonged standing is impossible. For amputees, heights of worktops may need to be lowered. For newly visually impaired people specially adapted cookers or microwaves with touch sensitive knobs are required. Patients with visual impairment may require the support of visual or mobility therapists from the local authority in order to access the wide range of special equipment and adaptations available. Deaf patients may require provision of visual alarms to tell them the door bell has been rung or the kettle is boiling.

Patients who need to be able to let in carers but cannot themselves access the front door may need a device to remotely open the front door or a key safe in a special security cupboard by the front door for which only the carers have the access code. Modern assistive technology can be of help to many at-risk elderly patients going home so that calls and information can be sent to carers if, for example, a patient has fallen on the floor or is otherwise in need of assistance. Many areas now have community teams who carry on from hospital or intermediate care, not only providing home personal care such as assistance with dressing and making meals, etc., but also encouraging independence so that after a few weeks patients can carry out many tasks independently in their own home.

With regards to nursing issues such as management of incontinence and stoma care, community nurses will need to carry out appropriate assessments, e.g. frequency/volume urine charts and regular toileting, or more advanced bladder re-education programmes. Some patients and their carers will need to be taught to manage a catheter using leg and night bags, and how to cope with bladder spasm, etc. (using antimuscarinics, cranberry juice and, rarely, bladder washouts usually using Solution G). Some female patients, such as the cognitively intact patient with a major orthopaedic problem who is unable to transfer without help at night-time, may benefit from the use of a slipper pan at night time. Other patients will need to manage faecal incontinence using regular bisacodyl suppositories or occasionally phosphate enemas three times a week combined as necessary with judicious doses of constipating agents such as low dose codeine 15 mg three times a day or loperamide 2 mg daily. Other patients will need be taught by nursing staff how to self-monitor diabetes using blood glucose sticks, and yet others how to manage home oxygen, use of nebulizers or inhalation aids, etc.

Equipment used in community settings

There are many items of equipment which can be used to help specific needs. Many of these have already been referred to above. It is helpful to be familiar with these in order to advise patients appropriately, though GPs would not be expected to know the specifics of the whole range of equipment. GPs will often have to prescribe footwear for patients, so it is useful to know about 'post-op sandals' (Colour plate 35) which are designed for patients with temporary bandages on their feet for whom no ordinary footwear is suitable. Doctors in rehabilitation need to know when made-to-measure/bespoke footwear is needed or when off-the-shelf footwear is satisfactory. Surgical footwear may be required for diabetic patients with neuropathic feet or for patients who have deformities of the feet with overlapping and/or subluxed toes, etc. Rehabilitationists need to understand about other orthoses such as various types of knee braces (often used to relieve painful osteoarthritis or for an unstable knee), ankle braces (for an unstable ankle; Colour plate 36), a Swedish knee cage (for hyperextension of the knee; Colour plate 37) and foot drop splints—when they should and should not be used. Knowing the appropriate hosiery to prescribe for patients with previous venous ulcers and understanding the importance of measurement of ankle/brachial systolic blood pressure index (0.6–0.8 is marginal ischaemia and <0.6 is critical ischaemia) is important. One needs to know which patients need below-the-knee stockings and which patients need full-length stockings and which grade of compression to use. For postural hypotension one needs to know that full-length stockings of at least grade 2 is necessary, or preferably use of support tights. Support stockings quickly lose their elasticity when stocking pullers are used, so other techniques such as rolling up the stockings and use of talc may be needed to apply support stockings.

Conclusion

There is a whole range of knowledge required to successfully rehabilitate people in community settings. Knowledge of the roles and skills of each member of the team, whether that be physiotherapist, speech therapist, dietician, psychologist, pharmacist, rehabilitation nurse or social worker is vital. There is insufficient space here to describe the roles and skills of each member of the team, which can only be learned by working in a rehabilitation setting. Team management skills are also important, as are good communication skills with patients and carers.

Promoting physical activity in older people

The health benefits of physical activity are so extensive that exercise is probably the most important self-help therapy available to the population. The evidence suggests that regular exercise reduces the risk of cardiovascular disease, type 2 diabetes, osteoporosis and certain cancers.[14] It also promotes mental wellbeing and helps people to manage their weight.[15] There is growing evidence of an association between regular physical activity and a reduced risk of death from all causes, and also of the potential savings for National Health Service (NHS) budgets to be made through effective exercise promotion for older adults. Among older people the beneficial effects of exercise on falls risk and on depression (itself a cause of disability) are substantial.

Falls are common events in people aged ≥65 years and, although most are not reported to GPs or to the emergency services, they can have serious consequences, including impaired function, loss of confidence in carrying out everyday activities like shopping or going out socially, loss of independence and autonomy, and even death. There is a growing body of evidence that interventions providing some form of regular exercise may be effective in preventing falls among older people and that healthcare costs can be reduced if falls are reduced.[16]

Depression is the single biggest cause of disability worldwide,[17] with 5% of the adult population having a major depressive disorder (see Chapter 22). Recent studies consistently support the effectiveness of physical exercise in reducing depressive symptoms, and increasing the level of activity has been found to have a beneficial and lasting effect on depression in its own right.

Exercise programmes targeting depression may also have an impact on coronary heart disease, risk since depression is associated with higher risks of heart disease.

Current recommendations are that people do ≥30 min of physical activity of moderate intensity on ≥5 days of the week.[18] However, surveys have consistently shown a high prevalence of physical inactivity in the UK population. Recent estimates suggest that around 6 out of 10 men and 7 out of 10 women are not active enough to benefit their health, and activity levels vary with age, gender, class and ethnicity.[15]

Clinical and commissioning imperatives

General practitioners therefore have powerful clinical reasons for wanting to master exercise promotion for all adults, as a primary prevention strategy for disability and disease in later life. They have similar reasons for wanting to promote gait stability, strength, stamina and suppleness for older adults in particular, because of the potential for secondary and tertiary prevention of falls and depression. Practice-based commissioners will have a special interest in the possible downstream savings to be made from upstream investment in exercise promotion.

The NHS is attempting to provide resources to promote physical activity in a variety of ways, including exercise referral schemes in primary care (also known as 'exercise on prescription' which usually involves referring patients to the local leisure centre). All GPs can recommend exercise as a preventive activity and as a therapeutic remedy for older people, and most GPs in Britain probably have access to some form of local exercise promotion programme that their patients can use.[19] The Fitness Industry Association estimates that there are ~600 exercise schemes in England that require referral by an appropriate professional to a service where, after a formalized process of assessment of the person's needs, a tailored physical activity programme is developed to meet that need, and the individual's progress monitored. Physical activity public health intervention guidance from the National Institute for Health and Clinical Excellence (NICE) in 2006 described four commonly used methods to increase physical activity: brief interventions in primary care, exercise referral schemes, pedometers, and community-based exercise programmes for walking and cycling.[15]

We know from the NICE review that exercise referral schemes can have positive effects on physical activity levels in the short term (6–12 weeks). However, such referral schemes are ineffective in increasing physical activity levels in the longer term (over 12 weeks) or over a longer timeframe (over 1 year). A recent systematic review compared 17 randomized controlled trials with different interventions designed to encourage sedentary, community-dwelling adults to do more physical activity.[20] Interventions varied widely and included counselling (individually or in groups), self-directed or prescribed, supervised or unsupervised, and home-based or facility-based physical activity. They were effective in the short and mid term, at least in middle age, and there were no significant increases in adverse events for intervention participants. Unfortunately, it is not yet clear which is the most effective individual intervention (e.g. home-based or facility-based) in increasing physical activity in the long term, or in older age groups.

Rules of thumb

The uncertainty about which approach works best for whom in the promotion of physical activity leaves GPs with a dilemma when facing older patients with declining functional capacity, and practice-based commissioners are left with little guidance about cost-effective investment in exercise promotion. We have six evidence-based 'rules of thumb' to help practitioners make clinical and investment decisions.

1) The EXERT (Exercise Evaluation Randomised Trial) trial, comparing leisure centre-based exercise on prescription, home-based walking and usual advice in primary care, was carried out in the UK and produced four important lessons for primary care. First, walking appears to be as effective as leisure centre classes and is cheaper. Second, efforts should be directed towards maintenance of increased activity, using proven reinforcement methods such as telephone support. Third, on cost-effectiveness grounds, assessment and advice alone from an exercise specialist (for example, in a leisure centre) may be appropriate to initiate physical activity. Finally, subsidized schemes may be best concentrated on patients at higher absolute risk, or with specific conditions for which particular exercise programmes may be beneficial.[21]

2) Self-monitoring of physical activity with expert feedback (e.g. from an exercise instructor, but potentially from a primary care professional) can be useful in increasing the weekly duration of overall physical activity in the short term.[22]

3) A primary care study from the USA suggests that exercise counselling with a prescription for walking at either a 'hard intensity' or a 'high frequency' produced significant long-term improvements in cardio-respiratory fitness.[23]

4) However, overly optimistic expectations of inexperienced exercisers may lead to disappointment and attrition. Interventions by primary care practitioners to ensure realistic expectations might increase the success of exercise promotion schemes and prevent potential negative effects of failure.[24]

5) The dialogue between the GP or practice nurse and the patient may be crucial to success. A trial conducted in general practice in New Zealand included the negotiation of activity goals and the writing of a 'green prescription' for exercise. Trained exercise specialists from a regional sports foundation gave follow-up telephone support for a 3 month period, and the outcomes suggested that systematic inclusion of the green prescription in routine primary health care would lead to health gain for older people[25] and represent better value for money than 'usual care'.[26]

6) Finally, relative frailty is not necessarily a barrier to exercise promotion, as referral for exercise has been shown to be feasible and effective in vulnerable older people on the borders of frailty.[27] The high level of adherence to the exercise programme, and the significant improvements in function achieved, may have been related to the siting of the exercise class in general practices. Location matters, because older people may experience significant barriers to uptake of exercise classes in leisure centres, and for many older people home exercise or group exercise in non-intimidating environments (e.g. community halls) may be more appealing, and result in higher uptake of exercise programmes and longer continuation of exercise.

Conclusion

The evidence base on how to promote physical activity among older people lags behind the clinical and economic rationales for doing so, but our knowledge about effective methods for increasing the activity of the older population is expanding rapidly. There is every reason to encourage older people to exercise regularly through simple advice and signposting to available exercise promotion schemes. The key to exercise promotion seems to be finding out what works for whom, and how. GPs know their older patients well, and have much to teach about what facilitates a change in exercise behaviour, what the obstacles to behaviour change really are, and how best to organize exercise as a therapy. Practice-based commissioners may have to take some investment risks with exercise promotion, but the potential economic gains to the health service make these risks worth considering.

References

1. Folstein MF, Folstein SE, McHugh PR. "Mini-mental state". A practical method for grading the cognitive state of patients for the clinician. *J Psychiat Res* 1975;12;189–98.

2. Royall DR, Cordes JA, Polk M. CLOX: an executive clock drawing task. *J Neurol Neurosurg Psychiat* 1998;64:588–94.

3. Zigmond AS, Snaith RP. The hospital anxiety and depression scale. *Acta Psychiat Scand* 1983;67:361–70.

4. Yesavage JA, Brink TL, Rose TL, *et al.* Development and validation of a geriatric depression rating scale: a preliminary report. *J Psychiat Res* 1983;17:37–49.

5. Mathias S, Nayak US, Issacs B. Balance in elderly patients: the "Get up and Go test". *Arch Phys Med Rehabil* 1986;67:387–9.

6. Albert ML. A simple test of visual neglect. *Neurology* 1973;23:658–664.

7. Department of Health. *National Service Framework for Older People.* London: DoH; 2001. Available at: http://www.dh.gov.uk/en/Publicationsandstatistics/Publications/PublicationsPolicyAndGuidance/DH_4003066

8. Kaambwa B, Bryan S, Barton P, *et al.* Costs and health outcomes of intermediate care: results from five UK case study sites. *Hlth Social Care Commun* 2008;16:573–81.

9. Fleming SA, Blake H, Gladman JR, *et al.* A randomised controlled trial of a care home rehabilitation service to reduce long-term institutionalisation for elderly people. *Age Ageing* 2004;33;384–90.

10. Forster A, Young J, Langhorn P. Systematic review of day hospital care for elderly people. *Br Med J* 1999;318:837–41.

11. Griffiths PD, Edwards MH, Forbes A, Harris RL, Richie G. Effectiveness of intermediate care in nursing-led in-patient units. *Cochrane Database Syst Rev* 2004;18(4):CD002214.

12. Miller P, Gladman JR, Cunliffe AL, Husbands SL, Dewey ME, Harwood RH. Economic analysis of an early discharge rehabilitation service for older people. *Age Ageing* 2005;34:274–80.

13. Young J, Robinson M, Chell S, *et al.* A whole system study of intermediate care services for older people. *Age Ageing* 2005;34:577–83.

14. Department of Health. *At Least Five a Week: Evidence on the Impact of Physical Activity and its Relationship to Health.* A Report from the Chief Medical Officer. London: DoH; 2004.

15. National Institute for Health and Clinical Excellence, Physical Activity Collaborating Centre. *A Rapid Review of the Effectiveness of Exercise Referral Schemes to Promote Physical Activity in Adults.* London: NICE; 2006.

16. National Institute for Clinical Excellence Guidelines. *Falls: The Assessment and Prevention of Falls in Older People.* London: NICE; 2004.

17. World Health Organization. *Mental Health and Work: Impact, Issues and Good Practices.* Geneva: WHO; 2000.

18. Department of Health. *Strategy Statement on Physical Activity.* London: DoH; 1996.

19. Department of Health. *Choosing Activity: A Physical Activity Action Plan.* London: DoH; 2005.

20. Hillsdon M, Foster C, Thorogood M. Interventions for promoting physical activity. *Cochrane Database Syst Rev* 2005;(1):CD003180.

21. Isaacs AJ, Critchley JA, See TS, *et al.* Exercise Evaluation Randomised Trial (EXERT): a randomised trial comparing GP referral for leisure centre-based exercise, community-based walking and advice only. *Health Technol Assessmt* 2007;11:1–165.

22. Aittasalo M, Miilunpalo S, Kukkonen-Harjula K, Pasanen M. A randomized intervention of physical activity promotion and patient self-monitoring in primary health care. *Prev Med* 2006;42:40–6.

23. Duncan GE, Anton SD, Sydeman SJ, *et al.* Prescribing exercise at varied levels of intensity and frequency: a randomized trial. *Arch Intern Med* 2005;165;2362–9.

24. Jones F, Harris P, Waller H, Coggins A. Adherence to an exercise prescription scheme: the role of expectations, self-efficacy, stage of change and psychological well-being. *Br J Health Psychol* 2005;10(Pt 3):359–78.

25. Kerse N, Elley CR, Robinson E, Arroll B. Is physical activity counseling effective for older people? A cluster randomized, controlled trial in primary care. *J Am Geriat Soc* 2005;53:1951–6.

26. Dalziel K, Segal L, Elley CR. Cost utility analysis of physical activity counselling in general practice. *Aust NZ J Public Health* 2006;30:57–63.

27. Dinan S, Lenihan P, Tenn T, Iliffe S. Is the promotion of physical activity in vulnerable, older people feasible and effective in general practice? *Br J Gen Pract* 2006;56(531):791–3.

Chapter 28

Social services, community care, and benefits

Paddy Goslyn and Garry Briggs

Introduction

This chapter comprises two sections: provision of a community care assessment; residential and nursing care criteria and funding.

Provision of a community care assessment

Background

The National Health Service and Community Care Act (1990) requires local authorities to assess the needs of adults who reside within a council's geographical boundary. The actual decision to provide a service is dependent on the individual person meeting the local authority's eligibility criteria.

Section 47 National Health Service & Community Care Act (1990), Section 47 states:

(1) … where it appears to a local authority that any person for whom they may provide or arrange for the provision of community care services may be in need of any such services, the authority—
  (a) shall carry out an assessment of his needs for those services; and
  (b) having regard to the results of that assessment, shall then decide whether his needs call for the provision by them of any such services.
(2) If at any time during the assessment of the needs of any person under subsection (1)(a) above it appears to a local authority that he is a disabled person, the authority—
  (a) shall proceed to make such a decision as to the services he requires as is mentioned in section 4 of the [1986c. 33.] Disabled Persons (Services, Consultation and Representation) Act 1986 without his requesting them to do so under that section; and
  (b) shall inform him that they will be doing so and of his rights under that Act.

The Department of Health provides general written guidance to local authorities on what a community care assessment should include (see 'The assessment process' below). *Fair Access to Care Guidance* sets out the core elements of an eligibility framework that all local authorities must adhere to. The framework consists of a general overview of what constitutes low, moderate, substantial and critical need.

The needs assessment methodology used by most local authorities loosely follows Abraham Maslow's theory on human hierarchy of need. Maslow was a psychologist who developed a framework for explaining human behaviour. In his book *Motivation and Personality*, Maslow proposed that there is a specific hierarchy of five needs and that each must be satisfied in an ascending order. 'Biological and psychological needs' such as warmth, food, drink and shelter

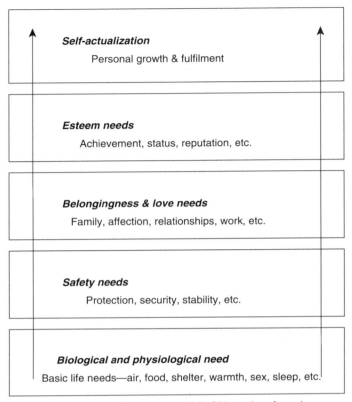

Fig. 28.1 Outline of Maslow's original five-stage model of hierarchy of need.

must be satisfied before higher, so-called 'esteem needs' such as achievement, reputation and status, can be met (Figure 28.1).[1]

Although Social Services assessments and eligibility criteria do not adhere to this model strictly, the basic principles are the same with biological, physiological and safety needs taking precedence over esteem and personal growth needs. An example of an eligibility matrix is shown in Table 28.1.

Even though local authorities have to apply an eligibility criteria framework, the level at which individuals' needs and their eligibility to services are matched can be locally determined, depending on available local resources. Therefore some local authorities provide services to people with moderate needs, whereas others only provide services to people with substantial or critical needs. Local authorities have to review their eligibility criteria annually.

The assessment process

Community care assessments take place in Social Services after a referral has been received or is taken at the point of contact with an individual or organization. Anyone can make a referral to Social Services. Local authorities now use either a 'one-stop shop' customer service model for facilitating the first point of contact with the council or a single point of entry. In the former, a customer services team take the basic details and pass them on to the appropriate directorate or team, or in the latter a 'single point of access' within a specific service area, e.g. community care or housing, and enquiries are directed through a contact number.

Table 28.1 Example of an eligibility matrix

	General health and disabling conditions	Communication and sensory impairment	Self-care and daily living	Risk and vulnerability
Critical	Health problems that are significant and life-threatening, person will be at risk without high levels of care, unlikely to be able to live independently.	Cannot live independently due to sensory or communication losses. Previous experience of exploitation or abuse or is at risk of exploitation or abuse and requires protection.	Person unable to care for self independently, needs high levels of assistance and would be at risk without it. Unable to care for family members without input.	Person has or could experience an abusive situation. Unable to protect self from harm or accidents. Degree of risk such that immediate intervention needed as risks to life.
Substantial	Substantial and regular care needed to sustain or promote independence due to levels of ill-health and disability.	Sensory impairment and communication difficulties of a high level requiring daily support in order to maintain safety and independence.	Person requires daily and substantial assistance to live independently and would be at risk without it.	May not be able to understand or manage risk levels or vulnerability and may be at risk of abuse. Action needed to reduce risk levels.
Moderate	Disability or health condition is causing difficulties. Some help is needed in the long or short term to maintain independence/reduce risks.	Some sensory/ communication difficulties posing a threat to independence and increasing risks. Low level regular input or short term rehabilitation may be required.	Person may need some assistance regularly to maintain independence, would be at some degree of risk without low level support.	Vulnerability issues identified and accepted by person. Action taken to reduce risk/ensure safety. Person able to take responsibility for own safety with help.

Most local authorities use a standard referral format. The referral gathers the initial basic information such as name, address, next of kin and carer, existing support and a basic outline of the presenting problem. If the client is known the referral is passed to the relevant team and current caseworker to carry out a review. If the client is new to the service then the referral will be progressed by a response and assessment team or access team who will carry out a community care assessment.

The assessment format for a community care assessment has not changed much since community care was introduced in 1993. The structure provides a framework for doing a holistic needs assessment on an individual. The assessor looks at the relevant aspects of the individual's life and the presenting needs. When all the needs are ascertained, the social worker uses the council's eligibility criteria to determine which of the presenting needs are eligible for the council to support.

The assessment process usually involves the completion of a set pro-forma but the format of this will vary between local authorities. However, if the 'single assessment process' (SAP) has been introduced the assessment format will be standardized and health and social care professionals will use the same basic paperwork for gathering general information. A 'contact' assessment is used to gather initial information and/or a more detailed 'common' assessment form is completed if at the point of contact it is obvious there are presenting needs that require immediate action. The initial assessment information can then be passed on to another professional. The sharing of information in this way prevents duplication by every professional who comes into contact with the service user. An additional specialist assessment is still completed by an appropriate professional if required, e.g. occupational therapist or physiotherapist or specialist nurse, etc.

Both community care and SAP assessments take into account most of the following areas, although there will be regional variations to the format and content:

- Risks.
- Social history and relevant relationships and life events.
- General health/medical condition(s).
- The wishes of people being assessed.
- Whether people have any particular physical difficulties, for example, problems with walking or climbing stairs.
- Sensory needs.
- Cognitive impairment.
- Mental health.
- Whether people have any particular housing needs.
- The sources of help to which people have access, such as carers, family or nearby friends, and their willingness to continue providing care.
- What needs these people who provide care may have.

A community care assessment is carried out by a qualified social worker or a non-qualified worker such as a case co-ordinator (some local authorities only employ qualified workers). The type of worker allocated is dependent on the complexity of the presenting problem. The level of risk to self or others dictates the speed at which assessments are carried out.

More than one person could be involved in a community care assessment, including social worker, GP or consultant, a nurse or district nurse a physiotherapist and an occupational therapist, etc. However, it is usually the social worker's role to co-ordinate the gathering of the relevant information recorded in the assessment and to discuss the identified needs and possible outcomes with the individual or their carer.

In order to achieve the best outcome in health and social care, good partnership working is required. A key part of the assessment and care management process includes working with health partners such as district nurses and community matrons.

District nurses play a crucial role in the primary health care team in supporting people's health needs in the community. They visit people in their own or in residential homes, providing health care for patients and supporting family members. As well as providing direct patient care, district nurses also have a teaching role, working with patients to enable them to care for themselves or with family members teaching them how to give basic health care to their relatives. District nurses play a vital role in keeping hospital admissions and readmissions to a minimum and ensuring that patients can return to their own homes as soon as possible.

The role of community matrons has developed through the pilot projects on long-term conditions for diabetes and chronic obstructive pulmonary disease. Community matrons are nurses who are case managers for patients with complex conditions and high intensity needs. They provide case management that is user/carer-led and they help to maximize choice and improve the quality of life for patients.

The community matron role is to assess physical, social and psychological needs, co-ordinate, manage and evaluate the package of care. This is a clinical role and community matrons will provide clinical care as appropriate.

Other professionals such as social workers can be case managers for patients with less complex needs and liaise with community matrons as required.

As part of primary care services the interlinked roles of district nursing, community matrons and social work provide a crucial professional support network for maintaining peoples' health and wellbeing in the community.

Carer assessment

A carer can be a family member or a friend who takes responsibility for looking after a disabled, ill or elderly person and who does not provide the care as part of a job or as a volunteer with a voluntary organization. Some carers provide care for a few hours a week, others for 24 h a day, every day. A carer does not have to be living with the person being cared for.

When the local authority is deciding what community care services the person being cared for will receive, the needs of a carer must be taken into account, unless the carer declines the offer of an assessment. A carer's assessment can also be carried out independent of an assessment being carried out for the person being cared for.

What happens after an assessment

Following a community care assessment, if services are going to be provided they must be set out in a care plan. The person assessed should be given a copy of the care plan, which will explain the following:

◆ The services which are to be provided, by whom, when and what will be achieved by providing them.

◆ A contact point to deal with problems about services.

◆ Information on how to ask for a review of the services provided if circumstances change.

Services available in the community

Following a community care assessment, there is a wide range of community care services to which people may be entitled. There may be regional variations on what is provided, depending on local eligibility criteria. The following list gives only the main examples:

◆ A place in a care home.

◆ Home care services.

◆ Adaptations to the home.

◆ Meals.

◆ Day care.

Care homes

If people need long-term care, because they can no longer manage in their own home, one option may be moving into a care home. All care homes provide personal care. This could include help with washing, dressing or going to the toilet. Some care homes can also provide nursing care or specialist care for people with specific degenerative illnesses such as multiple sclerosis or motor neuron disease (see Chapter 26).

Home care services

Home care services generally provide help with personal tasks or essential daily living tasks, for example, bathing and washing, getting up and going to bed, going to the toilet, shopping and managing finances. The provision of home care involves someone coming to the individual's home at agreed times. This could be up to five times per day.

Aids to daily living and adaptations to the home

Aids to daily living are pieces of equipment that help people to remain independent. They are too numerous to list but the most common ones that people access are: raised toilet seats, bath aids such as bath seats or bath boards or even electric bath seats, chair raisers, bed raisers and specialized trolleys for aiding walking and carrying (see Chapter 27).

Adaptations to the home may be major or minor and can be particularly important in assisting people to remain independent in their own home. Major adaptations could include, for example, the installation of exterior ramps. Adaptations indoors could be a stair lift, a downstairs lavatory or the lowering of work tops in the kitchen. Minor adaptations might include hand rails for the stairs or in the bathroom or toilet.

An assessment for specialist pieces of equipment or an adaptation to the home is carried out by an occupational therapist. Financial assistance may be available for adaptation to the home via a disabled facilities grant from the local authority. If this is an option, specialist advice would be provided. If major work is undertaken specifically for a disabled person, the community charge on the property may be reduced.

Meals

The provision of meals as a community care service could mean a daily delivery of a meal or, in some areas, the delivery of a week's or month's supply of frozen meals. A meal could also be provided at a day centre or lunch club. In exceptional cases a main meal is sometimes prepared for an individual.

Personalization of health and social care

The information about the assessment process and services available is important as it places social care practice in a context. The way in which assessments are carried out and services are provided is changing. Social care is going through a major transformation. The current government has an agenda for the personalization of health and social care over the next few years. A framework for cross-sector reform was launched in December 2007 and the strategic direction is laid out in the publication *Putting People First 2007*. This focused on transforming people's experiences of local support and services, as well as highlighting how councils will redesign and reshape their systems over the next 3 years. Everyone, regardless of their level of need, in any setting, whether statutory services, third and community or private sector or by funding it themselves, will have choice and control over how that support is delivered—confident that services are of high quality, are safe, and promote their own individual requirement for independence, well-being, and dignity.[2]

To provide care in the way that has been envisaged requires a major change in the organization of assessments and in the delivery of services across the continuum of care. A whole-systems approach will need to be developed ranging from local joint strategic needs assessments between local authorities, Primary Care Trusts (PCTs), and National Health Service (NHS) providers, and linking to other local needs assessments that will inform a wider sustainable community strategy.

The change in the way services are provided puts people in the centre of the process. Some of the headings and themes mentioned in this chapter on what pertains to an assessment will still exist but they will be answered by the service user, with support from a professional or other person if required. The outcomes from the assessment and the types of services provided will be led by the service user within a set budget. This process is called Self Directed Support (SDS). At the heart of all the change is the service user. Over the last 2 years, 'in control' pilot schemes have been developing the process and systems for SDS; 'direct payments' and 'individualized budgets' are a means of delivering SDS. A self- or shared assessment process produces agreed outcomes. The cost of care services is rationalized via a resource allocation system whereby a points system equates each need from the assessment with a monetary value. Where the service user is able to manage the process, assessments will be user-led with the professional guiding the individual through the process; the responsibility for achieving the appropriate outcome will be shared.

Service users will have the choice of organizing their own social care and services. The organization of the provision of care will be available, if required, from the local authority or independent brokerage. The service user will no longer have to have their needs meet through mainstream service provision—they will be able to employ their own carer or purchase services from the wider community. The types of services or items purchased can be very diverse, all they have to do is meet the agreed outcome from the assessment and remain within the allocated budget.

Local authorities in the UK are at different stages of the implementation of SDS but a target of 30% of all service users in social care to be provided with SDS by 2011 has been set by the government.

Residential and nursing care criteria and funding

Introduction

Health and social care services work in partnership to provide advice and assistance to help vulnerable adults live their lives to the full. The aim is to encourage and enable people to live as independently as possible in their own homes or in a homely environment with support if and when they need it. Whatever the personal situation, finding the right services to meet someone's needs is important—it may be older people finding it difficult to look after themselves at home; they may have been ill or in hospital and need some support until they recover; they may also have a physical, sensory or learning disability, a mental health problem or substance misuse issues.

This chapter aims to provide information about care and support services where the possibility of need for residential or nursing care is identified. It includes details on who can get help; what kind of help is available; how to apply for it and what happens when someone applies. Contact details of useful voluntary support organizations are also listed.

Who can get help?

If an older person is having difficulties managing everyday tasks they may be entitled to help from adult social services.

In line with government guidance *Fair Access to Care Services*, social services will assess, plan and provide care for adults who have needs that fall within the agreed criteria. The eligibility criteria consist of two bands: critical and substantial. It must, however, be remembered that there can be variations between local authority social services' interpretations.

Choosing a residential or nursing home

Residential care homes aim to provide the same level of care and attention received at home from a caring relative. Residential homes have staff that will help with personal care, such as getting up, washing, dressing, and going to the toilet. Each residential home generally offers care to people with a similar condition or problem; a physical disability, a learning disability, mental health problems, or to older people with physical disabilities or mental health problems. Meals are provided and there are often outings and other activities. Residential homes do not, however, provide care for people who require nursing support.

Nursing homes also offer care to people with a similar condition or problem but specialize in providing nursing care for persons suffering from illness, injury or infirmity—the kind of care that requires the skills of a qualified nurse. Nursing homes are required by law to have a qualified nurse on duty 24 h a day.

Care homes registered as both residential and nursing homes are known as 'dual registration'. Some people may choose such a home so that if their condition deteriorates they do not need to change homes.

This also enables a couple with differing needs to stay together in the same home. Both residential and nursing care homes are registered and inspected by the Commission of Social Care Inspection (CSCI) who can provide an inspection report on any home on request. The CSCI can be contacted as follows:

Internet: http://www.csci.org.uk

E-mail for enquiries: Enquiries@csci.gsi.gov.uk

Telephone: 0845 015 0120

What to look for in a care home

Individuals need to be sure that the home meets all their needs and would be somewhere that they would enjoy living. The following questions may be helpful:

◆ What personal possessions can be brought to the home?

◆ Are special diets catered for?

◆ When are meal times and can food be obtained 'out of hours'?

◆ Are there social activities and outings?

◆ Can family and friends stay?

◆ What arrangements are made for medical support?

◆ Are there opportunities for religious worship?

◆ What will the cost be and what does this include?

This list is not exhaustive. Individual patients need to ask questions about things that are important to them. If there is a social care worker assisting with the move to a care home, they will be able to obtain all the information needed to allow the correct decision to be made (see Chapter 26).

Help from Social Services

Moving into a care home is a big life change. It is important that the individuals feel that it is the right thing to do. Social Services can help them choose the right home by giving comprehensive lists of homes in the local area and advice on the admission process.

Whether older people intend to pay their own home fees, or think that they may require financial support from Social Services: please note that they must meet the eligibility criteria for support (see section 1). All Social Service Departments have information brochures on *Social Care for Adults* and it is advisable that this information should be consulted before choosing a home.

If the older person needs help with paying fees, and it has been agreed that a care home place is best for them, then a social care worker will be allocated. An agreement that a person's needs can best be met in a care home is taken by Social Services, usually by means of a panel. This process can differ between areas. For example: DAN Panel (Decisions Around Need) agrees the criteria; DAR (Decision Around Resources) agrees the funding and placement. The operational protocol may be different between local areas.

If fees are to be paid for the home, and it has been agreed that a care home is the appropriate placement, your patient has the legal right to choose any home provided that:

◆ a place is available;

◆ the home is suitable for their care needs;

◆ contact with the chosen home can be made; and

◆ the home does not cost more than Social Services usually pay for the care needed, or if it does, someone can pay the difference.

Social services staff can help an individual chose a residential or nursing home. They will help to complete the relevant paperwork and make a contract with the home to plan for the admission. However, they may have to wait until Social Services can agree their choice of home or a vacancy occurs.

How much will it cost?

The weekly charge for accommodation is determined by Social Services according to financial details supplied; the assessment is based on policies agreed by government. If the placement is in nursing care, part of the fees may be paid by the NHS under 'continuing care' criteria. If continuing care funding is to be applied for, this will be recognized and is integral to the overall assessment process. The leaflet *NHS Funded Nursing Care in Nursing Homes* is also helpful. There are variations across the UK on funding criteria and these are explained below.

NHS-funded nursing care in England and Wales

In England, 'nursing home co-ordinator' is the equivalent of 'care home co-ordinator' in Wales; and local PCT is the equivalent of Health Board in Wales.

Older people living in a care home in England or Wales may be eligible for help with the cost of their nursing care. Before entering a care home an assessment is required from the local PCT. If the PCT agrees that nursing care is needed, it organizes an assessment by a registered nurse. If they agree that nursing care is needed, the NHS will pay an amount directly to the care home towards the cost of nursing care.

◆ If individuals pay their own fees they may see a reduction in how much they have to pay.

◆ If fees are paid by the local council the NHS will still contribute towards the cost of nursing care, but the amount the individual pays will not be affected.

◆ If the individual pays part of the fees and the local council pays part of the fees, there may be a reduction. Advice can be obtained from SeniorLine on 0808 800 6565.

In England, the amount the NHS will contribute toward nursing care costs changed on 1 October 2007 to a flat rate of £101 per week for those people newly assessed as needing nursing care.

Transitional arrangements for existing claimants

Those people who have already been assessed as needing nursing care will be reassessed. For people who were previously assessed as needing the middle or lower rates of nursing care, and who are still assessed as needing this level of care, their care home will now receive the flat rate of £101 per week for their care.

For people who were previously assessed as needing the higher rate of nursing care, and who still need this level of care, their care home will continue to receive the higher rate of £139 per week.

For those living in Wales, the care home will receive a flat rate of £117.66 per week towards fees.

Individuals assessed by an NHS nurse will receive regular reviews of their nursing care needs. The reviews should take place within 3 months of initial assessment and then yearly. If, at any time, nursing needs change, the care home should notify the NHS nursing home co-ordinator at the local PCT.

If the nurse decides that nursing care is not required, the NHS will not be obliged to pay for it, and neither will the local council. Those wishing to go into a care home offering a high level of nursing care can only do so if they agree to pay for the nursing aspect of care themselves. Those who disagree with the level of nursing care that they have been assessed as needing can ask to be referred to the PCT continuing care panel for a review. If still dissatisfied, they can ask the Healthcare Commission for a further review. If patients are entering nursing care for a period of <6 weeks they will not need assessment by an NHS nurse. For the remaining part of their fees, covering personal care and accommodation costs, they will still be assessed under the rules as stated in *Rules on Savings and Capital*. The Department of Health published advice on nursing care bands on 4 March 2009, confirming the annual increase in the level of NHS contribution towards the cost of a place in a care home with nursing for those people assessed as requiring the help of a registered nurse.

◆ For advice on how these rules will affect particular situations, call the SeniorLine number 0808 800 6565.

If patients are assessed as needing nursing care, it is worth checking whether they have been properly assessed for fully funded NHS care first – see 'NHS-funded nursing care in England and Wales' above.

Help with personal and nursing care in Scotland

Those paying all or part of their care home fees, and aged ≥65 years, may be eligible for help with the nursing and personal care part of their fees. Those aged <65 years will only get extra help with nursing fees.

First, care needs to be assessed by the local council. For those aged ≥65 years where the local council agrees that personal care is needed, it will pay £149 per week towards care. For those of any age requiring nursing care the council will pay an additional £67 per week. These payments will be made by the local council to the care home, leading to a reduction in the fees paid.

Personal care is defined as:

◆ Help with washing, bathing and showering.

◆ Help with managing continence including using continence equipment such as catheters and stomas.

◆ Assistance with eating, managing special diets and preparing specialist meals such as puréed food.

◆ Help to move around indoors.

◆ Help with simple treatments such as applying creams, lotions and dressings.

Nursing care is defined as:

◆ Care provided by a registered nurse or doctor.

Payment will still be required for normal accommodation costs which do not involve personal or nursing care, and finances will be assessed. The information in *Rules on Savings and Capital* is a guide to how much you are likely to be charged.

◆ For further advice contact SeniorLine on 0808 800 6565.

Nursing care contribution in Northern Ireland

Those individuals funding all or part of their nursing home fees may be able to get help with the cost of nursing care.

Assessment by a health and social care (HSC) trust nurse is required. If they agree that nursing care is needed, the local HSC trust will pay up to £100 per week towards care fees, depending on how much the individual is contributing towards the cost of the nursing home.

◆ For those paying the full cost of their fees and assessed as needing nursing care, the Health and Personal Social Services (HPSS) should contribute £100 towards the cost of the nursing home.

◆ If the HPSS is already making a contribution towards nursing home fees, that contribution will be increased to £100.

◆ If the HPSS is already contributing more than £100 towards nursing home fees, there will be no extra help and fees will remain the same.

◆ For more advice, call SeniorLine on 0808 808 7575.

Funding nursing home care

Sometimes the exact amount required to pay may still not be worked out (or assessed) before moving into a care home. In these circumstances Social Services will be involved and will explain what happens.

Please note that the value of the property (the property that was occupied before admission) will be excluded from the financial assessment for up to the first 12 weeks of the placement, this is known as '12 week property disregard' and is explained below along with the 'deferred payment' arrangement.

Twelve-week property disregard

Under the local authority system, the value of an assessable property will be disregarded for a period of up to 12 weeks from the date at which permanent care commenced.

This disregard rule was designed to provide individuals with savings below the upper capital limit, a period of grace before having to sell their assessable property to pay for care.

During the disregarded period, the individual will make a contribution based on the individual's income and other assets. The local authority is obliged to apply for any state benefits to which the resident is entitled and then top up the resultant income to their prevailing tariff rate for care in the area. For the disregarded period, the local authority contribution does not need to be repaid; but once that period has expired, the amount of support provided by the authority will accrue as a loan against the property to be repaid at a future date.

The local authority does allow the resident to retain a small element of their income for personal expenditure, currently £18.10 per week.

Should an individual choose to enter a care home which is more expensive than the local authority would normally pay for their assessed need, Section 54 of the Health and Social Care Act (2001) makes provision for residents to top up from their own resources during the 12 week disregard period. It should be noted that once this period has ended, the resident is no longer able to top up directly. The payment must be taken over by a third party, namely a family member, friend or charity who will be required to sign a contract or agreement confirming their ability to pay the top-up until the property has been sold.

Deferred payment agreement

Subject to the approval of their local authority, individuals who wish to postpone the sale of their assessable property can do so under the deferred payment agreement. The aim is to allow people with property, but without income and other assets sufficient to meet their full assessed contribution, to have a legal charge placed on their property to meet any shortfall for the duration of the exempt period.

Councils have the discretion over whether or not to agree to defer payments in individual cases, and a person may only enter into a deferred payment agreement once the 12 week property disregard period has been completed.

Individual agreements should be put in writing and should state categorically that residents or their estate will repay the full amount of the deferred contributions following the end of the exempt period. This should then be signed by an authorized officer of the council and the resident, the holder of enduring power of attorney or a receiver appointed by order of the Court of Protection in the case of residents who lack capacity to act on their own behalf.

Deferred payments do not apply to individuals entering care on a temporary basis and should not be used in place of any other discretionary property disregards as set out in the *Charging for Residential Accommodation Guidelines*, for example, if the property is occupied by a spouse.

The contribution a resident is liable to pay is defined as:

> ... the difference between what a resident is assessed as being able to contribute from means tested income and assets including his former main home or only home and the amount he would be assessed as being able to contribute if his main or only home were not taken into account is then deferred.

Individuals who are refused a deferred payment will be notified of the reason in writing by the council and a copy given to the resident with information regarding how to complain or comment on the decision. Residents seeking deferred payments are advised by councils to seek independent financial advice.

Benefits Agency or Department of Works and Pensions (DWP)

Pension Credit

As an alternative to local authority funding, a package of support is available directly from the Benefits Agency or Department for Works and Pensions, which does not restrict receipt of Attendance Allowance and which may offer a higher overall benefit entitlement. This is subject to the review of Attendance Allowance with the new Pension Credit system as referred to previously. This option is accessed via the Pension Credit system which has replaced the Income Support system and is available to individuals aged ≥60 years.

Entitlement to benefit consists of two elements. The first is *Guarantee Credit* which ensures that individuals receive a minimum level of income, according to their needs and circumstances. This minimum level is known as the applicable amount and for someone in care, who is in receipt of Attendance Allowance, the amount is £149.60 per week. Anyone with an income below this figure will receive benefits up to this amount and thus the total income achievable, including higher rate Attendance Allowance, would be £208.40 per week.

In calculating the level of benefit, any savings are deemed to provide tariff income at the rate of £1 per week for every £500 of assets above £10,000. For individuals who are not resident in a care home, the capital disregard reduces to £6,000.

The second element is Savings Credit, which is available to individuals aged ≥65 years and is designed to benefit those who have a 'private income' above the basic State Pension. This income may be in the form of private pension or tariff income arising from savings. Individuals are entitled to receive Savings Credit for 60% of their income above the State Pension subject to a maximum limit of £15.51. This entitlement then reduces at the rate of 40% for any excess income above the individual's applicable amount.

♦ To claim, contact the Pension Credit Helpline on 0800 991234 or for more information see the CareAware Pension Credit bulletin.

Attendance allowance

This benefit is payable to everyone who has a care need, and it is payable irrespective of the total money or assets owned by the individual. There are two rates reflecting the levels of need, and the benefit is subject to a number of qualification requirements. The lower rate is £39.35 and the higher rate is £58.80. Both of these amounts are payable weekly. There is a fast track system for palliative care patients with a prognosis of <6 months: a DS1500 form is filled out by the patient's doctor (see Chapter 25).

♦ To claim, contact the Attendance Allowance Unit on 08457 123456 and for more information request the CareAware Attendance Allowance bulletin.

♦ Note that funding agreements/arrangements for care homes can be complex and it is important that Social Services' support and advice is sought. Also note that all payments shown in these sections are subject to change.

Paying for extras and personal expense allowance

Accommodation fees cover heating, lighting, food and all basic requirements. Personal expense allowance is for spending on daily items such as toiletries, clothes, leisure activities, outings, etc.

All personal expense requirements will be explained before the placement starts. A review of the placement will be carried out by Social Services in the first 6 weeks and any concerns can be addressed at this time.

Privately funded residents

If an individual has in excess of the capital threshold, currently £23,000 (including money in the bank, building society, pensions, shares, insurance policies and the value of your property), there will be a liability that the full cost of the placement will need to be paid, except for the costs of Registered Nursing Care agreed by the NHS.

It is important to take professional advice, as there are various types of insurance schemes available to help patients pay for their care. These organizations will also help to ensure that people receive all their entitlements to state benefits.

Useful contacts

♦ Nursing Home Fees Agency: 0800 998 833
♦ CareAware: 08705 134925
♦ Care Direct: 0800 444 000
♦ Or make contact with your patient's Social Worker/Care Manager.

References

1. Maslow A. *Motivation and Personality*. New York: Harper; 1954.
2. Department of Health. *Putting People First: A Shared Vision and Commitment to the Transformation of Adult Social Care*. London: DoH; 2007. Available at: http://www.dh.gov.uk/en/SocialCare/ Socialcarereform/index.htm

The voluntary sector

Heather Mercer

Introduction

The term 'Third Sector' was introduced by the Government in June 2006 to describe the voluntary sector, when the first 'Minister for the Third Sector', Ed Milliband, was appointed. In a speech to voluntary organizations 6 weeks later, he identified the importance of his Ministry in delivering the Government's agenda in partnership with the Third Sector by challenging the contributions of the private, public and Third Sectors on a range of fronts; by helping to deploy the talents of the Third Sector; and by demanding improvement in public services. The Minister's role was to break down the barriers that prevented Third Sector organizations from achieving their goals. However, the impact of voluntary action on health and social care had been identified by William Beveridge in 1948 when he spoke of the 'driving power of social conscience'.[1]

This focus and development of the Third Sector is needed because the founding principles of health and social care no longer reflect the demands made on services now, and many of these current demands could not have been predicted.

The Third Sector is diverse, active and passionate, encompassing voluntary and community groups, social enterprises, charities, co-operatives and mutuals. All embrace the core values of being non-governmental, value-driven organizations who reinvest their surpluses to further social, environmental or cultural objectives. This enables the sector to campaign for change, deliver public services, promote social enterprise and strengthen communities.[2–4]

The public health agenda to improve the health and wellbeing of older people is identified in the Department of Health's document *Choosing Health: Making Healthier Choices Easier*.[5] This shifts the balance of care and responsibility from the 'professional' to community-based initiatives. The Healthy Ageing programme is an example of this. The role of the Third Sector in supporting the Government's public health agenda has never been greater.

Policy reforms have focused on encouraging people to assume more responsibility for promoting and maintaining their own health. Wanless[6,7] highlighted the need to focus on prevention and the long-term determinants of health. The *National Service Framework* [NSF] *for Older People*[8] identifies targets for services and *A New Ambition for Old Age*[9] describes the next stage of implementing the NSF. The key themes relevant to general practice are: to challenge negative attitudes to older people in the health care system; the promotion of healthy ageing; and improved co-ordination of early support for frail older people. Government targets to tackle inequalities in socially disadvantaged areas require that life expectancy should rise more significantly in these areas by 2010. This should have a direct effect on life expectancy for the over-fifties.[10]

Theme: volunteering

Volunteering involves offering to perform a service of one's own free will. Within health and social care this normally involves doing charitable work without pay. Many volunteers are retired people who provide services in the community or day care centres.

Box 29.1 Five key advantages in recruiting older volunteers

◆ Maturity: older people are better able to understand the age-related problems of others because of their life experience.

◆ Skills: older people have developed all kinds of work-related or social skills.

◆ Availability: older people who are retired from paid work and have finished raising children may have more time and flexibility to participate.

◆ Loyalty: older people remain longer and spend more time with their organization than younger people.

◆ Numbers: older people comprise a growing proportion of the population.[14]

The concept of community and society has been challenged over the last two decades. Margaret Thatcher in 1987 said; 'There are individual men and women and there are families. And no government can do anything except through people, and people must look after themselves first. It is our duty to look after ourselves and then, also, to look after our neighbours'.[11] The changing demographic profile of society and local communities requires alternative approaches to supporting community care for an ageing and increasingly frail population. European legislation requires that all volunteers are trained in health and safety and key areas of governance, and those working with vulnerable people on a one-to-one basis undergo a Criminal Records Bureau check. This is a costly and challenging requirement, as it can deter many volunteers from coming forward; and for the organization it places an added burden on a diminishing funding base. Despite these challenges, the number of volunteers participating in health initiatives is increasing.[12] Many are older volunteers and Lambert et al.[13] identify that there are five key advantages in recruiting older volunteers (see Box 29.1).

Case Study   Local volunteering

'Ageing Well' was developed by Age Concern England in 1993,[15] in response to the national strategy of Health of the Nation targets,[16] as a programme for people aged >50 years to become more involved in local initiatives designed to improve the physical, social and emotional health and wellbeing of their peers.[13] Its aims are to raise expectations of good health in old age and to motivate people to maintain, sustain and improve their own health and that of their peers. Volunteers are trained as 'senior health mentors' and there are also trained 'peer health members' to support others on a regular basis. Using a holistic approach, the activities offered vary according to the skill sets of the volunteers and the needs of the community in which they are working. These range from exercise classes to yoga and Tai Chi, complementary therapies and cultural events. The evaluation of the initiative, after 13 years of activities, revealed how positive the experience was, not just for the recipients but also for the mentors and peer health members.

The two extracts below illustrate the volunteers' positive and negative comments:

'People are depressed, they're isolated, they're lonely. They've got no shop, no way of getting out .... They don't want to move ... all these things add to the feeling of depression and isolation and if you can take those people out of their homes and bring them to the centre they can meet their friends. How can you measure that? What would these people be like if you left them in their homes, day in, day out? You would be adding to an already over-burdened health authority.' [FG2][13]

'When they come from the same background they actually communicate with people of their own age. I think they would listen to them a little bit more. It's also to do with experience and knowledge and knowing that they went through the same thing.' [AWM2][13]

Commenting on the impact the project had on her, one volunteer said,

> 'It's gone downhill [i.e. her health] because I have never been so busy, I am working 60 to 70 hours a week and I haven't got time for me to do things, so I would say that it has impacted in that I am more than aware of what we should be doing but I am my own worst enemy. I will go and skip lunch because I am so busy I forget to have it, and I am not doing regular exercise.' [FG2][13]

This study identifies the benefit to older, more isolated people, in participating in external activities to promote health and wellbeing. It also had a predominately positive effect on older volunteers who gained from the interaction and leadership of planned activities. It highlights how volunteers can become important in health promotion activities in the community, because they have the time, experience and the credibility with their peers.

Theme: social care

General practice predominately relies on the social care sector to liaise and deliver care within the Third Sector. There are many Third Sector organizations available to support individual health conditions, and it would be unreasonable to expect every general practitioner (GP) to have a contact number for a specific organization. They rely on the effectiveness of local area agreements to ensure that frail older people are supported in the community. Practices with a community matron[5] or a nominated older persons nurse may have this information to hand, but unless the patient is referred to the nurse, patients could still slip through the net of targeted, specialist Third Sector support. Those that tend to be missed are the middle income, moderately disabled who can survive at home because of the support of their carers, neighbours and volunteers.

The role of carers in supporting older people in the community is significant. The Government is aware of their contribution and the additional risks they run while caring, which include risks to physical and emotional health and wellbeing, and social isolation. The rights of carers are enshrined in the Carers [Recognition and Service] Act (1995)[17] and the Carers [Equal Opportunities] Act (2004).[18]

Case Study   Dementia care

Mrs J, aged 91 years with chronic emphysema, is caring for her husband, aged 96 years with dementia. He attends a day hospital once a week but she refuses all other support as Mr J becomes agitated when strangers are in the house. Her family are concerned that she needs a break, but Social Services have a 6 month waiting list for respite care. Whilst she is waiting for a respite bed she hurts her back lifting her husband out of the bath.

This is not an unfamiliar case in general practice and yet the Third Sector may have been able to support her. Crossroads[19] and befriending services (Joseph Rowntree Foundation)[20] can establish ongoing relationships with such families and win over the trust of people unhappy at having 'strangers in the house', because volunteers tend to remain constant over longer periods than some care staff who work shifts and may frequently move employment.

Within social care, these changes include the move towards personal budgets (which may or may not involve someone actually handling their allocated funds through a direct payment). In the meantime, the evaluation of the Individual Budgets pilot (which incorporated other funding streams in addition to the social care spend) was published in October 2008.[21]

The ways in which, and the speed at which, different local authorities are responding to this agenda vary significantly. Some local authorities appear completely to have revised their initial thinking even since the beginning of 2008. Many of the providers offering services will be from the Third Sector.

Theme: key areas of Third Sector involvement

The Third Sector has a significant role in supporting health care professionals to maintain vulnerable older people in their own homes and communities. These include support for: poverty and deprivation; mobility; feet; social exclusion; end of life care; protection of vulnerable adults; assistive technology.

Poverty and deprivation

Poverty among pensioners has been falling since 1996/97, from 29% of all pensioners in 1996/97 to 17% in 2005/06. Poverty is most commonly defined as those households living with 60% of median income (adjusting for the size of household). The rate of reduction has been particularly great since 2002/03 and pensioners are now less likely to be living in low income households than non-pensioners. The most significant fall has been among single pensioners where the proportion has dropped to 17% from 39% in 1996/97. Single female pensioners and older pensioner couples aged >75 years are the most likely to be in low income. Apart from Inner London (where it is much higher), the proportion of pensioners living in low income households is similar in all regions.

Case Study   West Hackney

West Hackney is estimated to be the fifth most deprived local authority in the 2004 Multiple Deprivation Index.[22]

Ethnic diversity is wider than anywhere else in Inner London or England and Wales, and the number who do not speak English fluently is high and increases among older members of the community.

A study was undertaken by local agencies to inform the health needs of the community. The groups involved were from Age Concern Hackney, Enabling Projects Consultancy, Turkish Community Outreach and Interpreting, Anchor Staying Put, the Community Resource team, the Mobile Library service and the Older People's Reference Group Advisory Group. There were five main conclusions of the study:

1) The need for a befriending service among older, housebound people whose social networks were reduced because of their progressive ill health.

2) Making benefits 'health checks' as older and more vulnerable people struggled to complete forms to apply for benefits.

3) Owner occupiers had special issues in trying to repair or renovate their homes to match their health needs. Such tasks required administrative skills as well as money to achieve these needs.

4) The Turkish speakers identified a need for help with the integration process. Local English language classes were needed not to 'pass exams' but simply to aid everyday activities.

5) Turkish speakers wanted 'escorted trips' so they could see and understand more about the England in which they were living.

Addressing all five needs would significantly improve the health and wellbeing of the community but this information would not normally be available in general practice.

Mobility

Case study

The challenge of maintaining mobility with increasing age and progressive long-term conditions is recognized by older people and health care professionals. The growing interest in low level preventive services and social rehabilitation, which aims to reduce re-admission to hospital or long term care, underpins the NSF for Older People and the concept of intermediate care. In 2003 the University of Birmingham evaluated a five-centre rehabilitation programme run by Age Concern across the UK. Although it was evaluated as a successful project, there were inherent difficulties in recruiting volunteers to support the project. Also, during the life of the project no local service contracts were awarded. The researchers concluded that, although the projects were 'successful in helping many older people to gain confidence and motivation to overcome personal and environmental barriers', the real benefit was in 'its contribution to a general service ethos and its application as part of other services, such as day services and hospital discharge services, rather than as a "stand alone" service'.[23]

Feet

Case study

Foot care becomes increasingly difficult for older people to maintain as their mobility becomes compromised. For many groups, good foot care is essential to prevent complications from vascular disease or infection. But indirect age discrimination is evident in some areas where there are long waiting lists for podiatry services, where exclusion criteria prevent older people from accessing NHS podiatry services or where only private podiatrists offer a nail-cutting service.

Age Concern Oxford and County,[24] in partnership with Oxfordshire NHS Podiatry Service, as the training partner, trained volunteers to deliver foot care in three GP surgeries, on the two health buses and at 'the Corner', a drop-in lunch venue run by Oxford City Council and other voluntary organizations which provides social and physical wellbeing opportunities to tackle social exclusion. The service is registered with the Commission for Social Care Inspection.[25] The outcomes of the service were the delivery of accessible and affordable foot care to >1000 older people annually, both in their own home and at other sites. The volunteers also carried out falls risk assessments with clients and signposted the vulnerable to the County Falls Service; provided access to all the services offered by Age Concern and directed clients to other services; and fulfilled a social function by providing a 'listening ear' to vulnerable clients who might not otherwise have been assessed and referred on appropriately. The Joseph Rowntree Foundation[20] and IDeA[26] identified this as an example of best practice.

Social exclusion

In 2006 the Government undertook the English Longitudinal Study on Ageing.[27] In 2008, Age Concern, the largest organization working for older people in England, published a report highlighting the seriousness of social exclusion for older people.[28] It identified that over a million older people, including one in five people aged >80 years, are shut out from society and ignored by Government policy. Severe exclusion among older people is a significant and pressing problem that will not disappear without urgent Government action.[28]

It shows that severe exclusion is about more than money, crossing the boundaries of social class, race, gender and financial status. New research for the charity also reveals that the risk of exclusion increases with age—leaving many older people without access to things that most people take for granted, such as a decent home, close friends and regular company, stimulating activity and access to local services (see Box 29.2).

The report also profiles four groups of older people at high risk of social exclusion, and outlines simple, low-cost proposals to improve their situation. Proposals include introducing local programmes to enhance social contact for people who are aged >80 years and living alone; improved support services for people who are recently bereaved; nationwide 'handyperson' schemes for people who are living in unfit housing; and improved support for independent advocacy for people who have limited capacity to make their own decisions.

Box 29.2 'Out of Sight, Out of Mind': key research findings[a]

- ◆ 56% of severely excluded people aged >50 years are in poor health.
- ◆ 40% of severely excluded people aged >50 years are lonely.
- ◆ 45% of men and 34% of women aged >80 years who live alone are lonely, as are 62% of recently bereaved older people.
- ◆ People aged 50–64 years are eight times more likely to be severely socially excluded if they rent their home privately than if they own it or pay a mortgage.
- ◆ 25% of people aged >80 years living in their own homes have significant memory problems: of these, one in four (26%) are severely excluded.

[a] Age Concern England.[29]

End of life care

Ever since the introduction of the National Cancer Plan,[30] the Government has been aware that the choice of 'place to die' is frequently denied patients and their families. Causal factors range from lack of specialized knowledge, out of hours services and hospice beds which are full. The Government's *End of Life Care Strategy*[31] seeks to bring together researchers and commissioners of care to create an 'intelligence network'. Interestingly, it is the Third Sector that is charged with improving end of life care.

The King's Fund and Marie Curie Cancer Care are extending their partnership to improve end of life care. From September 2008, The King's Fund Director of Development will take up a shared post between the two organisations. He will work to develop the contribution of both organizations to the further improvement of end of life services across the UK.

Protection of vulnerable adults

The only charity working exclusively to protect, and prevent the abuse of, vulnerable older adults is Action on Elder Abuse (AEA). The debate about elder abuse has fallen behind because of the paramount need to protect vulnerable children. AEA seeks to influence public policy and promote awareness and discourse around a difficult and challenging subject. It produces a Domiciliary Care Pack providing real-life scenarios of abuse and gives invaluable guidance on how to tackle it. It is appropriate for settings in all four nations of the UK. The pack is compatible with National Vocational Qualification level 2 work and can be taken as an optional module for care staff or family members.

Comic Relief has funded a website project that is jointly managed by AEA[32] and the Practitioners' Alliance for Vulnerable Adults. The project gathers examples of good practice from local authorities, service providers, advocates, service users, etc. and provides practical approaches to the dissemination of best practice around the country to inform and encourage improved service outcomes for vulnerable adults.

Assistive technology

Many disabled people in the community are being encouraged to take responsibility for their own self-care. The Department of Health has identified the positive impact of self-care in promoting positive health and wellbeing,[33] thereby reducing the impact on services. Voluntary sector providers, e.g. the Disabled Living Foundation, offer advice and individually tailored consultations[34] related to the most suitable aids for individuals to buy.

The greatest challenge lies in ensuring that individuals receive information about the technologies available to meet their holistic needs and preferences. About 75% of 'high tech' (computer-related) assistive technology is abandoned due to lack of available training and support.[35] Many individuals are unaware of the risks they carry after purchasing assistive technology; this is particularly important when carers and volunteers also lack training in its use. Inappropriate choice or usage can lead to accidents, pressure sores and injuries to the user. Inadequate cleaning can lead to transmission of disease and poor maintenance to risk of fires. The marketing of assistive technology had led to selling of equipment over the internet. The assumption is made that retailers are alerting the buyer to the risks attached to the equipment. The British Healthcare Trades Association is encouraging retailers to take a more responsible approach to selling, and Age Concern England is currently working with Boots plc to develop an agreed code of conduct.

Conclusion

In the new health and social care environment, all charities now have well-established governance practices and many are closely embedded into the delivery of services through local area agreements and service contracts. The benefits of the Third Sector, both for the recipients of care and for caregivers, cannot be underestimated.

References

1. Beveridge WH. *Voluntary Action: A Report of Methods*. London: Allen & Unwin; 1948.
2. Cabinet Office, London: UK Government; 2008. Available at: http://www.cabinetoffice.gov.uk/thirdsector.aspx
3. House of Commons Select Committee. *Public Services and the Third Sector: Rhetoric and Reality*. London: Stationery Office; 2008.
4. National Audit Office. *Working with the Third Sector*. London: Stationery Office; 2005.
5. Department of Health. *Choosing Health: Making Healthier Choices Easier*. London: DoH; 2004.
6. Wanless D. *Securing our Future Health: Taking a Long-Term View. Final Report*. London: HM Treasury; 2002.
7. Wanless D. *Securing Good Health for the Whole Population. Final Report*. London: HM Treasury; 2004.
8. Department of Health. *National Service Framework for Older People*. London: DoH; 2001.
9. Department of Health. *A New Ambition for Old Age*. London: DoH; 2006.
10. Department of Health. *Tackling Health Inequalities: A Programme for Action*. London: DoH; 2003.
11. Thatcher M. Speech to Conservative Party Conference, 9 October 1987.
12. Jones H. *Volunteering for Health. Research report produced for the Welsh Assembly Government*. Cardiff: Welsh Assembly; 2004.
13. Lambert S, Granville G, Lewis J, Merrell J, Taylor C. *Age Concern's 'Ageing Well' programme in England and Wales. Final Evaluation Report*. London: Age Concern; 2007.
14. Community Service Volunteers. *The Time of Your Life*. London: CSV/Retired and Senior Volunteers Programme; 2001.
15. Age Concern England. *Ageing Well*. London: ACE; 1993.
16. Department of Health. *Health of the Nation*. London: DoH; 1992.
17. HM Government. Carers [Recognition and Service] Act. London: Stationery Office; 1995.
18. HM Government. Carers [Equal Opportunities] Act. London: Stationery Office; 2004.
19. Crossroads. *New Standing Commission for Carers*. London: Crossroads; 2007.
20. Joseph Rowntree Foundation. *That Little Bit of Help*. York: Joseph Rowntree Foundation; 1998.
21. Available at: http://individualbudgets.csip.org.uk/dynamic/dohpage3.jsp.

22. Department for Communities and Local Government. *Multiple Deprivation Index*. 2004. Available at: http://www.communities.gov.uk/archived/general- content/communities/indicesofdeprivation/216309/

23. Age Concern England. *Research Briefing Number 4. So Much More Than Just Walking*. London: Age Concern England; 2003.

24. Age Concern England. *Needs Must*. London: Age Concern England Feet for Purpose. Oxford: Age Concern Oxford and County; 2007.

25. Commission for Social Care Inspection. *Registered Services Directory*. 2008. Available at: http://www.csci.org.uk/registeredservicesdirectory/RSSearch Detail.asp?ID=000

26. IDeA. *Suitcase Studies, lessons in good procurement practice*. London: 2008. Available at: IDeA http://www.idea.gov.uk/idk/aio/615947

27. Social Exclusion Unit. *The Social Exclusion of Older People: Evidence from the First Wave of the English Longitudinal Study on Ageing*. London: Stationery Office; 2006.

28. Department for Communities and Local Government. *English House Condition Survey 2005 Annual Report*. London: Stationery Office; 2007.

29. Age Concern England. *Out of Sight, Out of Mind*. London: Age Concern England; 2008.

30. Department of Health. *The National Cancer Plan*. London: Stationery Office; 2000.

31. Department of Health. *End of Life Care Strategy*. London: Stationery Office; 2008.

32. Comic Relief. *Action on Elder Abuse*. 2008. Available at: mhtml:http://www.elderabuse.org.uk/Mainpages/Elder%20Ab use.mht

33. Department of Health. *Supporting People with Long Term Conditions to Self Care: A Guide to Developing Local Strategies and Good Practice*. London: DoH; 2006.

34. Mandalatum M. *Going to Market—Equipment and Products for Disabled and Older People*. London: Jessica Kingsley & Kogan Page (for the Disabled Living Centres Council, London); 1996.

35. Microsoft. *Enable Ireland and Microsoft*. High Tech Assistive Technology Training Service; 2006. Available at: http://www.microsoft.com/Ireland/

Index

Managing Older People in Primary Care

We wish to express our gratitude to a number of people, including our families, but especially to Mrs Julie Farwell whose secretarial skills were essential to ensure the completion of the book and the sanity of the editors.